Common Eye Diseases
and their Management

Nicholas R. Galloway
Winfried M. K. Amoaku
Peter H. Galloway
Andrew C. Browning

Common Eye Diseases and their Management

Fifth Edition

 Springer

Nicholas R. Galloway
Nottingham, UK

Peter H. Galloway
St James University Hospital Leeds
Wetherby, UK

Winfried M. K. Amoaku
University of Nottingham and
Nottingham University Hospital
Queen's Medical Centre
Nottingham, UK

Andrew C. Browning
University Hospital
Royal Victoria Infirmary
Newcastle upon Tyne, UK

ISBN 978-3-031-08452-2   ISBN 978-3-031-08450-8   (eBook)
https://doi.org/10.1007/978-3-031-08450-8

This Springer imprint is published by the registered company Springer Nature Switzerland AG
The registered company address is: Gewerbestrasse 11, 6330 Cham, Switzerland

Preface to the Second Edition

Like the first edition, this textbook is intended primarily for medical students, but it is also aimed at all those involved in the primary care of eye disease, including general practitioners, nurses and optometrists. The need for the primary care practitioner to be well informed about common eye conditions is even more important today than when the first edition was produced. A recent survey from North London has shown that 30% of a sample of the population aged 65 and over are visually impaired in both eyes and a large proportion of those with treatable eye conditions were not in touch with eye services. It is clear that better strategies for managing problems of eyesight need to be set up. One obvious strategy is the improved education of those conducting primary care and it is hoped that this book will contribute to this. For this second edition, I am grateful for the help of my coauthor Winfried Amoaku, whose personal experience in teaching medical students here in Nottingham has been invaluable. His expertise in the management of macular disease, now a major cause of sensory deprivation in the elderly, is also evident in these chapters.

The format of the book has not changed but some of the chapters have been expanded. For example, there is now a section dealing with the eye complications of acquired immune deficiency syndrome (AIDS). This problem barely existed at the time of the first edition. Cataract surgery has changed a great deal in this short time and is becoming one of the commonest major surgical procedures to be performed in a hospital. The management of glaucoma has also changed with the introduction of a range of new medications. Our aim has been to keep the original problem-oriented layout and to keep it as a book to read rather than a book to look at. There are a number of good atlases on eye disease and some of these are mentioned in the section at the end on further reading. Although the title of the book is "Common Eye Diseases", some less common conditions are mentioned and it is hoped that the reader will gain some overall impression of the incidence of different eye diseases.

Nottingham, UK   Nicholas R. Galloway
Nottingham, UK   Winfried M. K. Amoaku
Leeds, UK   Peter H. Galloway
Newcastle upon Tyne, UK   Andrew C. Browning

Preface to the Third Edition

It is a pleasure to welcome two new authors who have contributed to the third edition of "Common Eye Diseases": Peter Galloway and Andrew Browning. Six years have passed since the last edition but even in this relatively short time there have been significant advances in the diagnosis and management of eye disease and an update has become necessary. Each author has taken a block of chapters for revision and, where needed, illustrations have been added or removed. Apart from the four main authors, I am indebted to Mr Roland Ling for his invaluable work on the chapter on the retina and once again to Professor Rubinstein for his help with the chapter on contact lenses.

The original aims of the book have not been changed. It remains as a textbook for medical students and those starting a career in ophthalmology, but also for those in primary care who are likely to deal with eye problems, including nurses, optometrists and general practitioners.

It has been the intention to keep explanations as simple and nontechnical as possible without losing scientific accuracy; more detailed accounts should be sought in the larger textbooks. An updated reference list for further reading is given at the end of the book. An internet version of this edition is being planned and, in order to keep down the retail price, some financial help is needed. For this we are grateful for the interest of Pfizer Ltd, whose policy of educational support has allowed this edition to go forward at its present low price.

Nottingham, UK   Nicholas R. Galloway
Nottingham, UK   Winfried M. K. Amoaku
Leeds, UK   Peter H. Galloway
Newcastle upon Tyne, UK   Andrew C. Browning

Preface to the Fourth Edition

Nearly ten years have passed since the third edition of this book was published, and once again it is a pleasure to welcome the same three other authors and proceed with our fourth edition.

Over the past ten years, there have been a number of important advances in the field of clinical ophthalmology. Of great impact has been the newer treatments available for the management of macular degeneration as will be seen in the chapter on the ageing eye. Improvements in the surgery of glaucoma and cataract have also been developed.

Apart from the scientific advances, a quiet revolution has occurred with the advent of the digital age. Understanding and informing the patient has become a more important part of medical practice and with the availability of information the patients themselves are better informed. This textbook is now produced as an ebook, and most of the chapters are preceded by a summary. At the end of many of the chapters is a list of questions to be answered relating to the content of the chapter.

Most of the original illustrations have been retained and some have been added.

Once again, this book is aimed at medical students, trainee ophthalmologist and general practitioners but also anyone involved in the primary care of eye conditions especially optometrists.

Nottingham, UK   Nicholas R. Galloway
Nottingham, UK   Winfried M. K. Amoaku
Leeds, UK   Peter H. Galloway
Newcastle upon Tyne, UK   Andrew C. Browning

Preface to the Fifth Edition

Six years have now passed since the last edition of this book was published, and once again it is a pleasure to welcome my three colleagues as co-authors. Apart from minor adjustments to the text, important changes have been made relating to two advancing fields in the specialty. These can be found in the chapters on Genetics and Macular Degeneration. As before the book is aimed at trainee Ophthalmologists but also those working in association with Eye departments including Orthoptists, Optometrists, Specialist Nurses, and research workers in other medical specialties.

The rise of the internet over the past 6 years has changed the practice of Ophthalmology and trainees rely more on internet reference than textbooks. This is evidenced by the popularity of the e version of the last edition. As before there are no references in the text but an up-to-date list of further reading is provided at the end of the book.

Nottingham, UK   Nicholas R. Galloway
Nottingham, UK   Winfried M. K. Amoaku
Leeds, UK   Peter H. Galloway
Newcastle upon Tyne, UK   Andrew C. Browning

Acknowledgements

Once again, I am grateful for all the help from those involved with the early editions of this book, especially from my secretary at that time, Ann Padgett and Geoffrey Lythe, who drew many of the illustrations. Since I have been retired from full-time practice for many years, I am especially indebted to my three co-authors who have been very much involved in clinical work during the recent difficult times, and yet have found time to do a thorough update of the book. Thanks are also due to all those at Springer who have been involved with the production of this fifth edition.

Contents

Part I   Introducing the Eye

1   The Scope of Ophthalmology 3
Patient Communication. 4
Historical Background 4
Making a Career in Ophthalmology 5

2   Basic Anatomy and Physiology of the Eye 7
Introduction. 7
Basic Structure of the Eye and Supporting Structures 7
The Globe 7
The Outer Layer of the Eye 8
The Middle Layer 9
The Inner Layer. 10
Blood Supply 11
The Optic Nerve 12
The Visual Pathway. 13
The Eyelids. 13
The Lacrimal Apparatus 14
The Extraocular Muscles 14
Physiology of the Eye. 14
The Eyelids. 14
The Tear Film 14
The Cornea 15
The Aqueous Humour. 15
The Vitreous Body 15
The Lens 16
The Ciliary Body. 16
Accommodation 16
The Retina. 16
Summary. 17

3   Examination of the Eye 19
How to Find Out What a Patient Can See. 19
Visual Acuity. 20
Visual Field. 21
Colour Vision 21
Spectacles 22

How to Start Examining an Eye   22
    Evaluating the Pupil   22
    External Eye and Lids.   23
    The Globe   23
How to Use the Ophthalmoscope   25
    Other Tests Available in an Eye Department   27

Part II   Primary Eye Care Problems

4   Long Sight, Short Sight   31

5   Common Diseases of the Eyelids   35
The Watering Eye   35
    Impaired Drainage of Tears.   35
    Excessive Secretion of Tears.   38
The Dry Eye   38
    Causes of Dry Eye   38
    Signs   39
    Management of the Dry Eye.   39
Deformities of the Eyelids   39
    The Normal Eyelid   39
    Epicanthus.   40
    Entropion.   40
    Ectropion.   40
    Lagophthalmos   41
    Blepharospasm   41
    Redundant Lid Skin   41
    Ptosis.   41
    Ingrowing Eyelashes (Trichiasis)   42
Infections of the Eyelids   42
    Meibomian Gland Infection   42
    Styes   43
    Blepharitis.   43
    Molluscum Contagiosum   44
    Orbital Cellulitis   44
    Allergic Disease of the Eyelids.   44
Lid Tumours   44
    Benign Tumours   44
    Malignant Tumours.   46
Lid Injuries   46

6   Common Diseases of the Conjunctiva and Cornea   49
Subconjunctival Haemorrhage   49
Conjunctivitis   49
    Symptoms   50
    Signs   50
    Microscopy   50
    Conjunctival Culture.   50
    Causes.   51

Bacterial Conjunctivitis. 51
Chlamydia Conjunctivitis 52
Trachoma 52
Adenoviral Conjunctivitis. 52
Herpes Simplex Conjunctivitis 53
Acute Haemorrhagic Conjunctivitis 53
Other Infective Agents 53
Allergic Conjunctivitis 53
Secondary Conjunctivitis 54
Corneal Foreign Body. 56
Signs and Symptoms. 56
Treatment 57
Corneal Ulceration 58
Types of Corneal Ulcer. 58
Corneal Dystrophies 62
Corneal Degenerations 62
Corneal Oedema 63
Absent Corneal Sensation. 63
Herpes Zoster Ophthalmicus (Shingles of the Eye) 64

7 The Red Eye. 67
Red Eye Which Is Not Painful and Sees Normally. 68
Subconjunctival Haemorrhage 68
Conjunctivitis 68
Episcleritis. 69
Red Painful Eye Which May See Normally 69
Scleritis. 69
Red Painful Eye Which Cannot See 70
Acute Glaucoma 70
Acute Iritis 70
Acute Keratitis 71
Neovascular Glaucoma. 71

8 Failing Vision. 73
Failing Vision in Eyes Which Look Normal. 73
When the Fundus Is Normal. 73
When the Fundus Is Abnormal 74
In Relation to Systemic Disease 74
Sudden Loss of Vision in One Eye 75
Treatable Causes of Failing Vision 75
Untreatable Causes of Failing Vision 76

9 Headache 79
History. 79
Classification. 80
Cerebrospinal Fluid. 80
Blood Vessels 80
Blood. 81
Nerves 81
Bones. 82

Meninges.   82
The Eyes   82
Pain Referred from Other Sites.   83
Drugs.   83
Post-traumatic Headache   84

10   Contact Lenses   85
Types.   85
Side-Effects.   86
Indications.   86
Cosmetic   86
Therapeutic   87

Part III   Problems of the Eye Surgeon

11   Cataract   91
The Lens   91
Aetiology.   92
Age   92
Diabetes.   93
Secondary   93
Trauma   93
Congenital Factors   94
Toxicity   94
Symptoms   94
Signs   95
Reduced Visual Acuity   95
Findings of Ophthalmoscopy   95
Findings on Slit Lamp Microscopy.   96
Other Important Signs.   96
Management   97
When to Operate.   98
Age of the Patient   98
Traumatic Cataract   99
The Cataract Operation.   99
Time Spent in Hospital   100
Convalescence.   100
Summary.   101

12   Glaucoma.   103
Normal Intraocular Pressure.   103
Maintenance of Intraocular Pressure   103
Measurement of Intraocular Pressure.   104
Clinical Types of Glaucoma   104
Primary Open Angle Glaucoma   104
Normal Pressure Glaucoma (NPG).   110
Acute Angle Closure Glaucoma   110
Secondary Glaucoma   114
Congenital or Developmental Glaucoma   115

13 Retinal Detachment 117
     Incidence... 117
     Pathogenesis 118
     Classification.. 118
          Rhegmatogenous Retinal Detachment 118
          Tractional Retinal Detachment....................... 118
          Exudative Retinal Detachment 119
     Rhegmatogenous Retinal Detachment 119
          The Presence of Breaks in Retinal Detachment 119
          Retinal Degeneration 119
          The Vitreous 119
          Posterior Vitreous Detachment....................... 120
          Retinal Breaks Formation........................... 120
          Mechanism of Rhegmatogenous Retinal Detachment 120
          Rhegmatogenous Retinal Detachment Associated with Trauma 120
     Signs and Symptoms of Retinal Tear and Retinal Detachment ... 120
          Flashes ('Photopsiae')............................. 121
          Floaters 121
          Shadow 121
     Traction Retinal Detachment 121
     Exudative Retinal Detachment 122
     Management of Rhegmatogenous Retinal Detachment 122
          Prophylaxis.................................... 122
          Retinal Surgery 122
          Prognosis...................................... 124

14 Squint... 125
     Types of Squint...................................... 127
          Squint in Childhood 127
          Squint in Adults................................. 131
          Ocular Muscle Imbalance........................... 133
     Summary... 134

15 Tumours of the Eye and Adnexae 135
     The Globe 135
          Choroidal Melanoma 135
          Choroidal Metastases 136
          Retinoblastoma.................................. 136
          Melanoma of the Iris.............................. 137
     The Eyelids... 137
          Benign Tumours 137
     Malignant Tumours of the Eyelids 139
     The Conjunctiva 140
          Benign Lesions 140
          Malignant Lesions................................ 141
     The Orbit... 141
     Exophthalmos and Proptosis............................. 142
          Causes of Proptosis............................... 142
          Assessment of Proptosis 143
     Summary... 143

16   Ocular Trauma   145
   Injuries to the Globe   145
      Contusion   145
      Perforation.   148
      Intraocular Foreign Body   148
      Sympathetic Ophthalmia.   149
   Injuries to the Eyelids   149
   Injuries to the Orbit.   150
   Radiational Injuries.   150
   Chemical Injuries   151
   Summary.   151

Part IV   Problems of the Medical Ophthalmologist

17   Testing Visual Acuity.   155
   Introduction.   155
      Measuring for Spectacles   159
      Objective Refraction   160
      Subjective Refraction   160
      Automated Refraction.   160
   Summary.   161

18   The Inflamed Eye   163
   The Role of Autoimmunity in Uveitis   163
   Anterior Uveitis   164
      Symptoms   164
      Signs   165
      Complications   166
      Causes   166
      Management   167
      Heterochromic Iridocyclitis (Fuch's)   168
   Intermediate Uveitis (Pars Planitis)   168
      Treatment and Management   168
   Posterior Uveitis   168
      Symptoms   169
      Signs   169
      Causes   170
      Management   170
      Specific Uveitis Entities   170
      Behcet's Disease   172
      Birdshot chorioretinopathy   174
      Sympathetic Ophthalmia.   174
      Other Causes   175
   Endophthalmitis and Panophthalmitis   175
   Episcleritis and Scleritis   176
   Summary.   177

19 The Ageing Eye 179

Changes in the Eyes with Age 180

The External Eye.. 180

The Globe 180

Eye Disease in the Elderly 181

Age Related Macular Degeneration 182

Cataract... 193

Glaucoma 193

Deformities of the Eyelids 194

Temporal Arteritis...................................... 194

Stroke 195

Summary.. 196

20 The Child's Eye... 197

How the Normal Features Differ from Those in an Adult 197

How to Examine a Child's Eye............................. 198

Screening of Children's Eyes 199

Congenital Eye Defects................................... 199

Lacrimal Obstruction 199

Epicanthus... 199

Ptosis... 199

Congenital Nystagmus 199

Structural Abnormalities of the Globe 200

Other Eye Conditions in Childhood 201

Abnormalities of Refraction............................. 201

Squint 201

Amblyopia of Disuse 202

Leucocoria... 202

Retinopathy of Prematurity............................. 202

Ophthalmia Neonatorum................................. 202

Uveitis.. 203

Optic Atrophy 203

Juvenile Retinal and Macular Degenerations 203

The Phakomatoses 203

Summary.. 204

21 Systemic Disease and the Eye............................ 205

Introduction.. 205

Diabetes Mellitus 206

Eyelids.. 206

Ocular Movements 206

Cornea and Conjunctiva 207

Anterior Chamber...................................... 207

Iris... 207

Lens... 207

Retina and Vitreous.................................... 208

Background Retinopathy 208

The Pre-Proliferative Stage.............................. 209

Proliferative Retinopathy 209
Diabetic Maculopathy.................................. 210
Treatment 210
Treatments for DMO.................................. 213
Treatments for Proliferative Diabetic Eye Disease........... 214
Prognosis.. 215
Thyroid Eye Disease...................................... 215
Management 217
Hypertension.. 218
The Effect of Age on the Retinal Blood Vessels............. 218
The Effects of Raised Blood Pressure on the Retinal Vessels... 218
'Malignant' Hypertension.............................. 218
Retinal Vascular Occlusions 220
Management 220
Retinal Artery Occlusions................................. 221
Ischaemic Optic Neuropathy............................... 223
Anaemia 223
The Leukaemias 225
Sickle Cell Disease 227
Onchocerciasis 229
Extraocular Features.................................. 229
Ocular Features...................................... 229
Management 229
Acquired Immune Deficiency Syndrome (AIDS).............. 230
Ocular Manifestations of Coronavirus (Covid-19)............. 232
Ocular Manifestations of Ebola Virus Disease 234
Connective Tissue Disease 234
Mucocutaneous Diseases 235
Summary... 236

22   **Neuro-Ophthalmology** 237
The Optic Disc 237
Normal Disc 237
Congenital Disc Anomalies............................. 238
Pale Disc 239
Swelling of the Optic Disc 241
Multiple Sclerosis....................................... 243
Ocular Findings...................................... 243
Defects in the Visual Fields............................... 244
Abnormalities of the Pupil 246
The Abnormally Dilated Pupil 247
The Abnormally Constricted Pupil....................... 247
Double Vision 248
Assessment of Eye Movements in Diplopia................ 248
Causes of Diplopia 249
Summary... 250

23 Genetics and the Eye. 253
Basic Genetic Mechanisms. 254
Autosomal Recessive Inheritance. 255
    Autosomal Dominant Inheritance. 256
    Sex-Linked Recessive Inheritance 256
    Mitochondrial Inheritance. 258
Digenic or Polygenic Inheritance 258
    Chromosomal Abnormalities 259
    Multifactorial Diseases 259
Gene Therapy 259
Summary. 260

24 Drugs and the Eye. 261
Introduction. 261
Treatment of Infection 262
Drops Which Widen the Pupil. 262
    Parasympathetic Antagonists 262
    Sympathetic Agonist. 263
Drops Which Constrict the Pupil 263
Drugs in the Treatment of Open Angle Glaucoma 264
Drugs in the Treatment of Acute Angle Closure Glaucoma 265
Drugs in the Treatment of Allergic Eye Disease. 265
Local Anaesthesia in Ophthalmology. 265
Drugs and Contact Lenses 266
Artificial Tears. 266
Anti-Inflammatory Drugs and the Eye 266
Diagnostic Agents Used the Eye. 268
Corneal Protection in Unconscious Patients or Patients
with Exposed Eyes 268
Retinal Pharmacotherapy: Anti-Angiogenic Drugs
and the Eye, and Intraocular Steroids. 268
Vitreomacular Traction. 269
Damage to the Eyes by Drugs Administered Systemically 269
Summary. 270

Part V Visual Impairment

25 Blindness 273
Definition 273
Benefits for the Visually Handicapped 274
Standards of Vision for Various Occupations 274
Colour Blindness. 274
Incidence and Cause of Blindness 275
Aids for the Visually Impaired 275
Artificial Eyes. 276

Further Reading 279

Index. 281

Part I

Introducing the Eye

The Scope of Ophthalmology

Abstract

This chapter explains how the specialty has developed historically and what the aims of the Ophthalmologist might be. The current training programme for eye surgeons is outlined and some of the techniques used in everyday practice are described.

Although the eye and its surrounding structures would seem to provide an ideal anatomical and functional basis for specialisation, ophthalmology can no longer regard itself as a specialty on its own but more the heading for a group of sub-specialties. There are those who know all about the pigment epithelium of the retina and yet bow to those who have a special knowledge of the bipolar cells in the retina. Over the past 100 years the science has advanced at an unbelievable rate and with the increase in our knowledge has come the development of treatments and cures, which have had a great impact on our everyday lives.

The importance of the eye and its function is sometimes underrated, but a consideration of the part played by vision in our consciousness makes us soon realise its value. If we think of dreams, of memories, of photographs and of almost anything in our daily existence, it is difficult to express them without visual references. After a little careful consideration of the meaning of blindness, it is easy to sense the rational and irrational fears that our patients present to us in the clinic. Nevertheless in a modern European community the effects of blindness are not so apparent as in former years, and blind people tapping their way about the street or begging for food are less in evidence to remind us of the deprivation that they suffer. This is due to the effective application of preventive medicine and the efficacy of modern surgical techniques as well as better support from social services. However in the western world we have a new and increasing problem related to the increasing number of elderly people in the population. The problem is that of sensory deprivation due to degenerative disease. Degenerative changes in the eye are now a major cause of blindness and although support services are being developed and treatment is now available in many cases, there is still an increasing toll of visual impairment in the ageing population.

The broad and detailed scientific interest in the eye and vision is witnessed by the large number of journals, conferences and meetings that now exist, possibly more than in any other specialty. There are several hundred ophthalmological journals all contributing to the scientific literature on the subject and many are now accessible through the Internet or CD-ROM. As an organ of clinical specialisation, the eye does have a special advantage; it can be seen. Using the slit lamp microscope it is possible to examine living nerves including nervous system tissues and blood vessels in a manner that is not possible in other parts of the body without endoscopy or biopsy. So much are the component parts of the eye on display to the clinician that when a patient presents to a casualty department with symptoms, the explanation of the symptoms should be made evident by careful examination. Compare this with the vague aches and pains which present to the gastroenterologist or the neurologist, symptoms which may ultimately resolve without any cause being found for them. The student or newly qualified doctor must be warned that if the patient presents with eye symptoms and no abnormality can be found after examination, then he or she must look again as it is likely that something has been missed.

Most of the work of the ophthalmologist is necessarily centred on the globe of the eye itself and there are a number of conditions which are limited to this region without there being any apparent involvement of the rest of the body. Ophthalmology is usually classified as a surgical specialty but it provides a bridge between surgery and medicine. Most of the surgery is performed under the microscope and here the application of engineering principles in the design of finer and finer instruments has played an important part. There is overlap with the fields of the plastic surgeons and the neurosurgeons. On the medical side, the ophthalmologist has links with the physicians and particularly the diabetic specialists, dermatologists, paediatricians and cardiologists.

Patient Communication

Ophthalmologists are no different from any other doctors in that they must establish a good rapport with the patients and their relatives. It is important to give a diagnosis and establish a treatment plan and tell the patient the results of tests. Sometimes the question "What do you think the problem is?" can save time. These days language difficulties can be overcome by an interpreter in many hospitals and if necessary, when the patient is deaf, important points can be written down in large print. It is a good practice with the elderly to repeat the diagnosis three times in different ways because we know that many people forget what the doctor has said in the heat of the moment. A particularly taxing situation arises when a patient has to be told that they are losing their eyesight. Many blind people complain that "they were not told anything" meaning often that they were given no insight into the difficulties that they might encounter. Time is short in the clinic but many clinics now have an "ECLO" (Eye clinic liaison Officer) who can spend some time discussing the problems with the patient and tell them about possible visual aids, internet sites and patient groups.

Historical Background

In 1847 the English mathematician and inventor, Charles Babbage, showed a distinguished ophthalmologist his device for examining the inside of the eye, but unfortunately this was never exploited and it was not until 1851 that Hermann von Helmholtz published his classic description of his instrument, the ophthalmoscope. He developed the idea from his knowledge of optics and the fact that he had previously demonstrated the "red reflex" to medical students with a not dissimilar instrument. In principle he had, for the purposes of his demonstration, looked through a hole in a small mirror, which reflected light from a lamp into the subjects eye. This produced the red reflex in the pupil well known to photographers and night drivers and no doubt this fascinated medical students at that time. Helmholtz worked out that a similar device could be used to inspect the inside of the eye. According to correspondence of the time it took him about a week to learn the technique of examining in detail the structures within the eye and he wrote a letter to his father telling him that he had made a discovery that was "of the utmost importance to ophthalmology". Soon after this a mass of descriptive information on the optic fundus, that is the inside of the eye, appeared in the scientific literature and modern clinical ophthalmology was born. The changes in the eye associated with systemic diseases such as hypertension and anaemia became recognised. Several blinding conditions limited to the eye itself such as glaucoma and macula degeneration were also described at this time.

But we must not belittle developments, which had occurred before the invention of the ophthalmoscope. In the eighteenth century considerable advances had been made in the technique and instrumentation of cataract surgery, and the science of optics was being developed to enable the better correction of refractive errors in the eye. If we go back to the seventeenth century, the existing ophthalmological services were definitely limited as is revealed in the writings of the famous diarist, Samuel Pepys. Although we have no record of his eye condition other than his own, he did consult an oculist at the time and unfortunately received little comfort or effective treatment. His failing eyesight brought his diary to an abrupt end in spite of the use of 'special glasses' and the medicaments, which caused him great pain.

Although records of eye surgical techniques go back as far as 3000 years, modern eye surgery was largely developed thanks to the introduction of cocaine and then of general anaesthesia at the end of the nineteenth century. The use of eserine eyedrops to reduce the intraocular pressure in glaucoma was introduced at the same time, this being the forerunner of a number of different medical treatments, which are now available. Cataract surgery saw great advances at the beginning of the twentieth century with the introduction of techniques to remove the opaque lens of the eye either completely or by leaving the posterior capsule in situ. In the 1920s, successful attempts were being made to replace the detached retina, which had previously been an irreversible cause of blindness. Such early surgical techniques have now been developed to produce some of the most dramatic means of restoring sight. As a spin-off from the last war came a revolutionary idea of 'spare parts' surgery in the eye. The observation that crashed fighter pilots were able to tolerate small pieces of perspex in their eyes led to the use of acrylic intraocular implants, the cataractous lens of the eye being replaced by an artificial one. Such spare-part surgery has now become commonplace as will be seen in Chap. 11. The operating microscope was introduced in the 1960s, and with it came the development of fine suture materials and the use of instruments too small for manipulation with the naked eye. This in turn has led to small incision techniques and sutureless surgery, which has made the day case cataract operation a routine. Fifty years ago the vitreous was a surgical no-man's land but instruments have now been developed that can cut, aspirate and inject fluid simultaneously, all these procedures being carried out through fine bore needles. Membranes, blood or foreign bodies can now be removed from the vitreous as a routine. Much important eye disease is inherited and it is not surprising that very important advances have occurred recently in the field of ophthalmic genetics. The gene controlling the development of the eye has now been identified and perhaps the answer to the tragic problem of inherited degenerative retinal disease is on the horizon.

In the early days of the development of the speciality a number of specialised hospitals were built throughout Britain. The first of these was Moorfields Eye Hospital, founded largely to combat the epidemic of trachoma, which was prevalent in London at the time. Subsequently other eye hospitals appeared in the main cities of this country, often the result of pressures of local needs such as for example the treatment of industrial accidents. In recent years, there has been a tendency for eye departments to become incorporated within the larger district general hospital although individual eye hospitals remain.

Making a Career in Ophthalmology

Ophthalmology is a popular specialty and so the aspiring eye surgeon can expect considerable competition. There are certain essential requirements. Firstly an initial interest in physics and optics is helpful and most important is a considerable degree of manual dexterity. Good binocular vision goes along with the manual dexterity demanded by microscopic surgery. That is to say, if aiming for the surgical rather than the medical side of ophthalmology, the trainee should see well out of each eye and should be able to use the eyes together to give proper stereoscopic vision.

In many cases an interest in the subject is aroused in medical school by a mentor or a good teacher. By and large those who see ophthalmology as a soft option are not happy in their career. Those who, as most doctors do, set out to improve the lot of the patient, find the specialty very rewarding because it is undoubtedly extremely effective in this respect.

Once a medical graduate has completed the 2 foundation years he or she can apply for specialist training in Ophthalmology. This is a 7 year course, the first 2 years being spent working towards the FRCOphth pt1 examination. This requires a basic knowledge of the science and practice of the specialty. The trainee then continues with a more in depth learning of the specialist skills and techniques, following a curriculum set by the Royal College of Ophthalmologists and supervised at a local level. At the end of the 7 years the trainee takes the FRCOphth pt 2 examination. This leads to the acquisition of the certificate of completion of training (CCT). A CCT and FRCOphth pt 2 are needed when applying for a consultant post. Most trainees aim towards obtaining a consultant post but some especially those requiring more flexibility can apply for staff grade posts. For part time work where doctors are involved with other specialties or general practice then clinical assistant posts are available. Useful career advice can be found in the website of the Royal College of Ophthalmologists. Apart from advice and also provision of training, the College offers travel awards and scholarships and an e-portfolio is offered to trainees to record their training progression.

After reading this chapter you should be able to answer the following questions:

1. Name some of the techniques that are employed in Ophthalmology
2. What structured training is available?
3. When was eye surgery first employed
4. How is "spare parts surgery" applied to the eye.
5. Why is patient communication important in the specialty?

Basic Anatomy and Physiology of the Eye

2

Abstract

This chapter describes the anatomy of the eyeball, the visual pathway, and the ocular adnexae. It also provides a basic introduction to the physiology and functioning of the eye.

Introduction

The eye is the primary organ of vision. Each one of the two eyeballs is located in the orbit where it takes up about one-fifth of the orbital volume (Fig. 2.1). The remaining space is taken up by the extraocular muscles, fascia, fat, blood vessels, nerves and the lacrimal gland.

The eye is embryologically an extension of the central nervous system. It shares many common anatomical and physiological properties with the brain. Both are protected by bony walls, have firm fibrous coverings and a dual blood supply to the essential nervous layer. The eye and brain have internal cavities perfused by fluids of like composition and under equivalent pressures. As the retina and optic nerve are outgrowths from the brain, it is not surprising that the eye and central nervous system are affected by similar disease processes. The physician should constantly be alerted that many diseases can simultaneously or sequentially involve the eye and central nervous system.

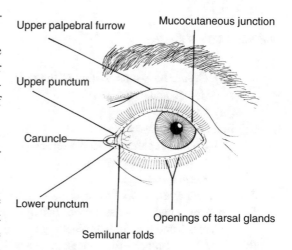

Fig. 2.1 Surface anatomy

Basic Structure of the Eye and Supporting Structures

The Globe

The eye has three coats or layers, three compartments and contains three different fluids (Fig. 2.2).

1. The three outer coats of the eye
   (a) Outer fibrous layer:
       (i) Cornea
       (ii) Sclera
       (iii) Lamina cribrosa
   (b) Middle vascular layer ('uveal tract'):
       (i) Iris

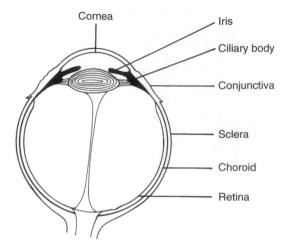

Fig. 2.2 Layers of the globe

    (ii) Ciliary body—consisting of the pars plicata and pars plana
    (iii) Choroid
  (c) Inner nervous layer:
    (i) Pigment epithelium of the retina
    (ii) Retinal photoreceptors
    (iii) Retinal neurons.
2. The three compartments of the eye
  (a) Anterior chamber—the space between the cornea and the iris-lens diaphragm.
  (b) Posterior chamber—the triangular space between the iris anteriorly, the lens and zonule posteriorly, and the ciliary body laterally.
  (c) Vitreous chamber—the space behind the lens and zonule.
3. The three intraocular fluids
  (a) Aqueous humour—a watery, optically clear solution of water and electrolytes similar to tissue fluids.
  (b) Vitreous humour—a transparent gel consisting of a three-dimensional network of collagen fibres, and the interspaces filled with polymerised hyaluronic acid molecules and water. The vitreous fills the space between the posterior surface of the lens, ciliary body and retina.
  (c) Blood—in addition to its usual functions, blood contributes to maintenance of intraocular pressure. Most of the blood is in the choroid. The choroidal blood flow

represents the largest blood flow/unit tissue in the body. The degree of de-saturation of efferent choroidal blood is relatively small and indicates that the choroidal vasculature has functions beyond retinal nutrition. The choroid serves as a heat-exchanger for the retina which absorbs energy as light strikes the retinal pigment epithelium.

Clinically, the eye may be considered to be composed of two segments:

1. Anterior segment—all structures from (and including) the lens forward
2. Posterior segment—all structures posterior to the lens.

The Outer Layer of the Eye

The **cornea** forms the anterior one-sixth of the outer coat of the eye. The posterior five-sixths of the outer coat is formed by the **sclera** and lamina cribrosa. The cornea is transparent, whereas the sclera, which is continuous with it, is white.

The cornea has five layers anterior posteriorly (Fig. 2.3):

1. Epithelium and its basement membrane—stratified squamous type of epithelium with five to six cell layers of regular arrangement.
2. Bowman's layer—homogeneous sheet of modified stroma.

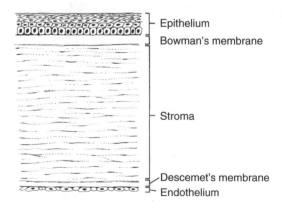

Fig. 2.3 The cornea

3. Stroma—consists of approximately 90% of total corneal thickness.

   It consists of lamellae of collagen, cells, and ground substance.
4. Descemet's membrane—the basement membrane of the endothelium.
5. Endothelium—a single layer of cells lining the inner surface of Descemet's membrane.

Recently (in 2013), another layer called the Dua layer has been described. This layer is distinct and located between the posterior stroma and the Descemet's membrane, and is strong and thought to be impervious to air.

In the region of the limbus, the epithelium on the outer surface of the cornea becomes continuous with that of the conjunctiva, a thin, loose, transparent, non-keratinising mucous membrane that covers the anterior part of the sclera, from which it is separated by loose connective tissue. Above and below, the conjunctiva is reflected onto the inner surface of the upper and lower lids. This mucous membrane, therefore, lines the posterior surface of the eyelids and there is a mucocutaneous junction on the lid margin. Although the conjunctiva is continuous, it can be divided descriptively into three parts: palpebral (tarsal), bulbar, and fornix conjunctiva.

The sclera consists of irregular lamellae of collagen fibres. Posteriorly, the external two-thirds of the sclera become continuous with the dural sheath of the optic nerve, while the inner one-third becomes the lamina cribrosa—the fenestrated layer of dense collagen fibres through which the nerve fibres pass from the retina to the optic nerve. The sclera is thickest posteriorly and thinnest beneath the insertions of the recti muscles. There is a layer of loose connective tissue deep to the conjunctiva, overlying the sclera, called the episclera.

The Middle Layer

The middle layer is highly vascular and called the uvea. If one were to peel the sclera away from this layer the remaining structure would look like a grape, as this middle layer, which is called the uvea, is heavily pigmented as well as being vascular. The anterior part of the uvea forms the bulk of the iris body and hence inflammation of the iris is called either anterior uveitis or iritis. The posterior part of the uvea is called the choroid, and the bit of the uvea joining the iris to the choroid is called the ciliary body or intermediate uvea.

The iris is the most anterior part of the uvea. It is a thin circular disc perforated centrally by the pupil. The anterior layer of the iris contains two muscles: the sphincter and dilator muscles. Contraction of the iris sphincter muscle constricts the pupil whilst contraction of the dilator pupillae muscle dilates the pupil.

The ciliary body is attached anteriorly to the iris and scleral spur; posteriorly it is continuous with the choroid and retinal pigment epithelium. The ciliary body is triangular in cross-section. The anterior side of the ciliary body is the shortest and borders the anterior chamber angle; it gives origin to the iris. The outer side of the triangle (mainly ciliary muscles) lies against the sclera. The inner side is divided into two zones: (1) the pars plicata forms the anterior 2 mm and is covered by ciliary processes (2) the pars plana constitutes the posterior 4.5 mm flattened portion of the CB. The pars plana is continuous with the choroid and retina.

The choroid consists of:

- Bruch's membrane—membrane on the external surface of the retinal pigment epithelium (RPE). It consists of the basement membrane of RPE cells and choriocapillaris. In between the two layers of basement membrane are the elastic and collagenous layers. Small localised thickenings of Bruch's membrane (which increase with age) are called drusen.
- The choriocapillaris—a network of capillaries supplying the RPE and outer retina.
- Layer of medium sized and larger choroidal blood vessels external to the choriocapillaris.
- Pigmented cells scattered in the choroid external to the choriocapillaris.

The Inner Layer

The inner layer of the eye, lining the inside of the choroid is called the retina, which consists of the retinal pigment epithelium and the neuroretina. This layer forms the retina posteriorly. Anteriorly the layer continuous with the retina comes to line the inner surface of the ciliary body and iris as a two-layered pigment epithelium. These same layers can be traced into the retina, which is composed of an outer pigment epithelium and an inner sensory part containing the rods and cones, bipolar cells, and ganglion cells (Fig. 2.4a). The junction of the retina and pars plana forms a scalloped edge and is called the ora serratta.

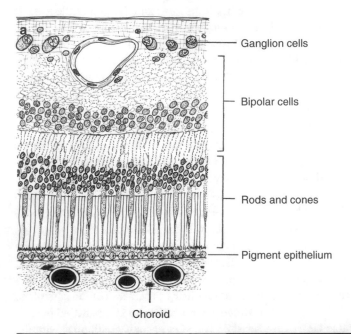

Ganglion cells

Bipolar cells

Rods and cones

Pigment epithelium

Choroid

Fig. 2.4 The retina: (**a**) diagrammatic representation of histology; (**b**) optical coherence tomography showing pseudo histology of the macula

The several layers of the retina from the outside to the inside:

- Pigment epithelium of the retina
- Rods and cones (photoreceptors)
- External limiting membrane
- Outer nuclear layer (nuclei of rods and cones with bipolar cells
- Inner nuclear layer (nuclei of bipolar cells)
- Inner plexiform layer (synapse of bipolar cells with ganglion cells)
- Ganglion cell layer
- Nerve figure layer
- Internal limiting membrane.

The anatomic macula is the area considered as the centre of the human retina and has a diameter of approximately 6 mm. It is oval shaped and extending from the temporal edge of the optic disc, and enclosed by the superior temporal and inferior temporal retinal blood vessels. The very central part of the macula is the foveola, measuring 0.35 mm in diameter, and is represented as a pit containing only cone photoreceptors, and is responsible for the high resolution, and colour vision of the eye. The anatomic fovea (referred to by some as the 'clinical macula') is larger with a size approximately the same as the optic disc. The inner retinal layers are displaced laterally in order to allow direct access to the cone photoreceptors without degradation that may occur otherwise. The different retinal layers in the macula may be viewed clinically in a pseudo-histological section provided by optical coherence tomography (OCT) clinically (Fig. 2.4b).

It is important to note that the photoreceptor cells are on the external side of the retina (i.e. further away from the vitreous). The relationship of the retinal elements can be understood most readily by following the formation of the optic cup. As the single-cell layer optic vesicle 'invaginates' to form the two-cell layers optic cup, the initially superficial cells become the inner layer of the cup. The pigment epithelium including the RPE develops from the outer layer of the cup, facing the photoreceptors across the now obliterated cavity of the optic vesicle. From the inner layer of the neurons of the retina differentiate.

Blood Supply

The blood supply of the globe is derived from three sources: the central retinal artery, the anterior ciliary arteries and the posterior ciliary arteries. All these are derived from the ophthalmic artery, which is a branch of the internal carotid artery. The central retinal artery runs in the optic nerve to reach the interior of the eye, and its branches spread out over the inner surface of the retina, with the branching capillaries supplying the inner half the neuroretina. The anterior ciliary arteries emerge from the insertion of the recti muscles and perforate the globe near the iris root to join an arterial circle in the ciliary body. The posterior ciliary arteries are the fine branches of the ophthalmic artery, which penetrate the posterior pole of the eye. Some of these supply the choroid and two or more larger vessels run anteriorly to reach the arterial circle in the ciliary body. The larger vessels are known as the long posterior ciliary arteries, and those supplying the choroid and peripapillary area are known as the short posterior ciliary arteries (Fig. 2.5). The branches of the central retinal artery are accompanied by an equivalent vein. However, the uvea

- Lacrimal gland
- Lacrimal artery
- Long posterior ciliary artery
- Optic nerve
- Ophthalmic artery
- Internal carotid artery

Fig. 2.5 Blood supply of the eye

(choroid, ciliary body, and iris are all drained by approximately four vortex veins in all. These vortex veins leave the posterior four quadrants of the globe and are familiar landmarks for the retinal surgeon.

The Optic Nerve

The retinal nerve fibres sweep across the innermost part of the retina to reach the optic disc (Fig. 2.6). These nerve fibres can be seen with the ophthalmoscope by carefully observing the way light is reflected off the inner surface of the retina (Fig. 2.7). The retinal vessels are also embedded on the inner surface of the retina. There is therefore a gap, which is the thickness of the transparent retina, between the retinal vessels and the stippled pigment epithelium. The optic nerve meets the posterior part of the globe slightly nasal to the posterior pole and very slightly above the horizontal meridian. Inside the eye this point is seen as the optic disc (or optic nerve head). There are no light-sensitive cells on the optic disc, and hence light falling ion this part of the fundus is not detected. This corresponds to the blind spot which anyone can find in their field of vision. The optic nerve is approximately 50 cm long, and contains about one million nerve fibres, each of which has a cell body in the ganglion cell layer of the retina.

Fig. 2.7 The normal fundus of (**a**) a Caucasian and (**b**) an African. The background is darker in the African owing to increased pigmentation in the retinal pigment epithelium (RPE). The nerve fibre layer is noticeable, especially along the superior and inferior temporal vascular arcades

Optic disc   Macula

Fig. 2.6 The optic fundus

The optic nerve fibres travel in bundles separated by fibrous tissue, and nerve is surrounded by the three sheaths: the pia, arachnoid and dura. Other cells types provide support within the optic nerve, including astrocytes, microglia and oligodendrocytes. Approximately 50% of the optic nerve fibres decussate at the optic chiasma. Most of the nerve fibres synapse in the lateral geniculate body, whist a few proceed to other centres including the pretectal nucleus.

Apart from the optic nerve, the posterior pole of the globe is also perforated by several long and short ciliary nerves. These contain parasympathetic, sympathetic and sensory fibres, which mainly supply muscles of the iris (dilator and sphincter) and ciliary body (ciliary muscles). Patients can experience pain when the iris is handled under inadequate local anaesthesia, and pain is also sometimes experienced during laser coagulation treatment of the chorio-retina—this would seem to prove the existence of sensory fibres in the iris and choroid. The cornea is extremely sensitive, but again, the only sensory endings are those for pain.

The Visual Pathway

The visual pathways include:

(a)	The retina	}	Common to visual and
	(i) Rods and cones	}	pupillary reflex
	(ii) Bipolar cells	}	pathways
	(iii) Ganglion cells	}	
(b)	Axons of the ganglion cells	}	
	(i) Nerve fibre layer of retina	}	
	(ii) Optic nerve	}	
	(iii) Optic chiasm	}	
	(iv) Optic tract	}	
(c)	Subcortical centres and relays		
	(i) Superior colliculus	Reflex control of eye movements	
	(ii) Pretectal nuclei nuclei/ Edinger-Westphal nucleus	Pupillary reflexes	
	(iii) Lateral geniculate body	Cortical relay (Visual pathway)	
(d)	Cortical connections	}	Vision and reflex eye
	(i) Optic radiations	}	movements
	(ii) Visual cortex (area 17)	}	
	(iii) Association areas (Areas 18 and 19)	}	
	(iv) Frontal eye field	Voluntary eye movements	

If the rods and cones are considered analogous to the sensory organs for touch, pressure, temperature, etc., then the bipolar cells may be compared to the first-order sensory neurons of the dorsal root ganglia, and the retinal ganglion cells to the second-order sensory neurons whose cell bodies lie within the spinal cord or medulla.

The pupillary light pathway is different (from the visual pathway). In brief, the pupillomotor nerve fibres leave the optic tract without synapsing in the lateral geniculate nucleus, but rather synapse in the pretectal nucleus of the midbrain. The interneurons to the Edinger-Westphal nucleus, and efferent pathways along the IIIrd cranial nerve are described in Chap. 22.

The Eyelids

The eyelids may be divided into anterior and posterior parts by the mucocutaneous junction—the grey line (Fig. 2.8). The eyelashes arise from hair follicles anterior to the grey line whilst the ducts of the meibomian glands (modified sebaceous glands) open behind the grey line. The meibomian glands are long and slender, and run parallel to each other perpendicular to the eyelid margin and are located in the tarsal plate of the eyelids. The tarsal plate gives stiffness to the eyelids and helps maintain its contour. The upper and lower tarsal plates are about 1 mm thick. The lower tar-

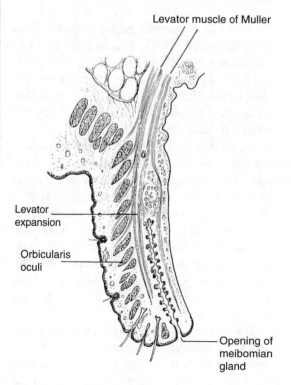

Levator muscle of Muller

Levator expansion

Orbicularis oculi

Opening of meibomian gland

Fig. 2.8 The eyelid (diagram)

sus measures about 5 mm in height whilst the upper tarsus measures about 10–12 mm.

The orbicularis oculi muscle lies between the skin and the tarsus and serves to close the eyelids. It is supplied by the facial nerve. The skin and subcutaneous tissue of the lids is very thin. The inner surface of the eyelids is lined by the palpebral conjunctiva.

The Lacrimal Apparatus

The major lacrimal gland occupies the superior temporal anterior portion of the orbit. It has ducts that open into the palpebral conjunctiva above the upper border of the upper tarsus.

Tears collect at the medial part of the palpebral fissure and pass through the puncta and the canaliculi into the lacrimal sac, which terminates in the nasolacrimal duct inferiorly. The nasolacrimal duct opens into the inferior meatus of the nose.

The Extraocular Muscles

There are six extraocular muscles which help to move the eyeball in different directions: the superior, inferior, medial and lateral recti, the superior and inferior obliques. All these muscles are supplied by the IIIrd cranial nerve except the lateral rectus (supplied by the VIth nerve) and superior oblique (IVth nerve).

All the extraocular muscles except the inferior oblique originate from a fibrous ring around the optic nerve (annulus of Zinn) at the orbital apex. The muscles fan out towards the eye to form a "muscle cone". All the recti muscles attach to the eyeball anterior to the equator whilst the oblique muscles attach behind the equator. The optic nerve, the ophthalmic blood vessels and the nerves to the extraocular muscles (except IVth nerve) are contained within the muscle cone (Fig. 2.9).

The levator palpebrae superioris is associated with the superior rectus. It arises from just above the annulus of Zinn, runs along the roof of the orbit overlying the superior rectus and attaches to the upper lid skin and anterior surface of the tarsal plate

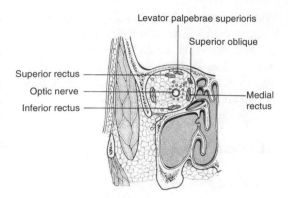

Fig. 2.9 Anatomy of the orbit

of the upper lid. Tenons capsule is a connective tissue covering which surrounds the eye and is continuous with the fascial covering of the muscles.

Physiology of the Eye

The primary function of the eye is to form a clear image of objects in our environment. These images are transmitted to the brain through the optic nerve and the posterior visual pathways. The various tissues of the eye and its adnexa are thus designed to facilitate this function.

The Eyelids

Functions include: (1) protection of the eye from mechanical trauma, extremes of temperature and bright light, and (2) maintenance of the normal pre-corneal tear film which is important for maintenance of corneal health and clarity.

Normal eyelid closure requires an intact nerve supply to the orbicularis oculi muscles (facial nerve). Eyelid opening is effected by the levator palpebrae superioris supplied by the IIIrd cranial nerve.

The Tear Film

The tear film consists of three layers: the mucoid, aqueous and oily layers.

The mucoid layer lies adjacent to the corneal epithelium. It improves the wetting properties of the tears. It is produced by the goblet cells in the conjunctival epithelium.

The watery (aqueous) layer is produced by the main lacrimal gland in the supero-temporal part of the orbit and accessory lacrimal glands found in the conjunctival stroma. This aqueous layer contains electrolytes, proteins, lysozyme, immunoglobulins, glucose and dissolved oxygen (from atmosphere).

The oily layer (superficial layer of the tear film) produced by meibomian glands—modified sebaceous gland of the eyelid margin. This oily layer helps maintain the vertical column of tears between the upper and lower lids and prevents excessive evaporation.

The tears normally flow away through a drainage system formed by the puncta (inferior and superior), canaliculi (inferior and superior), the common canaliculus, opening into the lacrimal sac, the naso-lacrimal duct (which drains into the nose).

The Cornea

The primary function of the cornea is refraction. In order to perform this function, the cornea requires:

(a) Transparency
(b) Smooth and regular surface
(c) Spherical curvature of proper refractive power
(d) Appropriate index of refraction

Corneal transparency is contributed to by anatomical and physiological factors.

Anatomical
– Absence of keratinisation of epithelium
– Tight packing of epithelial cells
– Mucus layer providing smooth lubricated surface
– Homogeneity of membranes—Bowman's and Descemet's
– Regular arrangement of corneal lamellae (parallel collagen fibres within each lamella with adjacent lamellae being perpendicular)
  Regularity produces a diffraction grating

– Paucity of corneal stromal cells, which are flattened within lamellae
  Interspaces: absence of blood vessels.

Physiological
Active dehydration of the cornea through Na+/HCO3− metabolic pump located in the corneal endothelium. This dehydration is supplemented by the physical barrier provided by the corneal epithelium and endothelium.

The Aqueous Humour

The aqueous humour is an optically clear solution of electrolytes (in water), which fills the space between the cornea and the lens. Normal volume is 0.3 ml. Its function is to nourish the lens and cornea, and maintain the intraocular pressure.

The Aqueous is formed by active secretion and ultra-filtration from the ciliary processes in the posterior chamber. The fluid enters the anterior chamber (AC) through the pupil, circulates in the AC and drains through the trabecular meshwork into the canal of Schlemm, the aqueous veins and the conjunctival episceral veins.

The aqueous normally contains a low concentration of proteins, but a higher concentration of ascorbic acid compared to plasma. Inflammation of the anterior uvea leads to leakage of proteins from the iris circulation into the aqueous (= plasmoid aqueous).

The Vitreous Body

The vitreous consists of a three dimensional network of collagen fibres with the interspaces filled with polymerised hyaluronic acid molecules, which are capable of holding large quantities of water. The vitreous does not normally flow but is percolated slowly by small amounts of aqueous. There is liquefaction of the jelly with age with bits breaking off to form floaters. This degeneration occurs at an earlier age in myopes.

The Lens

The lens, like the cornea, is transparent. It is avascular and depends on the aqueous for nourishment. It has a thick elastic capsule, which prevents molecules e.g., proteins moving into or out of it.

The lens continues to grow throughout life. New lens fibres (produced by the lens germinal epithelium, located at the lens equator) from the outer part (subcapsular) of the lens and move inwards towards the nucleus with age.

The lens is composed of 65% water and 35% protein. The water content of the lens decreases with age and, this along with the increasing thickness makes the lens becomes less pliable.

The lens is suspended from the ciliary body by the zonule, which arises from the ciliary body and inserts into the lens capsule near the equator.

The Ciliary Body

The ciliary muscle (within the ciliary body) is a mass of smooth muscle, which runs circumferentially inside the globe and is attached to the scleral spur anteriorly. It consists of two main parts:

(a) Longitudinal (meridional) fibres, which form the outer layers and arise from the scleral spur and insert into the choroid. Contraction of this part of the muscle exerts traction on the trabecular meshwork and also the choroid and retina.
(b) Circular fibres—form the inner part and run circumferentially. Contraction moves the ciliary processing inwards towards the centre of the pupil leading to relaxation of the zonules.

Accommodation

Accommodation is the process whereby relaxation of zonular fibres allows the lens to become more globular thereby increasing its refractive power. When the ciliary muscles relax, the zonu-lar fibres become taut and flatten the lens, reducing its refractive power. The contracting ciliary muscle is associated with constriction of the pupil and increased depth of focus.

Accommodation is a reflex initiated by visual blurring and/or awareness of proximity of the object of interest. The maximum amount of accommodation (amplitude of accommodation) is dependent upon the rigidity of the lens and contractility of the ciliary muscle. As the lens becomes more rigid with age (and contractions of the ciliary body reduce), accommodation decreases. Reading and other close work become impossible without optical correction—termed PRESBYOPIA.

The Retina

This is the 'photographic film' of the eye that converts light into electrical energy (transduction) for transmission to the brain.

It consists of two main parts:

(a) The neuroretina—all layers of the retina, which are derived from the inner layer of the embryological optic cup.
(b) The retinal pigment epithelium (RPE), which is derived from the outer layer of the optic cup. It is composed of a single layer of cells, which are fixed to Bruch's membrane. Bruch's membrane separates the outer retina from the choroid.

The retinal photoreceptors are located on the outer aspect of the neuroretina, an arrangement, which arose from inversion of the optic cup and allows close proximity between the photosensitive portion of the receptor cells and the opaque RPE cells, which reduce light scattering. The RPE also plays an important role in regeneration/recycling of photopigments of the eye and during light-dark adaptation.

In order for the light to reach the photoreceptors to form sharp images, all layers of the retina inner to the photoreceptors must be transparent. This transparency is contributed to by the absence of myelin fibres from the retinal neurones. The axons of the retina ganglion cells normally become myelinated only as they pass through the optic disc to enter the optic nerve.

There are two main types of photoreceptors in the retina—the rods and the cones. In the fovea centralis the only photoreceptors are cones, which are responsible for acute vision (visual details) and colour vision. Outside the fovea, rods become more abundant towards the retinal periphery. The rods are responsible for vision in poor (dim) light and for the wide field of vision.

The retinal capillary network (derived from the central retinal artery) extends no deeper than the inner nuclear layer and nourishes the neuroretina from inside up to part of the outer plexiform layer, as a multilayered vascular system. It is an end-arterial system. The choroid serves to nourish the RPE and the photoreceptors (by diffusion of nutrients). There are no blood vessels in the outer retina. The central fovea is completely avascular and depends on diffusion from the choroidal circulation for its nourishment. Thus normal functioning of the retina requires normal retinal and choroidal circulation. These different layers of the retinal and choroidal circulations are clearly demonstrated on optical coherence tomography angiography (OCT-A) (Fig. 2.10).

Retinal and Optic Nerve Transport. Like in most nerve fibres, there is movement of organelles contained in the cytoplasm between the nerve cell body and its terminal synapse. This is called axoplasmic transport, and can be in either direction: from cell body to synapse or vice versa. Rapid axoplasmic transport is energy consuming, and may therefore be interrupted by hypoxia or other injury. Such interruption of axoplasmic transport results in accumulation of organelles adjacent to the injury site. In the retinal nerve fibre layer, that is seen clinically as cotton wool spots. Another example of that phenomenon is seen in papilloedema (see Chap. 22).

Summary

- The eye is embryologically an extension of the central nervous system. It shares many common anatomical and physiological properties with the brain.
- The ocular adnexae and the orbit protect the eyeballs.
- The eyeball has three coats or layers (the corneo-sclera, uvea and, retina), three compartments (the anterior, and posterior chambers, and vitreous cavity), and contains three different fluids (aqueous humour, vitreous and blood within the vasculature).
- The cornea, and lens of the eye are avascular and clear normally, and are responsible for focusing light on the retina in order to allow clear vision.

Fig. 2.10 Normal OCT-A image report demonstrating retinal and choroidal vasculature vasculature. The top panel depicts images of the different vascular layers of the retina and choriocapllaris

- The cornea has a fixed curvature (and therefore fixed refractive power), whilst the lens changes its curvature (refractive power or focal length) through contraction and relaxation of the ciliary body by reflex depending on the location of objects, until presbyopia sets in.
- The retina is nourished from the retinal and choroidal circulations, both of which are derived from different branches of the ophthalmic artery.
- The visual pathway transmits the electrical signals generated in the retina to the occipital lobe which is responsible for our visual experiences. This pathway consists of the retina, optic nerve, optic chiasma, optic tract and radiation and the visual cortex and other cortical centres including the frontal eye fields. Some information is relayed in the subcortical centres that are responsible for cortical relay of the visual fibres, pupillary reflexes, and reflex control of eye movements. The frontal eye fields and areas 18 and 19 are responsible for coordinating voluntary and reflex eye movements.
- The pupillary light pathway is different from the visual pathway. The pupillary pathway and eye movements are described in Chap. 22.

Examination of the Eye

3

Abstract

As in all other medical examinations, examination of a patient with an eye problem should include history, physical examination and special investigation. The age as well as social history, including occupation of the patient should not be forgotten in such evaluation. A summary of such evaluation is provided in Table 3.1.

As in all other medical examinations, examination of a patient with an eye problem should include history, physical examination and special investigation. The age as well as social history, including occupation of the patient should not be forgotten in such evaluation. A summary of such cvaluation is provided in Table 3.1.

How to Find Out What a Patient Can See

One obvious way to measure sight is to ask the patient to identify letters, which are graded in size. This is the basis of the standard Snellen test for visual acuity (Fig. 3.1). This test only measures the function of a small area of retina at the posterior pole of the eye called the macula. If we stare fixedly at an object, for example a picture on the wall, and attempt to keep our eyes as still as possible, it soon becomes apparent that we can only appreciate detail in a small part of the centre of the field of vision. Everything around us is ill defined and yet we can detect the slightest twitch of a finger from the corner of our eyes. The macula region is specialised to detect fine detail, whereas the whole peripheral retina is concerned with the detection of shape and movement. In order to see, we use the peripheral retina to help us scan the field of view. The peripheral retina may be considered as equivalent to the TV cameraman who moves the camera around to the relevant views and allows the camera (or macula) to make sense of the scene. If the macula area is damaged by, for example, age related macular degeneration, then the patient may be unable to see even the largest print on the test type and yet have no difficulty in walking about the room. Navigational vision is largely dependent on the peripheral field of vision. On the other side of the coin, the patient with marked constriction of the peripheral field of vision but preservation of the central field may behave as though blind. The same patient could read the test chart down to the bottom *once he has found it*. This situation sometimes arises in patients with advanced open angle glaucoma.

It should be becoming clear that measuring the visual acuity, although very useful, is not an adequate measure of vision on its own. For a

Table 3.1 Summary of patient evaluation

History	
Age	
Ophthalmic:	
Subnormal vision	Duration. Difference between eyes
Disturbances of vision	Distortion, haloes, floaters, flashing lights, momentary losses of vision—field defects
Pain/discomfort	Increase/decrease change in appearance—discolouration
Change in lacrimation	Swelling/mass
Diplopia	Displacement
General medical:	Diabetes/hypertension/COAD/dysthyroid/connective tissue disease
Drugs	FH social/occupational
Examination	
VA: distance/near (with and without glasses)	
Colour vision	
Visual fields	
Orbit	Proptosis/enophthalmos
Ocular movements—conjugate and convergence	Eyelids and lacrimal apparatus
Pupils	Intraocular pressure
Position of eyes conjunctiva, cornea	
AC Iris Media—lens/vitreous Fundus—retina/choroid, optic disc	
Special investigations	
Fluorescein angiography	
Radiological and ultrasound	
Haematological/biochemical	
Bacteriological/immunological	
Diagnosis	
Anatomical	E.g., cataract
Aetiological	E.g., diabetes

Fig. 3.1 The Snellen chart

Visual Acuity

The familiar Snellen chart has one large letter at the top, which is designed to be just visible to a normal-sighted person at 60 m. The chart is viewed from a distance of 6 m. If a patient is just able to see this large letter, the vision is recorded as 6/60. Below the large letter are rows of smaller letters decreasing in size down to the bottom. The size of letter normally visible to a normal-sighted person at 6 m is usually on the second-to-bottom line. Patients reading this line are said to have a vision of 6/6. If a patient cannot read the top letter, he is taken nearer to the chart. If the top letter becomes visible at 3 m, the acuity is recorded as 3/60. If the letter is still not visible, the patient is asked if he can count fingers (recorded as "CF") and, failing this, if he can see hand movements ("HM"). Finally, if even hand movements are not seen, the ability to see a light is tested ("PL").

Young children and illiterates can be asked to do the "E" test in which they must orient a large wooden letter "E" so that it is the same way up as an indicated letter E on a chart. Perhaps better than this is the Stycar test (Fig. 3.2) in which the

proper clinical examination we need to assess the visual fields and colour vision. A number of other facets of visual function can also be measured, such as contrast sensitivity and dark adaptation.

Fig. 3.3 The Humphrey field analyser

Fig. 3.2 The Stycar test

child is asked to point at the letter on a card which is the same as the one held up at 6 m. Other ways of measuring visual acuity including the more detailed LogMAR assessment are discussed in Chap. 17. Validated smartphone apps (e.g. Peek Acuity from www.peekvision.org) can be used to learn about types of acuity, and to simulate different levels of vision. Such tests may be practical to test vision when a standardised eye clinic environment is not available.

Fig. 3.4 Ishihara plates for colour vision

Visual Field

Some measurements of the visual field can be made by sitting facing the patient and asking if the movement of one's fingers can be discerned. The patient is instructed to cover one eye with a hand and the observer also covers one of his eyes so that he can check the patient's field against his own. The test can be made more accurate by using a pin with a red head on it as a target. None of these confrontation methods can match the accuracy of formal perimetry. A number of specialised instruments of varying complexity are available. Using such equipment, the patient is presented with a number of different-sized targets in different parts of the visual field, and a map of the field of vision is charted. An accurate map of the visual field is often of great diagnostic importance. In the past it was customary to map out

the central part of the visual field using the Bjerrum screen, and the peripheral field using a perimeter. The Goldmann perimeter was then introduced, and this instrument allows both central and peripheral fields to be plotted out on one chart. The Humphrey field analyser is a further development in field testing. It provides an automated visual field recording system (Fig. 3.3). It also records the reliability of the patient by showing false positive and false negative errors. In practice this is very useful as poor reliability is often an explanation for poor performance.

Colour Vision

The Ishihara plates provide a popular and effective method for screening for colour vision defects (Fig. 3.4). The patient is presented with a series of plates on which are printed numerous coloured dots. The normally sighted subject will see numbers on the majority of the plates, whereas the colour-defective patient will fail to see many of the numbers. The test is easy to do and will effectively screen out the more common red-green deficiency found in 8% of the male population. There are other tests available that will measure blue-green defects, for example, the City University Test. Other tests, such as the Farnsworth 100 Hue test, are available for the more detailed analysis of colour vision.

Spectacles

Measurement of the visual acuity may not be valid unless the patient is wearing the correct spectacles. Some patients when asked to *read* a Snellen chart will put on their reading glasses. Since these glasses are designed for close work, the chart may be largely obscured and the uninitiated doctor might be surprised at the poor level of visual acuity (Fig. 3.5). If the glasses have been left at home, long sight or short sight can be largely overcome by asking the patient to view the chart through a pinhole. Similarly, an appropriate spectacle correction (near) must be worn when testing visual fields and colour vision. In an ophthalmic department a check of the spectacle prescription is a routine part of the initial examination. Figure 3.6 shows how the converging power of the optical media and the length of the eye are

mismatched to produce the need to wear spectacles (the dotted lines indicate the paths for rays of light without any corrective lens).

How to Start Examining an Eye

Evaluating the Pupil

Examination of the pupil is best performed in a dimly lit room.

Size and symmetry of pupils is assessed by asking the patient to fixate on a distant object such as a letter on the Snellen chart. A dim light is then directed on to the face from below so that both pupils can be seen simultaneously in the diffuse illumination. Normally, the two pupils in

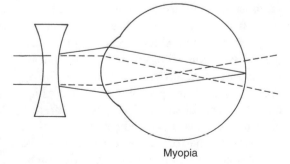

I borrowed my husband's glasses. . . .

Fig. 3.5 The uninitiated might be surprised at the poor level of visual acuity

Hypermetropia

Myopia

Fig. 3.6 Optical defects of the eye

any individual are of equal size, although slight differences in size may be observed in up to 20% of the population. Usually physiological unequal pupils (anisocoria) remain unaltered by changing the background illumination.

The pupil light reflex: A strong focal light is shone on the pupils, one after the other. The direct reaction as well as the consensual reaction (other pupil) are observed. If the afferent arc of the pupil pathway were normal the direct and consensual reactions would be equal.

The near response of the pupil: Ask the patient to gaze at a distant object (e.g. Snellen chart) then at a near object (e.g. his own finger tip just in front of his nose). Observe the pupils as the patient changes gaze from distant to near fixation and vice versa. Generally if the pupil light reflex is intact then the near reflex is normal.

External Eye and Lids

The eyelids should be inspected to make sure that the lid margins and puncta are correctly aligned against the globe and that there are no ingrowing lashes. Early basal cell carcinomas (also known as rodent ulcers) on eyelid skin can easily be missed, especially if obscured by cosmetics. The presence of ptosis should be noted and the ocular movements assessed by asking the patient to follow a finger upwards, downwards and to each side. Palpation of the skin around the eyes may reveal an orbital tumour or swollen lacrimal sac. Palpation with the end of a glass rod is sometimes useful to find points of tenderness when the lid is diffusely swollen. Such tenderness can indicate a primary infection of a lash root or the lacrimal sac. Both surfaces of the eyelids should be examined. The inside of the lower lid can easily be inspected by pulling down the skin of the lid with the index finger. The upper lid can be everted by asking the patient to look down, grasping the lashes gently between finger and thumb, and rolling the lid margins upwards and forwards over a cotton-wool bud or glass rod. The lid will usually remain in this everted position until the patient is asked to look up. Foreign bodies quite often lodge themselves under the upper lid and they can only be removed by this means. As a general rule, if a patient complains that there is something in his eye, there usually is, and if you find nothing, it is necessary to look again more closely or refer the patient for microscopic examination. A feeling of grittiness may be due to inflammation of the conjunctiva and this may be accompanied by evidence of purulent discharge in the lashes. The presence of tear overflow and excoriation of the skin in the outer canthus should also be noted.

The Globe

Much ophthalmic disease has been described and classified using the microscope. In spite of this, many of the important eye diseases can be diagnosed using a hand magnifier and an ophthalmoscope. At this point it is important to understand the principle of examining the eye with a focused beam of light. If a pencil of light is directed obliquely through the cornea and anterior chamber, it can be made to illuminate structures or abnormalities otherwise invisible. One might inspect the glass sides and water of a fish tank using a strong, focused torch in the same manner (Fig. 3.7). Many ophthalmoscopes incorporate a focused beam of light, which can be used for this purpose. A magnified image of the anterior segment of the eye can be viewed with a direct ophthalmoscope

Fig. 3.7 Focal illumination

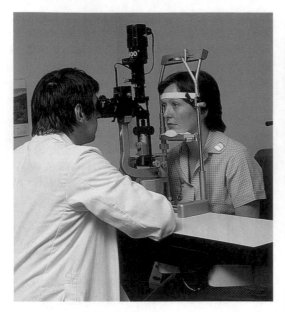

Fig. 3.8 Slit-lamp examination

held about 1/3 m away from the eye through a
+10 or +12 lens. The principle has been developed to a high degree in the slit lamp (Fig. 3.8).
This instrument allows a focused slit of light to
be shone through the eye, which can then be
examined by a binocular microscope. By this
means an optical section of the eye can be created. The method can be compared with making
a histological section where the slice of tissue
is made with a knife rather than a beam of light.
The slit lamp is sometimes called the biomicroscope. By means of such optical aids, the cornea must be carefully inspected for scars or
foreign bodies. The presence of vascular congestion around the corneal margin may be of
significance. Closer inspection of the iris may
show that it is atrophic or fixed by adhesions.
Turbidity or cells in the aqueous may be seen in
the beam of the inspection light. The lens and
anterior parts of the vitreous can be examined
by the same means.

Once the anterior segment of the eye has
been examined, the intraocular pressure is measured. The 'gold standard' method of measurement is to use the Goldmann tonometer
(Fig. 3.9), which relies on the principle of
'applanation'. In essence, the application of this

Fig. 3.9 The Goldmann tonometer

principle provides a derived measurement of
intraocular pressure by flattening a small known
area of cornea with a variable force. The amount
of force required to flatten a specific area is pro-
portional to the intraocular pressure reading,
and this is read from a dial. The readings provided by this measurement are highly reproduc-
ible and are given in millimetres of mercury
(mmHg).

Some optometrists however employ "air
puff" tonometers, which are more portable and
do not require attachment to a slit-lamp. These
instruments are excellent for screening but are
generally not as accurate as applanation tonometers. A convenient hand-held instrument (the
iCare® tonometer) is available (Fig. 3.10) and is
commonly used by ophthalmologists when a slit
lamp is not available. The iCare tonometer has
an advantage in that it is easy to learn to use, and
it can be used by allied health care profession-
als; with guidance, patients can also check their

Fig. 3.10 The iCare tonometer

own eye pressures at home using a home-use iCare.

At this stage, the pupil may be dilated for better examination of the fundi and optical media. A short-acting mydriatic is preferable e. g. Tropicamide 1% (Mydriacyl). These particular drops take effect after 10 min and take 2–4 h to wear off. Patients should be warned that their vision will be blurred and that they will be more sensitive to light over this period. Most people find that their ability to drive a car is unimpaired, but there is a potential medico-legal risk if the patient subsequently has a car accident. Once the pupils have been dilated, the eye can then be examined with the ophthalmoscope.

How to Use the Ophthalmoscope

Before the middle of the last century, nobody had seen the inside of a living eye and much of the science of medical ophthalmology was unknown. In 1851 Hermann Von Helmholtz introduced his ophthalmoscope and it rapidly became used in clinics dealing with ophthalmological problems. The task of Helmholtz was to devise a way of looking through the black pupil and at the same time illuminate the interior of the globe. He solved the problem by arranging to view the fundus of the eye through an angled piece of glass. A light projected from the side was reflected into the eye by total internal reflection. Most modern ophthalmoscopes employ an angled mirror with a small hole in it to achieve the same end. They also incorporate a series of lenses which can be interposed between the eye

of the patient and that of the observer, thereby overcoming any refractive problems which may defocus the view. These lenses are positioned by rotating a knurled wheel at the side of the ophthalmoscope. A number on the face of the instrument indicates the strength of the lens. When choosing an ophthalmoscope, it is worth remembering that large ones take larger batteries which last longer (or, better still, they may have rechargeable batteries); small ophthalmoscopes are handy for the pocket. Some ophthalmoscopes have a wider field of view than others and this is an advantage when learning to use the instrument.

If examining the patient's right eye, it is best to hold the ophthalmoscope in the right hand and view through one's own right eye. A left eye should be viewed with the left eye using the left hand (Fig. 3.11). It is best if the patient is seated and the doctor is standing. The first thing to observe is the red reflex, which simply refers to the general reddish colouring seen through the pupil. If viewed from about 30 cm away from the eye, very slight and subtle opacities or defects in the optical media may be seen, against the background of the red reflex. The patient's eye must always be brought into focus by rotating the lens wheel on the ophthalmoscope.

Having observed the red reflex, the eye can be approached closely and the focus of the ophthalmoscope adjusted so that fundus detail becomes visible. It is best to look for the optic disc first, remembering its position nasal to the posterior pole and slightly above the horizontal meridian.

Fig. 3.11 Direct ophthalmoscopy

The patient should be asked to look straight ahead at this point. The important points to note about the disc are the clarity of the margins, the colour, the nature of the central cup, the vessel entry and the presence or absence of haemorrhages. Once the disc has been examined carefully, the vessels from the disc can be followed. For example, the upper temporal branch vessels can be followed out to the periphery and back, then the lower temporal branch vessels, then the upper nasal and finally the lower nasal. Having examined the vessels, ask the patient to look directly at the ophthalmoscope light and the macular region should come into view. At first this may look unremarkable, like a minute dot of light which follows our own light. More careful examination will reveal that it has a yellowish colour. To obtain a very highly magnified view of the macular it is usually necessary to examine it with a special contact lens on the slip-lamp microscope, the Goldmann fundus lens. A fundus photograph is also very helpful. After viewing the macula the general fundus background should be observed. The appearance here depends upon the complexion of the patient: in a lightly pigmented subject it is possible to see through the stippled pigment epithelium and obtain an indefinite view of the choroidal vasculature. In heavily pigmented subjects, the pigment epithelium is uniformly black and prevents any view of the choroid, which lies behind it. Finally, the peripheral fundus can be inspected by asking the patient to look to the extremes of gaze and by refocusing the ophthalmoscope. Examining the peripheral fundus demands some special skill, even with the ordinary ophthalmoscope, but it is best seen using the triple mirror gonioscope. This is a modified contact lens which has an angled mirror attached to it. A view through this mirror is obtained using the slit-lamp microscope.

There are a number of other methods of examining the fundus. The ophthalmoscope described above is known as the direct ophthalmoscope. Shortly after the introduction of direct ophthalmoscopy, the indirect ophthalmoscope was introduced. If one examines an eye with the pupil dilated through a mirror with a hole in it, the patient being at arm's length from the observer and the mirror being held close to the observer's eye, then the red reflex is seen. If a convex lens is placed in the line of sight about 8 cm from the patient's eye, then, rather surprisingly, a clear wide field inverted view of the fundus is obtained. The view can be made binocular, and the binocular indirect ophthalmoscope is an essential tool of the retinal surgeon (Fig. 3.12). If we want a really magnified view of the fundus, then the slit-lamp microscope can be used. However, a special lens must be placed in front of the patient's eye, This may be in the form of the triple mirror contact lens (Fig. 3.13). In recent years it has become a routine practice to examine the fundus with the slit lamp and strong convex lenses e.g. VOLK +60, +78 or +90DS

Fig. 3.12   Indirect ophthalmoscopy

Fig. 3.13   The Goldmann triple mirror

Fig. 3.14 Fluorescein angiogram of normal fundus

Fig. 3.15 Indocyanine green angiography of normal fundus

aspheric lenses. These high power convex lenses provide inverted reversed images like the indirect ophthalmoscope. Another useful way of examining the fundus is by means of fundus photography. The photographs provide a permanent record of the fundus. A special type of fundus photograph known as a fluorescein angiogram shows up the retinal vessels, including the capillaries, in great detail. The technique involves taking repeated photographs in rapid succession after the injection of the dye fluorescein into the antecubital vein. The dye in the vessels is selectively photographed by using filters in the camera (Fig. 3.14). Indocyanine green angiography (ICG) is more useful in assessing the choroidal circulation since ICG-A fluorescence is transmitted through the retinal pigment epithelium (compared to fluorescein) (Fig. 3.15).

Video filming is becoming an important method for observing changing events in the fundus and it is now possible to view a real time image of the optic fundus on a TV screen using the scanning laser ophthalmoscope. This type of equipment will undoubtedly become a routine tool for the ophthalmologist.

Other Tests Available in an Eye Department

Several special tests are available to measure the ability of the eyes to work together. A department known as the Orthoptic Department is usually set aside within the eye clinic for making these tests. When there is a defect of the ocular movements,

this can be monitored by means of the Hess chart (see chapter on squint, Chap. 14). The ability to use the eyes together is measured on the synoptophore, and any tendency of one eye to turn out or in can also be carefully measured with prisms of differing strengths combined with a cover test to check the size of deviation in dioptres. The use of contact lenses and also of intraocular implants has demanded more accurate measurements of the cornea and of the length of the eye. A keratometer is an instrument for measuring the curvature of the cornea, and the length of the eye can now be accurately measured by ultrasound. If one eye appears to protrude forwards and one wishes to monitor the position of the globes relative to the orbital margin, then an exophthalmometer is used (Fig. 3.16). X-rays of the eye and orbit are still used. An X-ray is essential if an intraocular foreign body is suspected and it is useful for detecting bony abnormalities in the walls of the orbit due to tumours. Computerised tomography scanning (CT scan) has become an important diagnostic technique, especially for lesions in the orbit (Fig. 3.17) particularly those involving bony tissues. This specialised Xray has surpassed plain xrays for most ophthalmic purposes. Magnetic resonance imaging (MRI) is more useful in assessing soft tissues of the orbit and cranium. Ultrasonography (B scan ultrasound) is a technique used to visualise the poste-

Fig. 3.16 The exophthalmometer

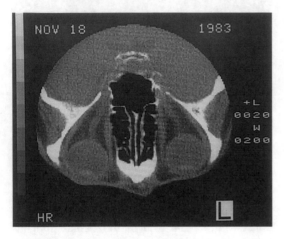

Fig. 3.17 Computed tomography (CT) scan of eyes and orbit (normal)

rior segment especially when then view is obscured by opaque media (e.g. cataract or vitreous haemorrhage). Electroretinography provides a measure of the electrical changes which take place in the retina when the eye is exposed to light. It can indicate retinal function in the same way that the electrocardiogram indicates cardiac function. The visually evoked potential (VEP) is a measure of minute electrical changes over the back of the scalp which occur when the eyes are stimulated with a flashing light. This test has been shown to be useful in detecting previous damage to the optic nerve in patients with suspected multiple sclerosis.

A variety of imaging devices are in widespread use now both in hospitals and in the community setting. For example, digital fundus cameras are used for diabetic retinal screening and optic disc. Ocular Coherence Tomography (OCT) is used for glaucoma monitoring (Fig. 3.18), whilst macula OCT is used for detecting and managing macula disease.

Fig. 3.18 Ocular coherence tomography

Part II

Primary Eye Care Problems

Long Sight, Short Sight

4

Abstract

In this chapter the optical problems caused by abnormality of the size of the eyeball are discussed and the confusion caused by the lay terms "long sight" and "short sight" is explained. The physical changes in the eye associated with refractive error as well as some of the associated eye diseases are described.

It is useful to distinguish between long sighted and short sighted patients as you will see later in this chapter but straight away we come across a problem with terminology. Think of the "short sighted" old man who cannot see to read without glasses and at the same time the "short sighted" young lady who cannot see clearly in the distance. The term "short sight" is used in these instances unwittingly by the layman to mean two different situations; it can either mean *presbyopia* (due to diminished focussing power with ageing as in the case of the old man) or it can mean *myopia* (due to a larger eyeball as in the case of the young lady).

Leaving aside presbyopia for the time being we need to realise that the myopic person has physically larger than normal eyes with an anteroposterior diameter of more than 24 mm and by contrast the hypermetropic person has smaller than usual eyes with an anteroposterior diameter of less than 24 mm. To obtain a clear image, this abnormal length of the eye needs optical correction with a lens to bring light rays to a focus on the retina. The hypermetropic (or longsighted person) requires a convex lens to converge the rays whereas the myopic person requires a concave lens to make light rays diverge before reaching the eye.

Glasses with convex lenses in them make the eyes look bigger and glasses with concave lenses in them make the eyes look smaller. Figure 4.1 shows a longsighted (hypermetropic) subject whose glasses seem to enlarge the eyes and Fig. 4.2 shows a shortsighted (myopic) subject. The clinical importance of all this is that with a little practice we can tell the difference at a glance as the patient enters the room. This often helps with the diagnosis because certain eye diseases are associated with myopia and others with hypermetropia.

The nature of the spectacle correction can be verified by moving the lens in the glasses from side to side in front of one's hand. If the hand appears to move in the opposite direction to that of the movement of the spectacle lens, it is convex (Fig. 4.3). The spectacles of the myopic patient contain concave or diverging lenses and, if these are moved to and fro in front of one's hand, the hand appears to move in the same direction as the movement. As a further clue, when we look at the

Fig. 4.1 A long-sighted person

Fig. 4.2 A short-sighted person

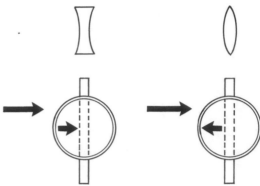

Fig. 4.3 Concave lens "with"; convex lens "against". Try this for yourself in the clinic

Here again let us remind ourselves that hypermetropia and myopia have nothing to do with presbyopia which is the failure of the eyes to focus on near objects which appears in middle age. This is nothing to do with the length of the eyeball but is related to a diminished ability to change the shape of the lens. It is corrected in otherwise normal eyes by using a convex lens. Obviously myopes, hypermetropes and those with no refractive error are all susceptible to presbyopia.

When we examine hypermetropic and myopic eyes with the ophthalmoscope we find that there are physical differences between the two. The optic disc of the hypermetrope tends to be smaller and pinker and in extreme cases especially in children, the disc can appear to be swollen when in fact it is quite normal. By contrast the optic disc of the myope is larger and paler with well defined margins and can be mistaken for an atrophic disc.

Hypermetropia is associated with certain eye condition notably narrow angle glaucoma and childhood amblyopia of disuse. Myopia is associated with others particularly retinal detachment cataract and myopic retinal degeneration. You must be aware though that whereas refractive errors are extremely common, these particular conditions are relatively rare in the general population. Table 4.1 shows a more comprehensive list of these associations.

Having observed the nature of the spectacle lenses we have now made a small step towards diagnosing the eye condition. If the patient is hypermetrope from a slight angle, the line of the cheek goes out behind the magnifying lenses and vice versa for the myope (see Figs. 4.1 and 4.2).

Table 4.1   Eye disease and refractive error

Myopia ('short sight')	Hypermetropia ('long sight')
CONDITIONS ASSOCIATED WITH MYOPIA	CONDITIONS ASSOCIATED WITH HYPERMETROPIA
Retinal detachment	
Macula haemorrhages	Narrow angle glaucoma
Cataract	Concomitant squint
Myopic chorio-retinal degeneration	Amblyopia of disuse
Down's syndrome	
Keratoconus (conical cornea)	
CONDITIONS CAUSING MYOPIA	CONDITIONS CAUSING HYPERMETROPIA
Large eye	Small eye
Cataract	Retinal detachment
Diabetes mellitus	Orbital tumours
Accommodation spasm, or 'pseudomyopia'	Macula oedema
Congenital glaucoma	

middle aged and complaining of evening headaches, seeing haloes around street lights and at the same time blurring of vision then narrow angle glaucoma is the wrong diagnosis if the patient is myopic. It could well be the right diagnosis if the patient is hypermetropic. If the patient in Fig. 4.2 were to be complaining of the sudden appearance of black spots combined with seeing flashes of light he may be about to have a retinal detachment.

If we take note of whether a patient is long sighted or short sighted at an early stage, then this information can influence the type of questions that are best asked when taking a history.

Finally it is worth remembering that the myopic patient can see objects close at hand and read without glasses at any age whereas the hypermetropic patient has to focus to see at all distances. If the hypermetrope has good focussing power (i.e. the younger subject) then the distance vision may be clear without glasses but when hypermetropia is more severe the unaided vision is poor at all ranges.

You should be able to answer the following questions after reading this chapter:

1. Is the myopic eye larger or smaller than normal and how does this affect the eyesight?
2. What is presbyopia
3. How can you tell whether someone is myopic or hypermetropic?
4. What eye conditions are more common in myopic eyes?
5. How do convex and concave lenses affect light rays?

Abstract

In this chapter the causes and treatment of the watering eye and the dry eye are described. The various common deformities of the eyelids are then considered and subsequently the commoner infections, tumours and injuries seen in the eyelids.

The Watering Eye

Quite often patients present at the clinic or surgery complaining of watering eyes. It may be the golfer whose glasses keep misting up on the fairway or the housewife who is embarrassed by tears dropping onto the food when cooking, or it may be the 6-month old baby whose eyes have watered and discharged since birth. Sometimes an elderly patient may complain of watering eyes when on examination there is no evidence of tear excess but the vision has been made blurred by cataracts. Some degree of tear overflow is of course quite normal in windy weather, and the anxious patient may over-emphasize this; it is important to assess the actual amount of overflow by asking the patient whether it occurs all the time both in and out of doors.

An eye may water because the tears cannot drain away adequately or because there is excessive secretion of tears.

Impaired Drainage of Tears

Normally the tears drain through 2 min openings at the inner end of the lid margins known as the upper and lower lacrimal puncta.

The Lacrimal Passageway

Most of the tears drain through the lower punctum. The puncta mark the opening of the lacrimal canaliculi and these small tubes conduct tears medially to the common canaliculus and thence into the tear sac (Fig. 5.1). The tear sac is con-

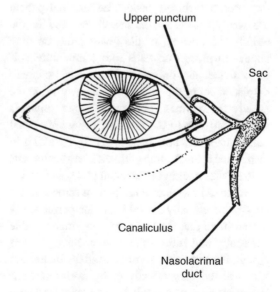

Fig. 5.1 The lacrimal passageway

Fig. 5.3 Ectropion

Fig. 5.2 Bilateral entropion. The inwardly turned lower eyelids are largely obscured by purulent discharge

nected directly to the nasolacrimal duct, which opens into the inferior meatus of the nose below the inferior turbinate bone. The lacrimal puncta are easily visible to the naked eye and in the elderly the opening of the lower punctum may appear to project upwards like a miniature volcano. Inadequate drainage of tears may be due to displacement of the punctum; the lower lid in the elderly sometimes becomes turned inwards (entropion) due to the fact that the whole tarsal plate rotates on a horizontal axis (Fig. 5.2). This in turn is due to slackening of the fascial attachments of the lower margin of the tarsal plate. At first the eyelid turns in whenever the patient screws up the eyes but eventually the lid becomes permanently turned in so that the lashes are no longer visible externally and rub on the cornea. Such patients complain of watering sore eyes and the matter can be corrected very effectively by eyelid surgery. Entropion may also result from scarring and contracture of the conjunctiva on the inner surface of the eyelid.

Not only may the punctum become turned inwards, but it may also be turned outwards. Sometimes the eversion may be very slight but enough to cause problems. Sometimes the patient may have been using eyedrops, which combined with the overflow of tears causes excoriation and contracture of the skin of the lower eyelid. This leads to further eversion or ectropion of the lower eyelid (Fig. 5.3). Often the ectropion arises as the result of increasing laxity of the skin in the elderly but it may also be due to scarring and contracture of the skin due to trauma (cicatricial ectropion). Ectropion may be corrected very effectively by suitable lid surgery.

Drainage of tears along the lacrimal canaliculi depends to some extent on the muscular action of certain fibres of the orbicularis oculi muscle. This band of fibres encloses the lacrimal sac and it is thought that the walls of the sac are thereby stretched, producing slight suction along the canaliculi. Whatever the exact mechanism, when the orbicularis muscle is paralyzed the tear flow is impaired even if the position of the punctum is normal. Sometimes patients who have suffered a Bell's palsy may complain of a watering eye even though they appear to have otherwise made a complete recovery.

Misplacement of the drainage channels, particularly of the punctum, may thus affect the outflow of tears, but perhaps more commonly the drainage channel itself becomes blocked. In young infants with lacrimal obstruction the blockage is usually at the lower end of the naso-lacrimal duct and takes the form of a plug of mucus or a residual embryological septum which has failed to become naturally perforated. In these cases there is nearly always some purulent discharge which may be expressed from the tear sac by gentle pressure with the index finger over the medial palpebral ligament. The mother is shown how to express this material once or twice daily and is instructed to instil antibiotic drops three or four times daily. This treatment alone may resolve the problem and many cases may undoubtedly resolve spontaneously. Sometimes it is necessary to syringe and probe the tear duct under sedation or a brief anaesthetic. Usually one waits until the child is at least 9 months old before considering probing. In adults the obstruction is more often in the common canaliculus or nasolacrimal duct. In these cases the tear duct can be syringed after the instillation of local anaesthetic drops. This procedure is simple though it must be done with care to avoid damaging the canaliculus, and even if the obstruction is not cleared it can allow the surgeon to identify the site of the obstruction. Sometimes a permanent obstruction is identified at the lower end of the nasolacrimal duct, which can be relieved by surgery under general anaesthesia or the more

recently introduced laser treatment applied through the nose. The initial investigation of lacrimal obstruction entails syringing and if this does not give the information required, it is possible to display the tear duct by x-ray using a radio-opaque contrast medium. This is injected into the lower canaliculus with a lacrimal syringe (Fig. 5.4). The technique is known as dacryocystography.

Acute Dacryocystitis

Sometimes the lacrimal sac may become infected. This may occur in either children or adults but is more common in adult females. The condition may present initially as a watering eye and, in its early stages, the diagnosis may be missed if the tear sac is not gently palpated and found to be tender. Subsequently there is marked swelling and tenderness at the inner canthus and eventually the abscess may point and burst. In its early stages the condition can be aborted by the use of local and systemic antibiotics, but once an abscess has formed this may point and burst on the skin surface. Surgical incision and drainage of a lacrimal abscess can lead to the formation of a lacrimal fistula (Fig. 5.5).

Very rarely, the lacrimal canaliculi may become infected by the fungus Actinomycosis and a small telltale bead of pus can be expressed from the punctum. The condition is very resistant to ordinary treatment with local antibiotics, and

Fig. 5.4 Dacryocystogram (With acknowledgement to Mr R. Welham)

Fig. 5.5 Acute dacryocystitis (With acknowledgement to Mr R. Welham)

Fig. 5.6 Diagnostic use of lacrimal syringing. (1) Obstruction in canaliculus shown by regurgitation of saline back through punctum. (2) Common canaliculus obstruction shown by return of saline through upper punctum. (3) Obstruction in nasolacrimal duct shown by filling of lacrimal sac

is best treated by opening up the punctum with a fine knife specially designed for the purpose— the procedure being called canaliculotomy—and then irrigating the canaliculi and tear duct with a suitable antibiotic.

The diagnosis of lacrimal obstruction therefore depends firstly on an examination of the eyelids, secondly on syringing the tear ducts, and then if necessary dacryocystography. Figure 5.6 illustrates the diagnostic use of lacrimal syringing.

Excessive Secretion of Tears

A wide range of conditions affecting the eye may cause an excessive production of tears, from acute glaucoma to a corneal abscess, but these do not usually present as a watering eye since the other symptoms such as pain or visual loss are more evident to the patient. Occasionally the unwary doctor may be caught out by an irritative lesion on the cornea, which mimics the more commonplace lacrimal obstruction. For example a small corneal foreign body or an ingrowing eyelash may present in this way. Not uncommonly, a loose lash may float into the lower lacrimal canaliculus where it may become lodged causing chronic irritation at the inner canthus. Its removal after weeks of discomfort produces instant relief and gratitude.

The Dry Eye

A patient may complain of dryness of the eyes simply because the conjunctiva is inflamed, but when the tear film really is defective the patient may complain of soreness and irritation rather than dryness. The diagnosis of a dry eye depends on a careful examination and it is quite erroneous to assume that the tear film is inadequate simply because the patient complains of dryness, or even if the symptoms appear to be improved by artificial tears.

The normal tear film consists of three layers and the integrity of this film is essential for comfort and more important for good vision. The anterior or outermost layer is formed by the oily secretion of the Meibomian glands and the layer next to the cornea is mucinous to allow proper wetting by the watery component of the tears which lies sandwiched between the two. This three layered film is constantly maintained by the act of blinking.

Causes of Dry Eye

- Systemic disease with lacrimal gland involvement.
    Sarcoidosis
    Rheumatoid arthritis (Sjogren's syndrome)
- Trachoma (Chlamydial conjunctivitis and keratitis—see next chapter)
- Neuroparalytic keratitis
- Exposure keratitis
- Other rare causes

Signs

Slit Lamp Examination

In a normal subject the tear film is evident as a rim of fluid along the lid margin and a deficiency of this may be seen by direct examination. Prolonged deficiency of tears may be associated with the presence of filaments—microscopic strands of mucus and epithelial cells, which stain well with Rose Bengal. Punctate staining of the corneal epithelium is also seen after applying a drop of fluorescein. In some dry eye syndromes, for example ocular pemphigoid and Stevens Johnson syndrome, keratinisation of the cornea and conjunctiva with the formation of contracting adhesions between the opposed surfaces of the conjunctiva occurs. A similar change is apparent following chemical or thermal burns of the eyes.

Schirmer's Test

One end of a special filter paper strip is placed between the globe and the lower eyelid. The other end projects forward and the time taken for the tears to wet the projecting strip is measured. The test is not a very accurate measure of tear secretion but it provides a useful guide (Fig. 5.7).

Tear Film Break-Up Time

Using the slit lamp microscope, the time for the tear film to break up when the patient stops blinking is measured. This test is sometimes used as an index of mucin deficiency.

Management of the Dry Eye

This, of course, depends on the cause of the dry eye and the underlying systemic cause may require treatment in the first place. Artificial tear drops are a mainstay in treatment and various types are available, their use depending on which component of the tear film is defective. In severe cases it may be necessary to consider temporary or permanent occlusion of the lacrimal puncta.

Deformities of the Eyelids

The Normal Eyelid

Figure 5.8 is a diagram of the normal eyelids in cross section. The lids contain two antagonistic voluntary muscles; the more superficial orbicularis oculi, supplied by the seventh cranial nerve, which closes the eye, and the tendon of the levator palpebrae superioris supplied by the third cra-

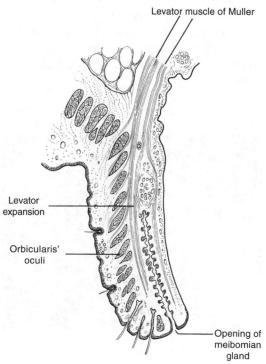

Fig. 5.8 Cross-section of a normal eyelid

Fig. 5.7 Schirmer's test

nial nerve, which opens the eye. We must not forget that there is also some smooth muscle in the upper and lower eyelids, which has clinical importance apart from its influence on facial expression when the subject is under stress. Loss of tone in this muscle accounts for the slight ptosis seen in Horner's syndrome; increased tone is seen in thyrotoxic eye disease. These muscles (that in the upper lid is known as Muller's muscle) are attached to the skeleton of the lid which is the tarsal plate, a plate of fibrous tissue (not cartilage) which contains the Meibomian glands.

Epicanthus

Figure 5.9 shows that this is characterised by vertical folds of skin at the inner canthus. These folds are seen quite commonly in otherwise quite normal infants and they gradually disappear as the facial bones develop. Children with epicanthus may appear to the uninitiated to be squinting and this can cause considerable parental anxiety. It is important to explain that the squint is simply an optical illusion once the absence of any true deviation of the eyes has been confirmed. Epicanthus persists into adult life in Mongolian races, and occasionally it is seen in European adults. It may also be associated with other eyelid deformities.

Fig. 5.9 Epicanthus

Entropion

This is an inturning of the eyelid. The common form is the inturning of the lower eyelid seen in elderly patients. Often the patient does not notice that the eyelid is inturned but complains of soreness and irritation. Closer inspection reveals the inturned eyelid, which can be restored to its normal position by slight downward pressure on the lower eyelid, only to turn in again when the patient forcibly closes the eyes. The inturned eyelashes tend to rub on the cornea and if neglected the condition can lead to corneal scarring and consequent loss of vision. The condition is often associated with muscular eyelids and sometimes seems to be precipitated by repeatedly screwing up the eyes. Slackening of the fascial sling of the lower eyelid with ageing combined with the action of the orbicularis muscle allows this to happen. This common type of entropion is called spastic entropion and it can be promptly cured without leaving a visible scar by minor eyelid surgery. Entropion may also be seen following scarring of the conjunctival surface of the eyelids and one must mention in particular the entropion of the upper eyelid caused by trachoma. This is very rare in Britain but still common in the Middle East and countries where trachoma is still rife.

Ectropion

This commonly seen outward turning of the lower eyelid in the elderly is eminently treatable and responds well to minor surgery. Senile ectropion may begin with slight separation of the lower eyelid from the globe, and the malposition of the punctum leads to overflow of tears and conjunctival infection. Irritation of the skin by the tears and rubbing of the eyes leads to skin contracture and further downward pulling of the eyelids. Like entropion, ectropion may be cicatricial and result from scarring of the skin of the eyelids. It may also follow a seventh cranial nerve palsy due to complete inaction of the orbicularis muscle; this is called paralytic ectropion.

Lagophthalmos

This is the term used to denote failure of proper closure of the eyelids due to inadequate blinking or lid deformity. In all these cases the cornea is inadequately lubricated and exposure keratitis may develop. If untreated this can lead to a serious situation; initially the cornea shows punctate staining when a drop of fluorescein is placed in the conjunctival sac and subsequently a corneal ulcer may appear. This in turn can lead to the spread of infection into the eye and without prompt treatment with antibiotics the eye may eventually be lost.

As a general principle it is important to realise that the sight may be lost simply because the eyes cannot blink. The principle applies especially to the unconscious or the anaesthetised patient where a disaster may be avoided by taping or padding the eyelids and applying an antibiotic ointment.

Blepharospasm

Slight involuntary twitching of the eyelids is very common and not usually considered to be of any pathological significance other than being a symptom of fatigue or sometimes of an anxiety state. The condition is termed 'myokymia'. True blepharospasm is rare. It may be unilateral or bilateral and may cause great inconvenience and worry to the patient. It tends slowly to become more marked over many years. A small proportion of patients eventually develops Parkinsonism. Cases of recent onset need to be investigated because they may be due to an intracranial space-taking lesion. In most cases though no underlying cause can be found. Patients with this type of blepharospasm (essential blepharospasm) can often be treated quite effectively by injecting small doses of botulinum toxin into the eyelids, but these need to be repeated every few months.

Redundant Lid Skin

Excessive skin on the eyelids is commonly seen in elderly people, often as a family characteristic. It may result from chronic oedema of the eyelids due, for example, to thyrotoxic eye disease or to renal disease. The problem is made worse in some cases by herniation of orbital fat through the orbital septum, and excision of the redundant skin and orbital fat may sometimes be necessary.

Ptosis

Drooping of one upper lid is an important clinical sign. In ophthalmic practice, ptosis in children is usually congenital and in adults is either congenital or due to a third cranial nerve palsy. These more common causes must always be kept in mind but there are a large number of other possible ones. When confronted with a patient, whose upper lid appears to droop, the first thing to decide is whether the eyelid really is drooping or whether the lid on the other side is retracted. The upper lid may droop because the eye is small and hypermetropic or shrunken from disease. Having eliminated the possibility of such 'pseudoptosis', the various other causes can be considered beginning on the skin of the eyelid—styes, meibomian cysts,—and advancing centrally through muscle—myasthenia gravis—along nerves—oculomotor palsy, Horner's syndrome—to the brainstem. Marked ptosis with the eye turned down and out and a dilated pupil is an oculomotor palsy whereas very slight ptosis, often not noticed by the patient nor sometimes by the doctor, is more likely to mean Horner's syndrome. This syndrome is due to damage to the sympathetic nervous supply to either upper or lower lids or both and is characterised by slight ptosis, small pupil, loss of sweating on the affected side of the face and slight enophthalmos (posterior displacement of the globe).

The management of ptosis depends on the cause and thus on accurate diagnosis. Surgical shortening of the levator tendon is effective in some cases of congenital ptosis and sometimes in long-standing third cranial nerve palsies. Before embarking on surgery it is important to exclude myasthenia gravis and corneal anaesthesia. Children with congenital ptosis need to be assessed very carefully before considering surgery. In young children ptosis surgery is indicated where the drooping lid threatens to cover the line of sight and where the ptosis causes an unacceptable backwards tilt of the head. In one rather strange type of congenital ptosis, the problem disappears when the mouth is opened and the patient may literally wink unavoidably when chewing. Careful consideration is needed before making the decision for surgery in these cases.

Causes of Ptosis

Pseudoptosis	small eye, atrophic eye, lid retraction on other side
Mechanical ptosis	inflammation, tumour, and excess skin
Myogenic ptosis	myasthenia gravis
Neurogenic ptosis	sympathetic—Horner's syndrome, IIIrd cranial nerve palsy, any lesion in the pathway of these, carcinoma of the lung may cause Horner's syndrome
Drugs	guanethidine eye drops cause ptosis
Congenital	ask for childhood photograph, ask for family history.

Ingrowing Eyelashes (Trichiasis)

The lashes may grow in an aberrant manner even though the eyelids themselves are in good position. This may be the result of chronic infection of the lid margins or may follow trauma. Sometimes one or two aberrant lashes appear for no apparent reason (Fig. 5.10). The lashes tend to rub on the cornea producing irritation and secondary infection. The condition is referred to as 'trichiasis'. When one or two lashes are found to be the cause of the patients discomfort, it is common practice simply to epilate them with epilating forceps. This produces instant relief, but often the relief is short-lived because the lashes regrow. At this stage the best treatment is to destroy the lash roots by electrolysis prior to epilation. Needless to say, before removing lashes it is essential to be familiar with the normal position

Fig. 5.10 Trichiasis. This ingrowing eyelash on the lower eyelid has been causing a sore eye for 3 months

of the lash line and to realise for example that hairs are normally present on the caruncle! When the lash line is grossly distorted by injury or disease, the rubbing of the lashes on the cornea can be prevented by fitting a protective contact lens or, if this measure proves impractical, it may be necessary to transpose or excise the lashes and their roots.

Infections of the Eyelids

Meibomian Gland Infection

The opening of the meibomian glands may become infected at any age resulting in meibomitis, seen initially as redness along the line of a gland when the eyelid is everted. A small abscess may then form with swelling and redness of the whole eyelid and this may point and burst either through the conjunctiva or less often through the skin. The orifice of a gland may become occluded and the gland then becomes distended and cystic (see Fig. 5.8). The retained secretions of the gland set up a granulating reaction and the cyst itself may become infected. The patient may complain of soreness and swelling of the eyelid which subsides leaving a pea-sized swelling, which can remain for several months and sometimes swells up again. During the stage of acute infection the best treatment is local heat preferably in the form of steam. This produces considerable relief and is preferable to the use of systemic or local antibiotics. Antibiotics may be required if the patient has several recurrences or if there are more generalized signs and symptoms. Once a pea-sized cyst remains in the tarsal plate, this can be promptly removed under a local anaesthetic unless the patient is a child in which case, if necessary, a general anaesthetic may be required. The method of removal involves everting the eyelid and incising the cyst through the conjunctiva and then curetting the contents. Postoperatively, local antibiotic drops or ointment are prescribed (Fig. 5.11).

Styes

These are distinct from meibomian infections, being the result of infection of the lash root. The eyelid may swell up and become painful and at this stage the site of the infection may be uncertain. However, a small yellow pointing area is eventually seen around the base of an eyelash.

Fig. 5.11 A meibomian cyst

Hot steaming again is effective treatment and once the pus is seen the eyelash can be gently epilated with resulting discharge and subsequent resolution of the infection.

Children aged from about 6–10 years sometimes seem to go through periods of their lives when they may be dogged by recurrent styes and meibomian infections, much to the distress of the parents. Under these conditions very frequent baths and hairwashing are advised and sometimes a long-term systemic antibiotic may be considered. Recurrent lid infections may raise the suspicion of diabetes mellitus but in practice this is rarely found to be an underlying cause.

Eyelid infections such as these very rarely cause any serious problems other than a day or two off work and it is extremely unusual for the infection to spread and cause orbital cellulitis. Recurrent swelling of the eyelid in spite of treatment may indicate the need for a lid biopsy because some malignant tumours may on rare occasions present in a deceptive manner.

Blepharitis

This refers to a chronic inflammation of the lid margins due to staphylococcal infection. The eyes become red rimmed and there is usually an accumulation of scales giving the appearance of fine dandruff on the lid margins. The condition is often associated with seborrhoea of the scalp. Sometimes it becomes complicated by recurrent styes or chronic infection of the meibomian glands. The eye itself is not usually involved although there may be a mild superficial punctate keratitis as evidenced by fine staining of the lower part of the cornea with fluorescein. In more sensitive patients the unsightly appearance may cause difficulties, but in more severe cases the discomfort and irritation may interfere with work. Severe recurrent infection may lead to irregular growth of the lashes and trichiasis.

In the management of these patients it is important to explain the chronic nature of the condition and the fact that certain individuals seem to be prone to it. Attention should be given to keeping the hair, face and hands as clean as possible and to avoid rubbing the eyes. When the scales are copious they can be gently removed with cotton wool moistened in sodium bicarbonate lotion twice daily. Dandruff of the scalp should also be treated with a suitable shampoo. A local antibiotic may be applied to the lid margins twice daily with good effect in many but not all cases. In severe cases with ulceration of the lid margin it may be necessary to consider prescribing a systemic antibiotic preferably after identifying the causative organism by taking a swab from the eyelids. Local steroids when combined with a local antibiotic are very effective treatment, but the prescriber must be aware of the dangers of using steroids on the eye and long term treatment with steroids should be avoided. Steroids should not be used without monitoring the intraocular pressure.

Molluscum Contagiosum

This is a viral infection usually seen in children. The lesions on the eyelids are discrete, slightly raised and umbilicated and usually multiple. There are also likely to be lesions elsewhere on the body, especially the hands and brothers or sisters may have the same problem. It is rare for the eye itself to be involved. In persistent cases, an effective form of treatment with children is careful curettage of each lesion under a general anaesthetic; in adults cryotherapy is used for individual lesions, especially if they are adjacent to the lid margin with the propensity to cause conjunctivitis.

Orbital Cellulitis

Although this is not strictly a lid infection it may be confused with severe meibomitis. The infection is deeper and the implications much more serious. In a child where the condition is more common, there is eyelid swelling, pyrexia and malaise and urgent referral to an ear nose and throat department is needed. This applies especially if there is diplopia or visual loss, and a scan will be required to decide whether surgical intervention is going to be needed to drain an infected sinus.

Allergic Disease of the Eyelids

This may present as one of two forms or a mixture of both. The more dramatic is acute allergic blepharitis in which the eyelids swell up rapidly often in response to contact with a plant or eyedrops. The cause must be found and eliminated and treatment with local steroids may be needed. It must be realized that the side effects from applying local steroids (raised intraocular pressure, cataract, aggravation of herpes simplex) can be more serious than the underlying problem. Chronic allergic blepharitis is seen in atopic individuals for example hay fever sufferers or patients with a history of eczema. The diagnosis may require histological examination of the conjunctival discharge. Drop treatment to alleviate symptoms includes mast cell stabilisers (such as lodoxamide) and histamine antagonists (such as emedastine), and these agents may take weeks to take effect. Patients with seasonal allergic conjunctivitis may require medication for a prolonged period over the spring and summer months each year.

Lid Tumours

Benign Tumours

Papilloma. Commonly seen on lids near or on the margin, these may be sessile or pedunculated, and are sometimes keratinised. These lesions are causes by the papilloma virus, and are easily excised but care must be taken if excision involves the lid margin Fig. 5.12.

Naevus. Flat brown spot on skin, may have hairs, very rarely becomes malignant.

Haemangioma. When seen as red 'strawberry mark' at or shortly after birth, may regress completely during first few years of life. The illustration shows a gross example of the rare cavernous haemangioma, which may be very disfiguring. This also may regress in a remarkable way (Fig. 5.13a, b) 'Port wine stain' is the name applied to the capillary haemangioma. This is usually unilateral and when the eyelids are involved there is a risk of association with congenital glaucoma, haemangioma of the choroid and haemangioma of the meninges on the ipsilateral side (Sturge Weber syndrome). Children with port wine stains involving the eyelids need full ophthalmological and neurological examinations.

Dermoid cyst. These quite commonly seen lumps are seen in or adjacent to the eyebrow. They feel cystic and are sometimes attached to bone. Typically they present in children as a minor cosmetic problem. The cysts are lined by keratinised epithelium and may contain dermal appendages and cholesterol. A scan may be needed before surgical removal and biopsy since some extend deeply into the skull.

Xanthelasma. Seen as yellowish plaques in skin; usually begin at medial end of lids. Associated rarely with diabetes, hypercholesterolaemia and histiocytosis. Usually no associated systemic disease.

Fig. 5.12 Lid margin papilloma

Fig. 5.13 (a) Large disfiguring haemangioma in infancy. (b) The same lesion, which in this case had remained untreated, showing spontaneous regression

Fig. 5.14 Cystic basal cell carcinoma that has extended to involve most of the upper eyelid

Malignant Tumours

Basal Cell Carcinoma. The most common malignant tumour of the lids, usually on the lower lid. It appears as a small lump, which tends to bleed forming a central crust with a slightly raised hard surround. The tumour is locally invasive only but should be excised to avoid spread into bone. Even large lesions may be approached surgically (Fig. 5.14) and "Mohs" micrographic surgery is recognized as a tissue-sparing gold standard approach in many centres. Radiotherapy is only very occasionally used with a greater risk of recurrence than formal surgical excision.

Squamous Cell Carcinoma. Tends to resemble basal cell carcinoma and biopsy is needed to differentiate. May also be mimicked by a benign self healing lesion known as keratoacanthoma.

Malignant Melanoma. A raised black pigmented lesion. Highly malignant; rare.

Lid Injuries

One of the commonest injuries to the eyelids is due to the presence of a foreign body under the eyelid—a subtarsal foreign body. A small particle of grit lodges near the lower margin of the lid, but to see it the lid must be everted. Every medical student should be familiar with the simple technique of lid eversion. This is performed by gently grasping the lashes of the upper lid

Fig. 5.15 Everting the upper eyelid

between finger and thumb and at the same time placing a glass rod horizontally across the lid. The eyelid is then gently everted by drawing the lid margin upwards and forwards. The manoeuvre is only achieved if the patient is asked to look down beforehand, and the everted lid is replaced by asking the patient to look upwards. If a small foreign body is seen, it is usually a simple matter to remove it using a cotton wool bud (Fig. 5.15).

Cuts on the eyelids may be caused by broken glass or sharp objects such as the ends of screwdrivers. The important thing here is to realise that cuts on the lid margin can leave the patient with a permanently watering eye if not sewn up with proper microscopic control and using very fine sutures. The lids may also be injured by chemical burns or flash burns. Exposure to ultra-violet light, as from a welder's arc or in snow blindness, may cause oedema and erythema of the eyelids.

This may appear after an hour or 2 but usually resolves spontaneously after about two days.

After reading this chapter you should be able to answer the following:

1. List the important causes of a watering eye.
2. What are the causes of a dry eye?
3. What are a. Entropion and b. Ectropion?
4. What are the causes of ptosis?
5. What is the commonest malignant tumour of the eyelids?
6. How can eyelid injuries cause permanent damage to the eyesight?

Common Diseases of the Conjunctiva and Cornea

Abstract

In this chapter the various types of conjunctivitis are dealt with in more detail. The important primary care problem of corneal foreign body is also described in detail and the diagnosis and management of corneal ulceration is outlined. Particular pathological changes in the cornea such as dystrophy, oedema, degenerations and loss of nerve supply are then described ending with a more detailed account of Herpes Zoster involvement of the eye.

Fig. 6.1 Subconjunctival haemorrhage

Subconjunctival Haemorrhage

This is common and tends to occur spontaneously or sometimes after straining, especially vomiting. Other less common causes should be born in mind as listed below. The eye becomes suddenly red and although the patient may experience a slight pricking, the condition is usually first noticed in the mirror or by a friend. The haemorrhage gradually absorbs in about 14 days and investigations usually fail to reveal any underlying cause. Very rarely, it is necessary to cauterise the site of bleeding if the haemorrhage is repeated so often that it becomes a nuisance to the patient (Fig. 6.1).

Conjunctivitis

Inflammation of the conjunctiva is extremely common in the general population and the general practitioner is often expected to find out the cause and treat this condition. If we consider that the conjunctiva is a mucous membrane, which is exposed during the waking hours to wind and weather more or less continuously, year in year out, then it is not surprising that this membrane is rather susceptible to inflammation. Furthermore, the conjunctiva can be compared with the lining of a joint, the eye being considered as an unusual type of ball and socket joint. The analogy takes on more meaning when the relation between conjunctivitis and some joint disease is seen.

There are a large number of different specific causes of conjunctivitis. Some of these are interesting but rare and it is important that the student obtains an idea of the relative importance and frequency of the different aetiological factors. In this chapter a more or less categorical list is given of the different causes. In the chapter on the red eye (Chap. 7) you will find a plan of approach to the red eye which deals with the relative importance and more common causes of conjunctivitis seen in day to day practice.

Although the conjunctiva is continuously exposed to infection, it has special protection from the tears, which contain immunoglobulins and lysozyme. The tears also help to wash away debris and foreign bodies and this protective action can explain the self-limiting nature of most types of conjunctivitis.

Symptoms

In all types of conjunctivitis the eye becomes red and feels irritable and gritty as if there were a foreign body under the lid. There is usually some discharge and if marked this may make the eyelids stick together in the mornings. Itchiness may also be present, especially in cases of allergic conjunctivitis. The discharge around the eyelids tends to make vision only intermittently blurred (if at all) and the patient may volunteer that blinking clears the sight.

Signs

Visual acuity is usually normal in conjunctivitis. The conjunctiva appears hyperaemic and there may be evidence of purulent discharge on the lid margins causing matting together of the eyelashes. The redness of the conjunctiva extends to the conjunctival fornices and is usually less marked at the limbus. When a rim of dilated vessels is seen around the cornea, the examiner must suspect a more serious inflammatory reaction within the eye. Apart from being red to a greater or lesser degree, the eyes also tend to water, but a dry eye may lead one to suspect conjunctivitis due to inadequate tear secretion. Drooping of one or both upper lids is a feature of some types of viral conjunctivitis and this may be accompanied by enlargement of the preauricular lymph nodes. The ophthalmologist should train himself to feel for the preauricular node as a routine part of the examination of such a case. Closer inspection of the conjunctiva may reveal numerous small papillae giving the surface a velvety look, or the papillae may be quite large. Giant papillae under the upper lids are a feature of spring catarrh, a form of allergic conjunctivitis. Close inspection of the conjunctiva may also reveal follicles or lymphoid hyperplasia. Being deep to the epithelium, they are small, pale, raised nodules and are commonly seen in viral conjunctivitis. Follicles under the upper lids are especially characteristic of trachoma.

Microscopy

The examination of a severe case of conjunctivitis of unknown cause is not complete until conjunctival scrapings have been taken. A drop of local anaesthetic is placed in the conjunctival sac and the surface of the conjunctiva at the site of maximal inflammation gently scraped with the blade of a sharp knife or a Kimura spatula. The material obtained is placed on a slide and stained with Gram's stain and Giemsa stain. The infecting organism may thus be revealed or the cell type in the exudate may indicate the underlying cause.

Conjunctival Culture

In most cases of conjunctivitis it may be good medical practice to take a culture from the conjunctival sac and the eyelid margin, but such a measure may not always be possible if a microbiological service is not near at hand. The cultures may be taken with sterile cotton tipped applicators and sent to the laboratory, in an appropriate medium, as soon as possible.

Causes

- Bacterial.
- Chlamydia.
- Viral.
- Other infective agents.
- Allergic.
- Secondary to lacrimal obstruction, corneal disease, lid deformities, degenerations and systemic disease.
- Unknown cause.

Bacterial Conjunctivitis

In Britain the commonest organisms to cause conjunctivitis are streptococcus pneumoniae, haemophilus and staphylococcus aureus. The last mentioned is normally associated with chronic lid infections, and the acute purulent conjunctivitis, known more familiarly as 'pink eye', is usually caused by the strep. pneumoniae. Chronic conjunctivitis may also be caused by Moraxella lacunata but this organism is rarely isolated from cases nowadays. An important but rare form of purulent conjunctivitis is that due to Neisseria gonorrhoeae; this is still an occasional cause of a severe type of conjunctivitis seen in the newborn babies of infected mothers. Untreated, the cornea also becomes infected, leading to perforation of the globe and permanent loss of vision. Purulent discharge, redness and severe oedema of the eyelids are features of the condition, which is generally known as ophthalmia neonatorum (Fig. 6.2). Ophthalmia neo-

Fig. 6.2 Ophthalmia neonatorum

natorum may also be caused by staphylococci and also chlamydia (see inclusion conjunctivitis of the newborn). The disease is notifiable and any infant with purulent discharge from the eyes, particularly between the 2nd and 12th day post partum, should be suspect. At one time, special blind schools were filled with children who had suffered ophthalmia neonatorum. An active campaign against this cause of blindness began at the end of the nineteenth century when Carl Crede introduced the principle of careful cleansing of the infant's eyes and the instillation of silver nitrate drops. Blindness from this cause has now disappeared in Britain but there is still a low incidence of ophthalmia neonatorum. Those affected require treatment with both antibiotic drops and intramuscular benzylpenicillin (a cephalosporin such as cefotaxime is an alternative). Both parents of the child should also be assessed.

Pink eye is the name given to the type of acute purulent conjunctivitis, which tends to spread rapidly through families or around schools. The eyes begin to itch and within an hour or 2 produce a sticky discharge, which causes the eyelids to stick together in the mornings. If the disease is mild, it can be treated by cleaning away the discharge with cotton wool, and it does not usually last longer than 3–5 days. More severe cases may warrant the prescription of antibiotic drops instilled hourly during the day for 3 days followed by four times daily for 5 days. A conjunctival culture should be taken prior to starting treatment. Common-sense precautions against spread of the infection should also be advised, although they are not always successful.

Attempts to culture bacteria from the conjunctival sac of cases of chronic conjunctivitis do not yield much more than commensal organisms.

One particular kind of chronic conjunctivitis in which the inflammation is sited mainly near to the inner and outer canthi is known as angular conjunctivitis with follicles on the superior tarsal conjunctiva. Another feature of this is the excoriation of the skin at the outer canthi from the overflow of infected tears. The clinical picture has been recognised in association with infection by the bacillus Moraxella lacunata. Often zinc sulphate drops and the application of zinc cream to the skin at the outer canthus are sufficient treatment in such cases. Tetracycline ointment may be more effective if it is felt that the long term use of an antibiotic is justified.

Chlamydia Conjunctivitis

The chlamydia comprise a group of "large viruses" which are sensitive to tetracycline and erythomycin and which cause relatively minor disability to the eyes in northern Europe and the United States when compared to the severe and widespread eye infection seen especially in Africa and the Middle East. Inclusion conjunctivitis ('inclusion blenorrhoea') is the milder form of chlamydial infection and is caused by serotype D to K of chlamydia trachomatis. The condition is usually but not always sexually transmitted. The conjunctivitis typically occurs 1 week after exposure. It may cause a more severe type of conjunctivitis in the newborn child, which can also involve the cornea. The infection is usually self-limiting but often has a prolonged course, lasting several months. The diagnosis depends on the results of conjunctival culture and examination of scrapings and the association of a follicular conjunctivitis with cervicitis or urethritis.

Chlamydial conjunctivitis responds to treatment with tetracycline. In children and adults tetracycline ointment should be used at least four times daily. In adults the treatment can be supplemented with systemic tetracycline, but this drug should not be used systemically in pregnant mothers or children under 7 years old. Azithromycin and other macrolide antibiotics are known to be particularly effective in treating systemic chlamydial infection; azithromycin may be given conveniently as a one-off dose. A referral to genitourinary medicine is advisable on presentation, as a screening measure, as reinfection from partners may trigger a recurrent infection.

Trachoma

Although a doctor practicing in Great Britain may rarely see a case of trachoma, and even

Fig. 6.3 Trachoma trichiasis of upper lid and corneal vascularisation (With acknowledgement to Professor D. Archer)

then only in immigrants. It is the commonest cause of blindness in the world and is hyperendemic in rural Africa, central and south America, Asia, Australia and the Middle East. It is spread by direct contact and perpetuated by poverty and unhygienic conditions. Trachoma is caused by chlamydia trachomatis serotypes A, B, C and affects under-privileged populations living in poor hygienic conditions. The disease begins with conjunctivitis, which, instead of resolving, becomes persistent, especially under the upper lid where scarring and distortion of the lid may result. The inflammatory reaction spreads to infiltrate the cornea from above and ultimately the cornea itself may become scarred and opaque (Fig. 6.3). At one time trachoma was common in Britain, especially after the Napoleonic wars at the end of the eighteenth century. It had been eliminated by improved hygienic conditions long before the introduction of antibiotics.

Adenoviral Conjunctivitis

Acute viral conjunctivitis is common. Several of the adenoviruses may cause it. Usually the eye symptoms follow an upper respiratory tract infection and, although nearly always bilateral, one eye may be infected before the other. The affected eye becomes red and discharges; characteristically the eyelids become thickened and the upper lid may droop. The

Fig. 6.4 Adenoviral keratoconjunctivitis

ophthalmologist's finger should feel for the telltale tender enlarged preauricular lymph node. In some cases the cornea becomes involved and subepithelial corneal opacities may appear and persist for several months (Fig. 6.4). If such opacities are situated in the line of sight, the vision may be impaired. There is no known effective treatment but it is usual to treat with an antibiotic drop to prevent secondary infection.

From time to time, epidemics of viral conjunctivitis occur and it is well recognised that spread may result from the use of improperly sterilised ophthalmic instruments or even contaminated solutions of eyedrops, and poor hand washing techniques.

Herpes Simplex Conjunctivitis

This is usually a unilateral follicular conjunctivitis with preauricular lymph node enlargement. In children it may be the only evidence of primary Herpes simplex infection.

Acute Haemorrhagic Conjunctivitis

Acute haemorrhagic conjunctivitis is caused by enterovirus 70 (picornavirus) and usually occurs in epidemics. The disease is hugely contagious but self-limiting.

Other Infective Agents

The conjunctiva may be affected by a wide variety of organisms, some of which are too rare to be considered here, and sometimes the infected conjunctiva is of secondary importance to more severe disease elsewhere in the rest of the body. Molluscum contagiosum is a virus infection, which causes small umbilicated nodules to appear on the skin of the lids and elsewhere on the body, especially the hands. It may be accompanied by conjunctivitis when there are lesions on the lid margin. The infection is usually easily eliminated by curetting each of the lesions. Infection from Phthirus pubis (the pubic louse) involving the lashes and lid margins may initially present as conjunctivitis but observation of nits on the lashes should give away the diagnosis.

Allergic Conjunctivitis

Several types of allergic reaction are seen on the conjunctiva and some of these also involve the cornea. They may be listed as follows:

Hay Fever Conjunctivitis
This is simply the commonly experienced red and watering eye that accompanies the sneezing bouts of the hay fever sufferer. The eyes are itchy and mildly injected and there may be conjunctival oedema. If treatment is needed, vasoconstrictors such as for example dilute adrenaline or antazoline drops may be helpful; sodium cromoglycate eyedrops may be used on a more long-term basis. Systemic antihistamines are of limited benefit in controlling the eye changes.

Atopic Conjunctivitis
Unfortunately patients with asthma and eczema may experience recurrent itching and irritation of the conjunctiva. Although atopic conjunctivitis tends to improve over a period of many years, it may result in repeated discomfort and anxiety for the patient, especially as the cornea may become involved, showing a superficial punctate keratitis or, in the worst cases, ulcer formation and scarring.

The diagnosis is usually evident from the history but conjunctival scrapings show the presence of eosinophils. Patients with atopic keratoconjunctivitis have a higher risk than normal for the development of Herpes simplex keratitis; the condition is also associated with the corneal dystrophy known as keratoconus or conical cornea. They are likely to develop skin infections and chronic eyelid infection by the staphylococcus. The recurrent itch and irritation (in the absence of infection) is relieved by applying local steroid drops, but in view of the long-term nature of the condition, these should be avoided if possible because of their side-effects. (Local steroids can cause glaucoma in predisposed individuals and aggravate Herpes simplex keratitis).

Vernal Conjunctivitis (Spring Catarrh)

Some children with an atopic history may develop a specific type of conjunctivitis characterised by the presence of giant papillae under the upper lid. The child tends to develop severely watering and itchy eyes in the early spring, which may interfere with schooling. Eversion of the upper lid reveals the raised papillae, which have been likened to cobblestones. In severe cases the cobblestones may coalesce to give rise to giant papillae (Fig. 6.5). Occasionally the cornea is also involved initially by punctate keratitis but sometimes it may become vascularised. It is often necessary to treat these cases with local steroids, for example prednisolone drops applied if needed every 2 h for a few days

Fig. 6.5 Vernal conjunctivitis (spring catarrh) papillary reaction

thus enabling the child to return to school. The dose can then be reduced as much as possible down to a maintenance dose over the worst part of the season. More severe cases may derive some benefit from topical cyclosporin drops, or eyelid injections of triamcinolone to control the inflammatory response. Less severe cases may respond well to sodium cromoglycate drops and these may be useful as a long-term measure. It is useful in preventing but not in controlling acute exacerbations. Other medications with a similar modest benefit in symptoms include lodoxamide (a mast cell stabilizer) and emedastine (a topical anti-histamine).

Secondary Conjunctivitis

Inflammation of the conjunctiva may often be secondary to other more important primary pathology. The following are some of the possible underlying causes of this type of conjunctivitis.

1. Lacrimal obstruction.
2. Corneal disease.
3. Lid deformities.
4. Degenerations.
5. Systemic disease.

Lacrimal obstruction may cause recurrent unilateral purulent conjunctivitis and it is important to consider this possibility in recalcitrant cases because early resolution may be achieved simply by syringing the tear ducts. Corneal ulceration from a variety of causes is often associated with conjunctivitis and here the treatment is aimed primarily at the cornea. Occasionally the presence of one of the two common acquired lid deformities, entropion and ectropion, may be the underlying cause. Sometimes the diagnosis may be missed, especially in the case of entropion when the deformity is not present all the time. Other lid deformities may also have the same effect. A special type of degenerative change is seen in the conjunctiva, which is more marked in hot, dry, dusty climates. It appears that the combination of lid movement in blinking, dryness and dustiness of the atmosphere and perhaps some abnormal factor in the patient's tears or tear production may lead to the heaping up of subconjunctival yellow elastic tissue which is often infiltrated with lymphocytes. The lesion is seen as a yellow plaque on the conjunctiva in the exposed area of the bulbar conjunctiva and usually on the nasal side. Such early degenerative changes are extremely common in all climates as a natural ageing phenomenon, but under suitable conditions the heaped-up tissue spreads into the cornea, drawing a triangular band of conjunctiva with it. The eye becomes irritable due to associated conjunctivitis and in worst cases the degenerative plaque extends across the cornea and affects the vision. The early stage of the condition, which is common and limited to a small area of the conjunctiva, is termed a pingueculum and the more advanced lesion spreading onto the cornea is known as a pterygium (Fig. 6.6). Pterygium is more common in Africa, India, Australia, China and the Middle East than in Europe. It is rarely seen in white races living in temperate climates. Treatment is by surgical excision if the cornea is significantly affected with progression towards the visual axis; antibiotic drops may be required if the conjunctiva is infected. Non-infective inflammation of pterygium is treated with topical steroids.

Finally when considering secondary causes of conjunctivitis one must be aware that redness and congestion of the conjunctiva with secondary infection may be an indicator of systemic disease. Examples of this are the red eye of renal failure

and gout and also polycythaemia rubra. The association of conjunctivitis, arthritis and non-specific urethritis makes up the triad of Reiter's syndrome. Some diseases cause abnormality of the tears and these have already been discussed with dry eye syndromes, the most common being rheumatoid arthritis. However there are other rarer diseases which upset the quality or production of tears such as sarcoidosis, pemphigus and Stevens-Johnson syndrome. Thyrotoxicosis is a more common systemic disease which is associated with conjunctivitis, but the other signs in the eye such as lid retraction, conjunctival oedema and proptosis are usually more evident. A rather persistent type of conjunctivitis is seen in patients with acne rosacea. Here, the diagnosis is usually, but not always, made evident by the appearance of the skin of the nose, cheeks and forehead, but the corneal lesions of rosacea are also quite characteristic (Fig. 6.7). The cornea becomes invaded from the periphery by wedge-shaped tongues of blood vessels associated with recurrent corneal ulceration. Severe rosacea keratoconjunctivitis

Fig. 6.7 Acne rosacea

Fig. 6.6 Pterygium

is seen less commonly now, perhaps because it responds well to treatment with the combination of systemic doxycycline, lubricants for associated dry-eye, and the judicious use of weak topical steroids. Usually it is also necessary to instruct the patient to clean the lids and perform 'lid hygeine', as such patients are often also affected by blepharitis.

Corneal Foreign Body

Small particles of grit or dust very commonly become embedded in the cornea and every casualty officer is aware of the increasing incidence of this occurrence on windy dry days. Small foreign bodies also become embedded as the result of using high-speed grinding tools without adequate protection of the eyes. The dentist's drill may also be a source of foreign bodies, but the most troublesome are those particles that have been heated by grinding or chiselling. It is important to have some understanding of the anatomy of the cornea if one is attempting to remove a corneal foreign body. One must realise, for example, that the surface epithelium can be stripped off from the underlying layer and can regrow and fill raw areas with extreme rapidity. Under suitable conditions the whole surface epithelium can reform in about 48 h. The layer underlying or posterior to the surface epithelium is known as Bowman's membrane and if this layer is damaged by the injury or cut into unnecessarily by over-zealous use of surgical instruments, then a

permanent scar may be left in the cornea. When the epithelium alone is involved there is usually no scar, and healing results in perfect restoration of the optical properties of the surface.

The stroma of the cornea is surprisingly tough, permitting some degree of boldness when removing deeply embedded foreign bodies. It should be remembered that if the cornea has been perforated, then the risk of intraocular infection or loss of aqueous dictates that the wound should be repaired under full sterile conditions in the operating theatre.

Signs and Symptoms

Patients usually know when a foreign body has gone into their eye and the history is clear cut—but not always. Occasionally the complaint is simply a red sore eye, which may have been present for some time. Spotting these corneal foreign bodies is really lesson number one in ocular examination. It involves employing the important basic principles of examining the anterior segment of the eye. Most foreign bodies can be seen without the use of the slit-lamp microscope if the eye is examined carefully and with a focused beam of light. Figure 6.8 demonstrates the great advantage of the focused beam, and in fact this very principle is used in slit-lamp microscopy. If the foreign body has been present for any length of time, there will be a ring of ciliary injection around the cornea due to the dilatation of the deeper episcleral capillaries, which

Fig. 6.8 Focal illumination of corneal foreign body

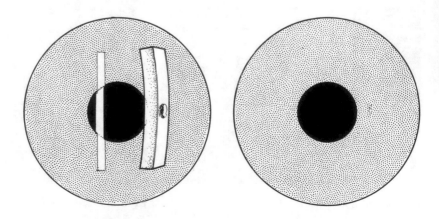

lie near the corneal margin. Ciliary injection is a sure warning sign of corneal or intraocular pathology.

Treatment

The aim of treatment is, of course, to remove the foreign body completely. Sometimes this is not as easy as it may seem, especially when a hot metal particle lies embedded in a 'rust ring'. In instances when it is clear that much digging is going to be needed, it may be prudent to leave the rust ring for 24 h, after which it becomes easier to remove. The procedure for removing a foreign body should be as follows: the patient lies down on a couch or dental chair and one or two drops of proparacaine hydrochloride 0.5% (Ophthaine) or a similar local anaesthetic are instilled onto the affected eye. A good light on a stand is needed, preferably one with a focused beam and the eyelids are held open with a speculum (Fig. 6.9). The doctor will also usually require some optical aid in the form of special magnifying spectacles, for example 'Bishop Harman's glasses' or the slit lamp microscope. Many foreign bodies can be easily removed with a cotton-wool bud (particularly those lodged under the upper lid), but otherwise at the slit lamp a 25 gauge orange needle angled nearly perpendicular to the plane of the iris may be used to lift off the foreign body. When the foreign body is more deeply embedded, a battery-powered handheld blunt tipped drill may be used to clean any rust deposits that remain,

Fig. 6.9 Removing corneal foreign body

again under the careful control of the slit-lamp microscope.

Once the foreign body has been removed, an antibiotic drop is placed in the eye and the lids are then splinted together by means of a firm pad. There is no doubt that the corneal epithelium heals more quickly if the eyelids are splinted in this way. It is usually advisable to see the patient the following day if possible to make sure that all is well, and if the damaged spot on the cornea is no longer staining with fluorescein, the pad can be left off. Antibiotic drops should be continued at least three times daily for a few days after the cornea has healed. The visual acuity of the patient should always be checked before final discharge.

There are one or two factors that should always be borne in mind when treating patients with corneal foreign bodies: in most instances healing takes place without any problem but, very rarely, the vision may be permanently impaired by scarring. Also on very rare occasions, the site of corneal damage becomes infected and if neglected the infection may enter the eye and cause endophthalmitis with total blindness of the affected eye. This is a well recognised tragedy, which should never happen in an age of antibiotics. Of course, if the eye has actually been perforated, endophthalmitis is a very frequent sequel in the absence of antibiotic treatment. One only has to examine old hospital case notes from the pre-antibiotic era to obtain proof of this.

It is important to remember that a perforating injury of the eye is a surgical emergency. Any doubt about the possibility of a perforating injury of the cornea can usually be resolved by examining it carefully with the slit-lamp microscope. One other factor to bear in mind is the possibility of a retained intraocular foreign body. Sometimes the patient may be quite unaware of such an injury and this may mislead the doctor into underestimating the serious nature of the problem. The answer for the doctor is 'when in doubt, x-ray', especially when a hammer and chisel or high-speed drill have been used. A retained intraocular foreign body may not set up an inflammatory reaction or irreversible degenerative changes until several weeks or even months have elapsed (Fig. 6.10).

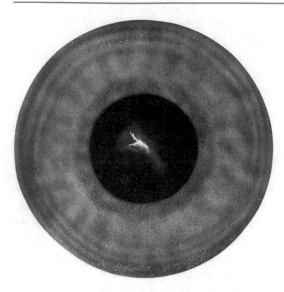

Fig. 6.10 Beware of the full-thickeness corneal scar, when in doubt do an X-ray

Corneal Ulceration

Corneal ulcers may arise spontaneously (primary) or they may result from some defect in the normal protective mechanism or sometimes they are part of a more generalised susceptibility to infection (secondary). The nerve endings in the cornea are pain-sensitive endings and a light touch is felt as a sharp pain. Furthermore, stimulation of these nerves causes a vigorous blink reflex and the eye begins to water excessively. A very effective protective mechanism is therefore brought into action, which tends to clear away infection or foreign bodies and warns the patient of trouble. In most instances of corneal ulceration the eye is painful, photophobic and waters. The conjunctiva is usually injected and there may be ciliary injection.

Types of Corneal Ulcer

Due to Direct Trauma

The corneal epithelium becomes disrupted and abraded by certain characteristic injuries. It is surprising how the same old story keeps repeating itself: the mother caught in the eye by the child's fingernail, the edge of a newspaper or the backlash from the branch of a tree. The injury is excruciatingly painful and the symptoms are often made much worse by the rapid eye movements of an anxious patient and sometimes by vigorous rubbing of the eye. The patient complains that there is something in the eye and once the diagnosis has been made it may be difficult to persuade the patient that there is no foreign body. A denuded area of cornea is seen which stains with fluorescein. It may not be possible to examine the patient until a drop of local anaesthetic has been instilled into the eye, but, as a general rule, local anaesthetic drops should not be used to treat a 'sore eye'. This is because healing is impaired and serious damage to the eye may result. Anaesthetic drops should only be used as a single-dose diagnostic measure in such cases. Treatment involves the instillation of a mydriatic such as homatropine 1% and an antibiotic ointment such as chloramphenicol 0.5% after which special care is needed to fix the eyelids. This is probably best achieved by directly sticking the eyelids together with two vertically placed short strips of micropore surgical tape. A pad is then placed over the closed eyelids. The patient is then given some analgesic tablets to take home and is advised to rest quietly until the eye is inspected the following day. The pad can be left off once the epithelium has healed over, but even then the patient should continue to instil an antibiotic ointment in the eye at night for several weeks. The reason for taking a little trouble over the management of a patient with a corneal abrasion is the recurrent nature of the condition. All too often after some months or even a few years, the patient begins to experience a sharp pain in the injured eye on waking in the morning. It is as if the cornea, or the weak part of the cornea, becomes stuck to the posterior surface of the upper lid during the night. The pain wears off after an hour or 2 and when the patient presents to the doctor there may be no obvious cause for the symptoms. In actual fact careful examination with the slit lamp reveals very minute cysts or white specks at the site of the original abrasion, indicating a weak area of attachment of the corneal epithelium. Severe recurrent corneal abrasion is best dealt with in an eye department where slit-lamp control is available.

Due to Bacteria

The commonest ulcer of this type is known as a 'marginal ulcer' (Fig. 6.11). The patient complains of a persistently red eye, which is moderately sore. Examination reveals conjunctival congestion, which is often mainly localised to an area adjacent to the corneal ulcer. The ulcer is often seen as a white crescentic patch near the corneal margin but there is usually but not always a small gap of clear cornea between it and the limbus (the corneoscleral junction). Such marginal ulcers are thought to be due to exotoxins from *Staphylococcus aureus*, mainly because they are often associated with *Staphylococcus aureus* blepharitis. On the other hand, it is not possible to grow the organism from the corneal lesion, and for this reason it is said that the infiltrated area is some form of allergic response to the infecting organism. Furthermore, these marginal ulcers respond very rapidly to treatment with a steroid-antibiotic mixture. It is essential that the usual precautions before applying local steroids to the eye are taken, that is to say, the possibility of Herpes simplex infection should be excluded and the intraocular pressure should be

monitored if the treatment is to continue on a more long-term basis.

A wide range of other bacteria are known to cause corneal ulceration, but, by and large, infections only occur as a secondary problem when the defences of the cornea are impaired (e.g. underlying corneal disease, trauma, dry eyes or contact lens wear).

There are three bacteria, which can produce corneal infection despite healthy epithelium: Neisseria gonorrhoea, Neisseria meningitidis and Corynebacterium diphtheriae. Pathogens most often associated with corneal infections, however, are staphylococcus aureus, streptococcus pneumoniae, pseudomonas aeruginosa and the Enterobacteria (E. coli, Proteus, and Klebsiella). Pseudomonas is an especially virulent bacterium as it can cause rapid corneal perforation if inadequately treated.

Usually there is pain, photophobia, watering and discharge in addition to redness. Examination reveals ciliary injection and a corneal defect, which may have a greyish base (infiltration). There is most often an associated (secondary) iritis, which may be severe giving rise to a hypopyon (layer of pus in the anterior chamber).

Management. Bacterial corneal ulcers are sight threatening and require urgent treatment. The causative organism needs to be identified by corneal scrapes. Appropriate antibiotics usually a combination of Gentamicin and Cefuroxime applied frequently in hospital provides a broad spectrum until the organisms are identified.

Due to Acanthamoeba

Acanthamoeba is a free-living genus of amoeba that has been increasingly associated with keratitis. The keratitis is usually chronic and may follow minor trauma. Contact lens wearers are particularly at risk of this infection.

Due to Viruses

Apart from other rare types of virus infection, there is one outstanding example of this—herpes simplex keratitis. The condition seems to be more common than it used to be, perhaps because the incidence of other types of corneal ulcer has become less with the more liberal use of local

Fig. 6.11 Marginal ulcer caused by bacterial infection

antibiotics on the eye. Every eye casualty department has a few patients with this debilitating condition, which may put a patient off work for many months. Fortunately it is only a few cases that have such a problem, and most instances of this common condition give rise to a week or 10 days of incapacity. Herpes simplex is thought to produce a primary infection in infants and younger children, which is transferred from the lips of the mother and may be subclinical. Sometimes a vesicular rash develops around the eyelids accompanied by fever and enlargement of the preauricular lymph nodes. Whatever the initial manifestation of the primary infection, it is thought that many members of the population harbour the virus in a latent form so that overt infection in an adult tends to appear in association with other illnesses. Most people are familiar with the cold sores that appear on the lips due to herpes simplex. Sometimes, after a cold, one eye becomes sore and irritable and inspection of the cornea shows the very characteristic corneal

changes of herpes simplex infection. A slightly raised granular, star-shaped or dendriform lesion is seen which takes up fluorescein (Fig. 6.12a). The virus can be cultivated from this lesion and the size of the dendriform figure is some guide to prognosis. A large lesion extending across the cornea, especially across the optical axis (i.e. the centre of the cornea), is likely to be the one which is going to give trouble and it is better that the patient should be warned about it at this stage. After a few days, or sometimes weeks, the epithelial lesion heals and at this point complete resolution may occur or an inflammatory reaction may appear in the stroma deep to the infected epithelium. The eye remains red and irritable to an incapacitating degree and further dendritic ulcers may subsequently appear. In worse cases the cornea may become anaesthetic so that although the eye may be more comfortable, the problems of a numb cornea are added to the original condition. Healing tends to occur with a vascular scar.

My eye seemed much better at first
on those steroid drops.

Fig. 6.12 (a) Dendritic ulcer of cornea. (b) Use of steroid drops in herpes simplex keratitis (With acknowledgement to Professor H. Dua). (c) Progression of herpes simplex keratitis following use of steroid eye drops

Treatment of Herpes Simplex Keratitis

Antiviral agents are usually the first line of treatment. Acyclovir in the form of an ointment is the treatment of choice supplemented by tablets in more severe cases. Early diagnosis and treatment seem to give the best chance of avoiding recurrences. The removal of virus-containing epithelial cells (debridement) is now indicated only in cases that are resistant to antiviral agents, where there is toxicity to the drugs, or there is difficulty in acquiring or applying the antiviral agents. After debridement, an antibiotic drop and a cycloplegic are instilled and a firm pad and bandage applied. Touching the debrided area with iodine is now obsolete. Following this procedure the eye may become very sore and the patient is given an analgesic. Often the corneal epithelium will heal after 48 h and the condition will be cured. Larger ulcers may not respond very satisfactorily to this treatment. Steroids should not be used in the treatment of dendritic ulcers of the cornea (Fig. 6.12b). It is well recognised that steroid drops enhance the replication of the herpes simplex virus (Fig. 6.12c). They reduce the local inflammatory reaction and may give the false impression that the eye is improving. However, persistent use of local steroids in such cases may result in corneal thinning and even corneal perforation. Once the dendritic ulcer has healed, residual stromal infiltration is then sometimes treated by carefully gauged doses of steroids, but this should be under strict ophthalmological supervision. In more severe cases, secondary iritis or secondary glaucoma may complicate the picture and require special treatment. The decision whether or not to apply a pad to the eye depends on the state of the corneal epithelium and also on the patient's response. In the worst cases it may be advisable to perform a tarsorrhaphy, that is to say, the lids are stitched together in such a way that they remain closed when the stitches are removed. An alternative is to induce drooping of the eyelid by an injection of botulinum toxin into the levator muscle.

Surprisingly, the keratitis seems to heal usually in 1–2 weeks when this is done and the patient may be able to return to work providing the work does not require the use of both eyes. When herpetic keratitis has taken its toll leaving a scarred cornea, the sight may eventually be restored again by a corneal graft. Unfortunately, recurrences still often occur and dendritic ulcers may appear on the graft.

Due to Damage to the Corneal Nerve Supply

When the ophthalmic division of the trigeminal nerve is damaged by disease or injury, the cornea may become numb and there is a high risk of corneal ulceration. Such neurotrophic ulcers are characteristically painless and easily become infected, with possible disastrous results. A tarsorrhaphy may be needed to save the eye but sometimes a soft contact lens may suffice provided the ulcer is not infected at the time. Before embarking on the treatment of an anaesthetic cornea, the cause should be established and this may involve a full neurological investigation.

Due to Exposure

When the normal 'windscreen wiper' mechanism of the lids is faulty, as, for example when the eyelids have been injured or in a case of facial palsy, then the surface of the cornea may dry and become ulcerated. The same problem occurs in the unconscious patient unless great care is taken to keep the eyelids closed. Most cases of Bell's palsy recover sufficiently quickly to prevent exposure keratitis, but when severe and when recovery is poor, a tarsorrhaphy, or at least treatment with an eyepad and local antibiotic ointment at night, may be needed. Botulinum toxin injection into the lid may obviate the need for surgery; this has the effect of dropping the upper lid for approximately 3 months, and is a useful temporizing measure in some cases. It is important to bear in mind that the same risk of corneal exposure is evident in patients with severe thyrotoxic exophthalmos.

Corneal Dystrophies

There are a number of specific corneal dystrophies, most of which are inherited and most of which cannot be diagnosed without the aid of the slit-lamp microscope. For this reason they will not be dealt with in any detail here. A list for reference is shown in Table 6.1.

Keratoconus (or conical cornea) is perhaps the commonest. It is still rare in the general population but is familiar to general practitioners looking after student populations because it tends to appear in this age group. The condition is bilateral and may be inherited as an autosomal recessive trait, although most patients do not have a positive family history. It should be suspected in patients who show a rapid change of refractive error, particularly if a large amount of myopic astigmatism suddenly appears. Often, but not always, there is an associated history of asthma and hay fever. The cornea shows central thinning and protrudes anteriorly. This may be observed with the naked eye by asking the patient to sit down and then standing behind him or her so that one can look down on the downturned eye. By holding up the upper lids one can make an estimate of the abnormal shape of the cornea by noting how the cornea shapes the lower lid. Alternatively, the patient's cornea can be observed using Placido's disc. This ingenious instrument is simply a disc with a hole in the centre of it through which one observes the patient's

Fig. 6.13 Keratoconus; Placido's disc image

cornea. On the patient's side of the disc is a series of concentric circles which can be seen by the observer reflected on the patient's cornea (Fig. 6.13). Distortion of these circles indicates the abnormal shape of the cornea. Of course, more accurate assessment of the cornea can be made by observing it with the slit-lamp microscope and still more information can be obtained by keratometry or corneal topography, that is, using an instrument to measure the curvature of the cornea in different meridians. Keratoconus tends to progress slowly and contact lenses may be very helpful. Sometimes a corneal graft is required. Less common corneal dystrophies include Fuch's endothelial, stromal and anterior dystrophies.

Table 6.1 Corneal dystrophies

Anterior dystrophies (corneal epithelium and Bowman's membrane):
Microcystic
Reis Buckler's
Stromal dystrophies:
Lattice
Macular
Granular
Posterior dystrophies (corneal endothelium and Descemet's membrane):
Fuch's
Posterior polymorphous
Ectatic dystrophies:
Keratoconus
Keratoglobus

Corneal Degenerations

Apart from the inherited corneal dystrophies, certain changes are often seen in the cornea with ageing such as arcus senilis and endothelial pigmentation. Band degeneration refers to a deposition of calcium salts in the anterior layers of the cornea. The calcification is first seen at the margin of the cornea in the 9 o'clock and 3 o'clock area, but it may gradually extend across the normally exposed part of the cornea. It is seen in cases of chronic iridocyclitis, in particular in patients with juvenile rheumatoid arthritis and also in those with sarcoidosis. In fact, band degeneration is seen in any eye, which has become degenerate or

Fig. 6.14 Band keratopathy

in cases of long-standing corneal disease (Fig. 6.14). Although band degeneration can, if sufficiently advanced, be diagnosed quite easily with the naked eye, most degenerative conditions of the cornea can only be diagnosed and classified under the microscope. Other corneal degenerations include Salzmann's nodular dystrophy and lipid keratopathies.

Corneal Oedema

To the naked eye, corneal oedema may not be very obvious but careful inspection will reveal a lack of lustre when the affected cornea is compared with that on the other side. The normal sparkle of the eye is no longer evident and the iris becomes less well defined. Microscopically a bedewed appearance is seen, minute droplets being evident in the epithelium. When the stroma is also involved this may seem misty and may be also infiltrated with inflammatory cells which are seen as powdery white dots. When the oedema is long standing the droplets in the epithelium coalesce to produce blisters or bullae.

The more important causes of corneal oedema are as follows.

1. Acute narrow angle glaucoma
2. Virus keratitis
3. Trauma
4. Contact lenses
5. Postoperative
6. Fuch's endothelial dystrophy

When the intraocular pressure is suddenly raised from any cause, the cornea becomes oedematous. The normal cornea needs to be relatively dehydrated in order to maintain its transparency, and the necessary level of dehydration seems to depend on active removal of water by the corneal endothelium as well as an adequate oxygen supply from the tears. The mechanism is impaired not only by raising the intraocular pressure, but also by infection or trauma. Senile degenerative changes may also be the sole underlying cause due to failure of the endothelial pumping mechanisms. Contact lenses, if ill fitting and worn for too long a period, may prevent adequate oxygen reaching the cornea, with resulting oedema.

The management of corneal oedema depends on the management of the underlying cause. Oedema due to endothelial damage may respond in its early stages to local steroids and sometimes a clear cornea may be maintained by the use of osmotic agents such as hypertonic saline or glycerol. Chronic corneal oedema tends to be painful and often acute episodes of pain occur when bullae rupture leaving exposed corneal nerves. In such cases it may be necessary to consider a tarsorrhaphy, or in some instances a corneal graft may prove beneficial. The pain of corneal oedema is a late symptom and in its early stages, oedema simply causes blurring of the vision and the appearance of coloured haloes around light bulbs. This is simply a 'bathroom window' effect. Patients with cataracts also see haloes, so that defects in other parts of the optical media of the eye may give a similar effect.

Absent Corneal Sensation

Corneal sensation is supplied by the fifth cranial nerve. About 70 nerve fibres are present in the superficial layers of the cornea and they can often be seen when the cornea is examined with the slit-lamp microscope. They appear as white threads running mainly radially. Asking the patient to gaze straight ahead then lightly touching the cornea with a fine wisp of cotton wool can assess corneal anaesthesia. Care must be taken not to touch the lid margins when doing this. The blink reflex is then noted and it is also important to ask the patient what has been felt. In the case of elderly people the blink reflex may be reduced, but a slight prick should be evident when the cornea is touched. Attempts to quantify corneal anaesthesia have led to the development of graded strengths of bristle, which can be applied to the cornea instead of cotton wool.

Corneal anaesthesia may result from a lesion at any point in the fifth cranial nerve from the cornea to the brainstem. In the cornea itself, Herpes simplex infection may ultimately result in anaesthesia. Herpes zoster is especially liable to lead to this problem and, because this condition may often be treated at home rather than in the ward, it will be considered in more detail here.

Fig. 6.15   Herpes zoster ophthalmicus

Herpes Zoster Ophthalmicus (Shingles of the Eye)

This is due to the varicella-zoster virus, the same virus that causes chickenpox. It is thought that the initial infection with the virus occurs with an attack of childhood chickenpox and that the virus remains in the body in a latent form, subsequently to manifest itself as Herpes zoster in some individuals. The virus appears to lodge in the Gasserian ganglion. The onset of the condition is heralded by headache and the appearance of one or two vesicles on the forehead. Over the next 3 or 4 days the vesicles multiply and appear on the distribution of one or all of the branches of the fifth cranial nerve. The patient may develop a raised temperature and usually experiences malaise and considerable pain. Sometimes a chickenpox-like rash appears over the rest of the body. The eye itself is most at risk when the upper division of the fifth nerve is involved. There may be vesicles on the lids and conjunctiva and, when the cornea is affected, punctate-staining areas are seen which become minute subepithelial opacities. After 4 days to a week, the infection reaches its peak; the eyelids on the affected side may be closed by swelling, and oedema of the lids may spread across to the other eye (Fig. 6.15). The vesicles become pustular and then form crusts

which are then shed over a period of 2 or 3 weeks. In most cases complete resolution occurs with remarkably little scarring of the skin considering the appearance in the acute stage. However, the cornea may be rendered permanently anaesthetic and the affected area of skin produces annoying paraesthesiae, amounting quite often to persistent very severe neuralgia which may dog the patient for many years. Other complications include extraocular muscle palsies or rarely, encephalitis. Iridocyclitis is fairly common and glaucoma may develop and lead to blindness if untreated. At present treatment in established cases is not very effective. Local steroids and acyclovir are given for the uveitis, and acetazolamide or topical beta-blockers for the glaucoma. It is however very important to realise that administration of systemic acyclovir or famciclovir early in the disease is known to reduce the severity of the neuralgia, but these medications need to be administered as soon as possible after the onset of symptoms for best effect. The disease still often has to run its course and the patient, who is usually elderly, may require much support and advice, especially when post-herpetic neuralgia is severe. It is accepted practice to treat the eye at risk with antibiotic drops and a weak mydriatic. Analgesics and sometimes antidepressants are also needed, often on a long-term basis. The recent introduction of a vaccine for herpes zoster has reduced the incidence by a third and if shingles occurs the disease is likely to be milder.

Other causes of corneal anaesthesia include surgical division of the fifth cranial nerve for trigeminal neuralgia or any space-occupying lesion along the nerve pathway. The possibility of exposure and drying of the cornea must always be borne in mind in the unconscious or the anaesthetised patient since corneal ulceration and infection will soon result if this is neglected.

Corneal anaesthesia due to nerve damage is nearly always permanent and, if it is complete, it may often be necessary to protect the eye by means of a tarsorrhaphy or botulinum toxin. Lesser degrees of corneal anaesthesia may be treated by instilling an antibiotic ointment at night and, if a more severe punctate keratitis develops, by padding the eye.

After reading this chapter you should be able to answer the following questions:

1. How do you manage acute conjunctivitis?
2. What organisms are known to cause conjunctivitis?
3. What are the complications of Herpes Simplex infection of the cornea?
4. What are the complications of Herpes Zoster in the eye?
5. What causes corneal oedema?
6. What particular corneal change is seen in sarcoidosis and juvenile rheumatoid arthritis?

The Red Eye

7

Abstract

This chapter describes how to deal with a patient presenting with a red eye and how to distinguish relatively mild conditions causing this with more serious ones. It is especially important to measure the patient's vision in these cases. A more detailed description of the individual diseases which cause the red eye is to be found in other chapters.

The covid 19 pandemic has given rise to widespread discussions and studies as to the value of virtual consultations in medical practice and a recent study of video consultations for the red eye in an emergency ophthalmology department has suggested that the safety of this practice compares favourably with face to face consultations. However the unplanned reattendance rate was higher after the virtual consultations in this study. Making an accurate diagnosis from the history alone becomes very important under these restricted conditions and greatly helped if possible by a relative or carer. However many ophthalmologists must feel that examining the eye without an ophthalmoscope must carry a high risk to the patient.

Redness of the eye is one of the commonest signs in ophthalmology, being a feature of a wide range of ophthalmological conditions, some of which are severe and sight threatening whereas some are mild and of little consequence. Occasionally the red eye may be the first sign of important systemic disease. It is important that every practicing doctor has an understanding of the differential diagnosis of this common sign, and a categorisation of the signs, symptoms and management of the red eye will now be made from the standpoint of the non-specialist general practitioner.

The simplest way of categorising these patients is in terms of their visual acuity. As a general rule, if the sight, as measured on the Snellen test chart and wearing appropriate glasses, is impaired, then the cause may be more serious. The presence or absence of pain is also of significance but as this depends in part on the pain threshold of the subject, it may be a misleading symptom. Disease of the conjunctiva alone is not usually painful whereas disease of the cornea or iris is generally very painful.

The red eye will therefore be considered under three headings: the red eye, which sees well and is not painful, and the red eye, which may or may not have visual impairment and is acutely painful and the red eye with pain and poor vision.

Red Eye Which Is Not Painful and Sees Normally

Subconjunctival Haemorrhage

Careful examination of the eye will easily confirm that its redness is due to blood rather than dilated blood vessels, and the redness may be noticed by someone other than the patient (see Fig. 6.1) The condition is common and resolves in about 10–14 days. It is extremely unusual for a blood dyscrasia to present with subconjunctival haemorrhages. Although vomiting or a bleeding tendency may also be rare causes, the normal practice is to reassure the patient rather than embark on extensive investigations, because the majority of cases are due to spontaneous bleeding from a conjunctival capillary. This may be spontaneous and can result from a sudden increase in venous pressure, for example after coughing or vomiting.

Conjunctivitis

Examination of the eye reveals inflammation, that is, dilatation of the conjunctival capillaries and larger blood vessels, associated with more or less discharge from the eye. The exact site of the inflammation should be noted and it is especially useful to note whether the deeper capillaries around the margin of the cornea are involved. The resulting pink flush encircling the cornea is called 'ciliary injection' and is a warning of corneal or intraocular inflammation. For clinical purposes it is useful to divide conjunctivitis into acute and chronic types.

Acute

This is usually infective and due to a bacterium; it is more common in young people. It may spread rapidly through families or schools without serious consequence other than a few days incapacity. When adults develop acute conjunctivitis it is worth searching for a possible underlying cause, especially a blocked tear duct when the condition is unilateral. Sometimes an ingrowing lash may be the cause or occasionally a free-floating eyelash lodges in the lacrimal punctum. The important symptoms of acute conjunctivitis are redness, irritation and sticking together of the eyelids in the mornings. Management entails finding the cause and using antibiotic drops if the symptoms are severe enough to warrant this. However, it must be remembered that the inadequate and intermittent use of antibiotic eyedrops may simply encourage growth of resistant organisms.

Chronic

This is a very common cause of the red eye and almost a daily problem in non-specialised ophthalmic practice. If we consider that the conjunctiva is a mucous membrane which is daily exposed to the elements, it is perhaps not surprising that after many years it tends to become chronically inflamed and irritable. The frequency and nuisance value of the symptoms are reflected in the large across-the-counter sales of various eyewashes and solutions aimed at relieving 'eyestrain' or 'tired eyes'. The symptoms of chronic conjunctivitis are therefore redness and irritation of the eyes with a minimal degree of discharge and sticking of the lids. If there is an allergic background, itching may also be a main feature. The chronically inflamed conjunctiva accumulates minute particles of calcium salts within the mucous glands. These conjunctival concretions are shed from time to time producing a feeling of grittiness.

When confronted with a patient with chronic conjunctivitis it is especially useful to keep in mind all the possible causes:

Checklist of Causes
Eyelids
Deformities such as entropion or ectropion
Displaced eyelashes
Chronic blepharitis

Refractive Error A proportion of patients who have never worn glasses and need them or who are wearing incorrectly prescribed or out-of-date glasses present with the features of chronic conjunctivitis, the symptoms being relieved by the proper use of spectacles. The cause is not clear but possibly related to rubbing the eyes.

Dry Eye Syndrome The possibility of a defect in the secretion of tears or mucus can only be confirmed by more elaborate tests, but this should be suspected in patients with rheumatoid arthritis or sarcoidosis.

Foreign Body Contact lenses and mascara particles are the commonest foreign bodies to cause chronic conjunctivitis.

Stress Often a period of stress seems to be closely related to the symptoms and perhaps eye rubbing is also the cause in these patients.

Allergy It is very unusual to be able to incriminate a specific allergen for chronic conjunctivitis, unlike allergic blepharitis. On the other hand, hay fever and asthma may be the background cause.

Infection Chronic conjunctivitis may begin as an acute infection, usually viral and usually following an upper respiratory tract infection.

Drugs The long -term use of adrenaline drops may cause dilatation of the conjunctival vessels and irritation in the eye. In 1974 it was shown that the B-blocking drug practolol (since withdrawn from the market) could cause a severe dry eye syndrome in rare instances. Since then there have been several reports of mild reactions to other available B-blockers, although such reactions are difficult to distinguish from chronic conjunctivitis from other causes.

Systemic Causes Congestive cardiac failure, renal failure, Reiter's disease, polycythaemia, gout, rosacea as well as other causes of orbital venous congestion such as orbital tumours may all be associated with vascular congestion and irritation of the conjunctiva. Migraine may also be associated with redness of the eye on one side and chronic alcoholism is a cause of bilateral conjunctival congestion.

Fig. 7.1 Episcleritis (With acknowledgement to Professor H. Dua)

Episcleritis

Sometimes the eye becomes red due to inflammation of the connective tissue underlying the conjunctiva, that is, the episclera. The condition may be localised or diffuse. There is no discharge and the eye is uncomfortable although not usually painful. The condition responds to sodium salicylate given systemically and to the administration of local steroids or non-steroid anti-inflammatory agents. The underlying cause is often never discovered, although there is a well recognised link with some joint and dermatological diseases, especially acne rosacea. Episcleritis tends to recur and may persist for several weeks producing a worrying cosmetic blemish in a young person (Fig. 7.1).

Red Painful Eye Which May See Normally

Scleritis

Inflammation of the sclera rather than the episclera is a less common cause of red eye. There is no discharge but the eye is painful. Vision is usu-

Fig. 7.3 Acute angle-closure glaucoma

Fig. 7.2 Scleritis

ally normal, unless the inflammation involves the posterior sclera. It is most often seen in association with rheumatoid arthritis and other collagen diseases and sometimes may become severe and progressive to the extent of causing perforation of the globe (Fig. 7.2). For this reason steroids must be administered with extreme care. Treatment normally is with systemically administered non-steroidal anti-inflammatory agents for example Froben tablets.

Fig. 7.4 Acute iritis. The pupil has been dilated with drops

Red Painful Eye Which Cannot See

It is worth emphasising again that the red painful eye with poor vision is likely to be a serious problem, often requiring urgent admission to hospital or at least intensive outpatient treatment as a sight-saving measure. The following are the principal causes.

Acute Glaucoma

The important feature here is that acute glaucoma occurs in long-sighted people and there is usually a previous history of headaches and seeing haloes round lights in the evenings. The raised intraocular pressure damages the iris sphincter and for this reason the pupil is semidilated. Oedema of the cornea causes the eye to lose its lustre and gives the iris a hazy appearance (Fig. 7.3). The eye is extremely tender and painful and the patient may be nauseated and vomiting. Immediate admission to hospital is essential where the intraocular pressure is first controlled medically and then bilateral laser iridotomies or surgical peripheral iridectomies performed to relieve pupil block. Mydriatics should not be given to patients with suspected narrow angle glaucoma, without consultation with an ophthalmologist.

Acute Iritis

The eye is painful, especially when attempting to view near objects, but the pain is never so severe as to cause vomiting. The cornea remains bright and the pupil tends to go into spasm and is smaller than on the normal side (Fig. 7.4). Acute iritis is seen from time to time mainly in the

20–40 age group, whereas acute glaucoma is unusual in this group. Unless severe and bilateral, acute iritis is treated on an outpatient basis with local steroids and mydriatic drops. Some expertise is needed in the use of the correct mydriatic, and systemic steroids should be avoided unless the sight is in jeopardy. Because the iris forms part of the uvea, acute iritis is the same as acute anterior uveitis. In many cases no systemic cause can be found but it is important to exclude the possibility of sarcoidosis or ankylosing spondylitis. The condition lasts for about 2 weeks but tends to recur over a period of years. After two or three recurrences there is a high risk of the development of cataract, although this may form slowly.

Acute Keratitis

The characteristic features are sharp pain, often described as a foreign body in the eye, marked watering of the eye, photophobia and difficulty in opening the affected eye. The clinical picture is very different from those of the above two conditions and the commonest causes are the Herpes simplex virus or trauma. The possibility of a perforating injury must always be borne in mind. Sometimes children are reticent about any history of injury for fear of incriminating a friend, but sometimes a small perforating injury is surprisingly painless. The treatment of acute keratitis has already been discussed in Chap. 6 and the management of corneal injuries will be considered in Chap. 16.

Neovascular Glaucoma

The elderly patient who presents with a blind and painful eye and who may also be diabetic should be suspected of having neovascular glaucoma. Often, a fairly well defined sequence of events enables the diagnosis to be inferred from the history, as in many cases secondary neovascular glaucoma arises following a central retinal vein occlusion. Following retinal vein occlusion, patients typically notice that the vision of one eye becomes blurred over several hours or days. Some elderly patients do not seek attention at this stage and some degree of spontaneous recovery may seem to occur before the onset of secondary glaucoma. Fortunately, only a modest proportion of cases develops this severe complication, which usually occurs, surprisingly enough, after 100 days, hence the term 'a hundred day glaucoma'. Once the intraocular pressure rises, the eye tends to become painful and eventually degenerates in the absence of treatment, and sometimes even in spite of treatment. This form of secondary glaucoma remains as one of the few indications for surgical removal of the eye, if measures to control the intraocular pressure are unsuccessful.

After reading this chapter you should be able to answer the following questions:

- What clinical features might make you decide to refer a patient with a red eye to a specialist?
- What are the causes of chronic conjunctivitis?
- How does neovascular glaucoma arise?

Failing Vision

8

Abstract

This chapter considers the main causes of failing vision when the eye looks outwardly normal either when the funds is normal ophthalmoscopically or when there are particular fundus changes. The relation of sight loss to systemic disease is also considered. Finally the more common conditions which respond well to treatment and those which up to now have been resistant to treatment are outlined.

Failing vision means that the sight as measured by the standard test type is worsening. The patient may say 'I can't see so well doctor' or they may feel that their spectacles need changing. Some patients may not notice visual loss especially if it is in one eye. Sometimes more specific symptoms are given; the vision may be blurred for example in a patient with cataract, or objects may appear distorted or straight lines bent if there is disease of the macular region of the retina. Disease of the macular may also make objects look larger or smaller. Double vision is an important symptom since it can be the result of a cranial nerve palsy but if monocular it may be due to cataract. Patients quite often complain of floating black spots. If these move slowly with eye movement they may be due to some disturbance of the vitreous gel in the centre of the eye. If they are accompanied by seeing flashing lights the possibility of damage to the retina needs to be kept in mind. 'Vitreous floaters' are very common and in most instances are of little pathological significance. Patients quite often notice haloes around lights and although this is typical of an attack of acute glaucoma haloes are also seen by patients with cataracts. Like many such symptoms they are best not asked for specifically. The question 'do you ever see haloes?' is likely to be followed by the answer 'yes'. Night blindness is another such symptom. No one can see too well in the dark but if a patient has noticed a definite worsening of his or her ability to see in dim light, then chronic glaucoma or an inherited retinal degeneration such as retinitis pigmentosa may be the cause.

Failing Vision in Eyes Which Look Normal

When the Fundus Is Normal

Very often a patient will present with a reduction of vision in one or both eyes and yet the eyes themselves look outwardly quite normal. In the case of a child, the parents may have noticed an apparent difficulty in reading or the vision may have been noticed to be poor at a routine school eye test. The next step is to decide whether the fundus is also normal but before dilating the pupil to allow fundus examination it is important to check the pupil reactions and to eliminate the possibility of refractive error. Once the possible need for glasses has been checked and the fundus examined then the presence of a normal fundus narrows the field down considerably. The likely diagnosis depends on the age of the patient. Infants with visual deterioration may require an examination under anaesthesia to exclude the possibility of a rare inherited retinal degeneration or other retinal disease. Other children, particularly those in the age group from 9 to 12 years, must first be suspected of some emotional upset, perhaps due to domestic upheaval or stress at school. This may make them reluctant to read the test type. Sometimes such children discover that exercising their own power of accommodation produces blurring of vision and they may present with accommodation spasm. The commonest cause of unilateral visual loss in children is amblyopia of disuse. This important cause of visual loss with a normal fundus is considered in more detail in the chapter on squint (Chap. 14). When, for any reason, one retina fails to receive a clear and correctly orientated image for a period of months or years during the time of visual development, then the sight of the eye remains impaired. The condition is treatable if caught before the visual reflexes are fully developed, that is, before the age of 8 years. Young adults who present with unilateral visual loss and normal fundi may, of course, have amblyopia of disuse and the condition may be confirmed by looking for a squint or a refractive error more marked on the affected side. We must also remember that retrobulbar neuritis presents in young people as sudden loss of vision on one side with aching behind the eye and a reduced pupil reaction on the affected side. This contrasts with amblyopia of disuse in which the pupil is normal. Migraine is another possibility to be considered in such patients.

Elderly patients who present with visual loss and normal fundi may give the history of a stroke and are found to have a homonymous hemianopic defect of the visual fields due to an embolus or thrombosis in the area of distribution of the posterior cerebral artery. Hysteria and malingering are also causes of unexplained visual loss, but these are extremely rare and it is important that the patient is investigated very carefully before such a diagnosis is made.

When the Fundus Is Abnormal

Quite a proportion of patients who complain of loss of vision with eyes that look normal on superficial inspection show changes on ophthalmoscopy. The three important potentially blinding but eminently treatable ophthalmological conditions must be born in mind: cataract, chronic glaucoma and retinal detachment. It is an unfortunate fact that the commonest cause of visual loss in the elderly is the one that is most resistant to treatment namely age related macular degeneration(AMD). AMD has been divided into the "wet" type and the "dry" type. The dry type is much more common but to date there is no effective treatment. On the other hand the wet type does respond well to recently introduced treatments as described in Chap. 19.

In Relation to Systemic Disease

The diseases described so far are limited to the eye itself, but disease elsewhere in the body can often first present as a visual problem. In this context we must remember what has been the commonest cause of blindness in young people—diabetic retinopathy, as well as the occasional case of severe hypertension. Intracranial causes of visual loss are perhaps less common in general practice and for this reason are easily missed. Intracranial tumours may present in an insidious manner, in particular the pituitary adenoma, and the diagnosis may be first suspected by careful plotting of the visual fields. In the case of the elderly patient who complains of visual deterioration in one eye, the ophthalmoscope all too commonly reveals age related macular degeneration but it is also common to find that the patient has suffered a thrombosis of the central retinal vein or one of its branches. Unlike the situation with a central retinal artery occlusion, which is less common, some vision is preserved with a central retinal vein thrombosis in spite of the dramatic haemorrhagic fundus appearance. Temporal arteritis is another important vascular cause of visual failure in the elderly.

Finally, there are a large number of less common conditions, only one or two of which will be mentioned at this point. At any age the ingestion of drugs may affect the eyesight but there are very few proven oculotoxic drugs still on the market. One important example is chloroquine. When a dose of 100 g in 1 year is exceeded there is a risk of retinotoxicity, which may not be reversible. Although age related macular degeneration is normally seen in the over sixties, the same problem may occur in younger people often with a recognised inheritance pattern. A completely different condition may also affect the macular region of young adults known as central serous retinopathy. This tends to resolve spontaneously after a few weeks although treatment by laser coagulation is occasionally needed. Unilateral progressive visual loss in young people may also be due to posterior uveitis, which is the same thing as choroiditis. The known causes and management of this condition will be discussed in a later chapter (See Chap. 18).

The more common causes of failing vision in a normal looking eye may be summarised as shown in Table 8.1.

Sudden Loss of Vision in One Eye

Table 8.2 shows the important causes of sudden visual loss in one eye only. Remember though that sometimes a longstanding condition in one eye may escape the notice of an elderly patient.

Patients with cataracts may notice that when washing the face and looking in the mirror and one hand is lowered there is sight loss in one eye. Typically the patient with a homonymous hemianopia describes the problem in the eye on the "blind side". As always it is very important to examine both eyes if possible with the pupils dilated once their reaction to light has been

Table 8.1 Reduced vision in a normal looking eye. Check list of likely causes

	Fundus normal	Fundus abnormal
Child	Refractive error	Cataract
	Disuse amblyopia	Macular degeneration
	Inherited retinal degeneration	Posterior uveitis
	Emotional stress	
Young adult	Refractive error	Diabetic retinopathy
	Retrobulbar neuritis	Retinal detachment
	Intracranial space occupying lesion	Macular disease
	Drug toxicity	Hypertension Posterior Uveitis
Elderly	Homonymous hemianopia	Macular degeneration
		Central vein thrombosis
		Chronic glaucoma
		Cataract
		Vitreous haemorrhage
		Temporal arteritis

Table 8.2 Sudden loss of vision in one eye

Diagnosis	Possible first line of referral
Central retinal vein thrombosis	Local eye department
Vitreous haemorrhage	Local eye department
Hemianopia	Stroke Unit (often described by patient as being in one eye)
Giant cell arteritis	Ophthalmologist/rheumatologist
Retinal detachment	Local eye department
Trauma	Local eye department

tested. As a general rule sudden loss of vision in one eye requires urgent referral to the local eye department.

Treatable Causes of Failing Vision

Nobody can deny that the practice of ophthalmology is highly effective. There are many eye diseases, which can be cured or arrested, and it is possible to restore the sight fully from total blindness. Many of the commoner causes of blindness especially in the third world are treatable. The most important treatable cause of visual failure in Britain is cataract, and of course no patient should be allowed to go blind from this cause although this does occasionally happen (Fig. 8.1). Retinal detachment is less common than cataract but it provides a situation where the sight may be lost completely and then be fully restored. For the best results, surgery must be carried out as soon as possible, before the retina becomes degenerate, whereas delay prior to cataract surgery does not usually affect the outcome of the operation. Acute glaucoma is another instance where the sight may be lost but restored by prompt treatment. The treatment of chronic glaucoma has less impression on the patient because it is aimed at preventing visual deterioration, although in sight saving terms it may be equally effective.

It is very easy to overlook the value of antibiotics in saving sight. Prior to their introduction, many more eyes had to be removed following injury and infection. Systemic and locally applied steroids also play a sight saving role in the management of temporal arteritis in the elderly and in the treatment of uveitis. In recent years the treatment of diabetic retinopathy has been greatly advanced by the combined effect of laser coagulation and scrupulous control of the diabetes. In the past, about half of the of the patients with the proliferative type of retinopathy would be expected to go blind over 5 years and many of these were young people at the height of their careers. The proper management of ocular trauma often has a great influence on the visual result, and the rare but dreaded complication of ocular perforating injuries—sympathetic ophthalmia—can now be effectively treated with systemic steroids. Amblyopia of disuse has already been mentioned; the treatment is undoubtedly effective in some cases but the results are disappointing if the diagnosis is made when the child is too old or when there is poor patient co-operation.

Untreatable Causes of Failing Vision

Ophthalmologists are sometimes asked if the sight can be restored to a blind eye and, as a general rule, one can say that if there is no perception of light in the eye, then it is unlikely that the sight can be improved irrespective of the cause. There are several ophthalmological conditions for which there is no known effective treatment and it is sometimes important that the patient is made aware of this at an early stage in order to avoid unnecessary anxiety, and so that suitable back up from the social services can be arranged. Most degenerative diseases of the retina fail to respond to treatment. If the retina is out of place, it can be replaced, but old retinae cannot be replaced with new. So far there has been no firm evidence that any drug can alter the course of inherited retinal degenerations such as retinitis pigmentosa, although useful information is beginning to appear about the biochemistry and genetics of these conditions. The dry type of age related macular degeneration tends to run a progressive course in spite of any attempts at treatment, and although most patients do not become completely

Fig. 8.1 The family thought it was just old age

blind, it accounts for loss of reading vision in many elderly people. Some myopic patients are susceptible to degeneration of the retina in later years; known as myopic chorioretinal degeneration, it may account for visual deterioration in myopes who have otherwise undergone successful cataract or retinal surgery.

Scarring of the retina following trauma is another cause of permanent and untreatable visual loss, but the most dramatic and irrevocable loss of vision occurs following traumatic section of the optic nerve. One must be careful here before dismissing the patient as untreatable because on rare occasions a contusion injury to the eye or orbit may result in a haemorrhage into the sheath of the optic nerve. Some degree of visual recovery may sometimes occur in these patients and it has been claimed that recovery may be helped by surgically opening the nerve sheath. There is one odd exception to this dramatic form of blindness which may follow optic nerve insult; visual loss due to optic neuritis. Patients with retrobulbar neuritis (optic neuritis) nearly always recover much of their vision again whether they receive treatment or not. The expla-

nation is that the visual loss is due to pressure from oedema rather than to damage to the nerve fibres themselves. It is hardly necessary to say that any neurological damage proximal to the optic nerve tends to produce permanent and untreatable visual loss, as exemplified by the homonymous hemianopic field defect which may follow a cerebrovascular accident.

Malignant tumours of the eye come into this category of untreatable causes of visual failure but in fact serious attempts are now being made to treat them with radiotherapy in specialised units and the prognosis appears to be improving in some cases.

After reading this chapter you should be able to answer the following:

- When the vision is failing in an otherwise normal appearing eye and a normal fundus what conditions might you suspect?
- What are the important treatable causes of failing vision?
- What is the commonest cause of blindness in young people?

Headache

9

Abstract

Although headache is a very common symptom it can sometimes indicate a serious underlying problem. In this chapter the important causes are considered with especial emphasis on th eye.

Headache must be one of the commonest symptoms, and few specialities escape from the diagnostic problems that it may present. We must begin with the realisation that more or less everyone suffers from headache at some time or other. In fact, the majority of headaches that present have no detectable cause and are often labelled psychogenic if there seems to be a background of stress. The implication is that the sufferer is perhaps exaggerating mild symptoms in order to gain sympathy from his or her spouse, or even perhaps the doctor. One must of course be extremely cautious about not accepting symptoms at their face value, and certainly cerebral tumours have been overlooked for this very reason. If the psychogenic headache is the commonest, then the headache due to raised intracranial pressure and a space-occupying lesion must be the most important. Between these two the whole spectrum of causes must be considered. It is essential, therefore, to memorise a permanent checklist in order that obvious causes are not omitted.

History

Often the history is the total disease in the absence of any physical signs and it is important to note the nature of the pain, the total duration and frequency of the pain, the time of day it occurs, and its relation to other events or the taking of analgesics. Headaches that are present 'all the time' and are described in fanciful terms tend not to have an organic basis; the patient with an organic headache is not usually smiling. The time of day may be important: raised intracranial pressure has the reputation of causing an early morning headache which is described as bursting or throbbing and which may be made worse by straining or coughing. We must always remember the triad of headache, vomiting and papilloedema in this respect, especially as the vomiting may not be accompanied by nausea, and is not necessarily mentioned by the patient. The family history should also be noted especially where there is a history of migraine.

Classification

When considering the different common causes of headache, an anatomical classification is a useful way of providing a reference list. The following should be considered by the examining doctor.

Cerebrospinal Fluid

A rise or fall from normal of the cerebrospinal fluid pressure is associated with headache. When the CSF pressure is raised the patient usually experiences a bursting pain, which may interrupt sleep or appear in the early morning. It tends to be intermittent and made worse by coughing or lying down. It may also, of course, be accompanied by papilloedema and vomiting, and another important symptom is blurring and transient obscurations of vision. The situation of the pain is usually diffuse rather than focal, but we must remember that a bursting headache made worse by coughing is sometimes described by otherwise healthy individuals. When the rise of intracranial pressure is due to a space-occupying lesion, signs of focal brain damage may also be present.

Blood Vessels

A variety of diseases involving the blood vessels may cause headache. The commonest is probably migraine. Classical migraine was thought to be due to an initial spasm followed by dilatation of the meningeal arteries, but more precise studies of the vasculature have failed to confirm this. There is usually a family history of the same problem showing dominant inheritance, and attacks may sometimes be precipitated by stress or taking certain foods such as cheese. Before the headache begins there is usually a visual aura characterised by a shimmering effect before one or both eyes which spreads across the vision, or the appearance of zigzag lines known as fortifications because of their resemblance to the silhouette of a

fortress. The visual disturbance may take the form of a hemianopic scotoma or, very rarely, of a formed hallucination but, whatever their nature, they tend to last for about 10–20 min and are followed by a headache which is centred above the eye and is described as a boring pain. The headache lasts for anytime between 1 and 24 h and then disperses. The patient may experience nausea and vomiting as the attack ends. Migraine may begin quite early in childhood and continue at regular intervals for many years. Migraines are more common in women and tend to improve at the time of the menopause. Atypical migraine can sometimes pose a diagnostic problem. The visual aura may appear by itself or the migraine attack may be accompanied by gastrointestinal symptoms or by ophthalmoplegia. The attack may be preceded by oliguria and fluid retention and be followed by a diuresis. Very rarely, a permanent hemianopic scotoma or ophthalmoplegia may result from an attack of migraine, but in these circumstances the original diagnosis must be reviewed very carefully. Of some importance is the fact that a history of migraine increases the risk of developing normal tension glaucoma 2–4 times. Interestingly migraine is one of the few risk factors for this condition.

There is some doubt as to whether essential hypertension causes headaches but there is no doubt that when the blood pressure becomes acutely raised, a severe headache may ensue, accompanied by blurring of vision. Any adults with headaches should have their blood pressure measured. Another form of headache associated with abnormality of the blood vessels is that due to an intracranial aneurysm of the internal carotid artery or one of its branches. The pain in this case is usually throbbing in nature and there may be other signs of a space occupying lesion at the apex of the orbit, for example, a cranial nerve palsy or a bruit heard with the stethoscope. In the case of elderly patients, the possibility of giant cell arteritis must always be kept in mind. This is an inflammation of the walls of many of the medium sized arteries in the body but it tends to affect the temporal arteries preferentially. The walls of the vessels become thickened by inflammatory cells and giant cells mainly in the media and there is fibrosis of the intima (Fig. 9.1). The lumen of the affected vessels becomes occluded. Affected patients are usually over the age of 70 and complain of tenderness of the scalp, especially over the temporal arteries, which may be seen and felt to be inflamed, and typically no pulse can be felt in them. The headache is made particularly bad by brushing the hair and other systemic symptoms include jaw claudication, weight loss, and malaise. The importance of this type of headache rests on the fact that the eye is involved in about 60% of cases and the patient may suddenly go blind in one eye and then a short time later go blind in the other. Patients with giant cell arteritis invariably have a raised ESR and CRP (typically the ESR is found to be above 70 mm/h) An ultrasound examination and or a temporal artery biopsy can be helpful to assist with the diagnosis particularly in those patients with indeterminate clinical findings. When giant cell arteritis is first considered as a diagnosis, it is advisable to start treatment with systemic steroids without delay before awaiting confirmatory diagnosis on histology. Steroid treatment is very effective in preventing blindness and is required usually for a 12–18 month period. Once instituted the response to treatment and the side effects should be very carefully monitored, preferably in coop-

Fig. 9.1 Cross-section of the temporal artery from patient with temporal arteritis. The artery is almost occluded. Note the large number of giant cells (With acknowledgement to Dr J. Lowe)

eration with a general physician with regular measurement of the ESR and other inflammatory markers. Other less common vascular causes of headache include intracranial angioma and subarachnoid or subdural haemorrhage.

Blood

Changes in the blood itself may also be associated with headache. It is easy to forget that anaemic patients often have headaches, which can be cured by treating the anaemia. Likewise, patients with polycythaemia may also complain of headache. Hypoglycaemia is another recognised cause; here the symptoms occur after strenuous exercise or insulin excess in a diabetic patient.

Nerves

Cluster headache. In many respects this type of headache resembles migraine although it is more common in men in the third or fourth decade. The word cluster refers to the timing of the attacks, which may be repeated several times over a few weeks followed by a period of remission for several months. The pain is described as being very severe and unilateral. There is conjunctival congestion and constriction of the pupil on the affected side, and the attack may last from minutes to hours. Tenderness over the side of the face and nasal discharge are also features. Raeder's paratrigeminal neuralgia probably merges with cluster headache, being described as severe ocular pain associated with meiosis and ptosis. Trigeminal neuralgia can be easily distinguished from these other forms of headache by its distribution over one or all of the terminal branches of the trigeminal nerve and the fact that the very severe pain is triggered by touching a part of the cheek or by chewing and swallowing. The pain is so severe that the patient may become suicidal, and surgical division of the trigeminal nerve at the level of the Gasserian ganglion has been a method of treatment.

Post herpetic neuralgia is an extremely debilitating form of headache experienced by elderly people after an attack of trigeminal herpes zoster. The pain seems to be more severe in the elderly and it may persist for many years. The cause of the headache is usually evident when one inspects the skin of the forehead, which is slightly whitened and scarred from the previous attack of herpes zoster. Apart from the use of analgesics, antidepressant drugs may also help, together with the application of local heat or vibration massage. Fortunately the prompt treatment of the original attack of herpes zoster at primary care level with systemic acyclovir does seem to be reducing the incidence of this troublesome condition.

Bones

Paget's Disease of bone. In this condition the bones of the head enlarge and grow abnormally, the abnormal growth being associated with headache and incidentally an increase in hat size. The eyes themselves may show optic atrophy, and close inspection of the fundi may reveal the curious appearance of wavy lines known as angioid streaks. Oxycephaly is a congenital defect of the skull due to premature closure of the sutures; patients sometimes complain of headache as well as visual loss due to optic nerve compression. Multiple myeloma is the name given to a malignant proliferation of plasma cells within the bone marrow. There is also an excessive production of immunoglobulins. Osteolytic bone lesions occur especially in the skull, and headache may be an accompaniment. The disease is more common in the elderly and is accompanied by a high ESR. Diagnosis is made by examining the urine for Bence Jones proteins and the serum for abnormal immunoglobulins. Disease of the cervical vertebrae is another cause of headache, due to the effect of spasm of the neck muscles. Relief of the pain by neck manipulation has been claimed but the exact diagnosis must be made before embarking on such treatment.

Meninges

It is presumed that the pain and headache, which accompany meningitis or encephalitis, are medi-ated through the sensory nerve supply to the meninges. The pain sensitive structures in the middle and anterior cranial fossa are supplied by the fifth cranial nerve, and inflammation may produce referred pain to the region of the eye.

The Eyes

The classical eye headache is that of subacute narrow angle glaucoma. Here the headache is an evening one, tends to be over one eye and is nearly always accompanied by blurring of vision and seeing coloured haloes around street lights. If the intraocular pressure is measured when the headache is present and is found to be normal, then it is unlikely that narrow angle glaucoma is the correct diagnosis. On the other hand, the diagnosis cannot be so easily excluded if the headache is absent at the time of examination. Patients with narrow angle glaucoma are long sighted—therefore beware the middle aged long sighted patient with evening headaches and blurring of vision. Chronic open angle glaucoma very rarely causes headache because the rise of intraocular pressure is too gradual and not great enough. The possibility should be born in mind when a patient experiences headaches following ocular trauma or eye surgery, that there may be secondary glaucoma. This type of glaucoma often responds well to treatment but if ignored may lead rapidly to blindness. Acute iritis is associated with headache but in practice rarely presents as such because the other ocular symptoms override this. Patients developing endophthalmitis complain of severe pain in the eye and headache, this being a particularly important symptom following cataract surgery.

It has been argued that refractive error does not cause headache, but nothing could be further from the truth. Refractive headache is most commonly seen in uncorrected hypermetropes, sometimes in children, but more commonly in adults aged 30–40 years who are beginning to have difficulty in accommodating through their long sightedness. For reasons of vanity, patients may have been deliberately avoiding the use of glasses and it may have to be explained to them that they have the choice of having headaches or wearing glasses. In the patient with no refractive error, the onset of presbyopia may be accompanied by headache, which is sometimes delayed until the morning after prolonged reading. An otherwise normal person aged 45 should be suspected of having presbyopic headaches. Uncorrected myopes do not usually complain of headaches. If the spectacle prescription is incorrect for any reason then a sensitive person may experience headache, but it is surprising how some people will tolerate an incorrect spectacle lens without complaint. Ocular muscle imbalance is an uncommon cause of headache but it is an important one because it can be corrected with considerable relief to the patient. Usually the patient shows a significant difference in refractive error between the two eyes and when the eyes are dissociated by such means as the cover test or the Maddox wing test, one eye tends to drift upwards or downwards. Relief of symptoms may be achieved by incorporating a prism into the spectacle lens or, if the deviation is marked by ocular muscle surgery. Horizontal imbalance of the ocular movements is less closely linked with headache, although there is a group of patients, usually young adults under stress, who seem unable to converge their eyes on near objects; instead they allow one eye to drift outwards when reading. Some elderly patients have the same problem but do not so often have associated headache. This so-called convergence insufficiency can be greatly improved by a course of convergence exercises and provides one of the few instances where exercises of the eye muscles have any therapeutic value.

Pain Referred from Other Sites

Sinusitis is well recognised as a common cause of headache and the patient with headache should be questioned about recent upper respiratory tract infections or a previous history of sinus disease. Tenderness over the affected sinus is an important sign. The headache tends to begin after rising in the morning and reaches a peak later in the morning. Pain from an infected tooth may be referred over the side of the face and cause some diagnostic confusion but it is usually worse when chewing or biting. Pain from a middle ear infection may cause similar problems. The temporomandibular joint is a recognised source of referred pain over the side of the face, and malfunctioning of the joint may result from incorrect jaw alignment or poorly fitting dentures.

Drugs

Over indulgence in alcohol is one of the three causes of morning headache; the other two being raised intracranial pressure and acute sinusitis. The diagnostic difficulty with alcoholism tends to be failure of the patient to admit or recognise excessive drinking. It may seem strange that such a patient should ever seek a doctor's opinion about headache, but alcoholics do sometimes seek an ophthalmological opinion for their symptoms without relating them to alcohol intake and perhaps urged on by an anxious relative or friend. Chronic poisoning by other drugs is too rare a cause of headache in ophthalmic practice to be considered here but it may have to be born in mind.

Post-traumatic Headache

Nearly all patients who have suffered a significant head injury complain of headaches. The pain may remain severe for many months and in the worst case may last a few years. Usually no obvious explanation can be found apart from the original injury. The severity of the headache may sometimes appear to be related to clinical depression following the injury but other causes of headache such as ocular muscle imbalance or raised intracranial pressure need to be excluded.

Contact Lenses

10

Abstract

The widespread use of contact lenses means that any one involved with eye care will find themselves confronted with more and more patients who have run into wearing problems of one kind or another. For this reason some of the likely emergency requirements are considered here.

Types

As long ago as 1912 a glass contact lens was being produced, but because of the manufacturing difficulties and wearing problems, the widespread use of this type of optical aid was delayed until the introduction of plastic scleral lenses in 1937. The obvious advantage of placing a lens directly on the cornea over the wearing of spectacles is the cosmetic one, but the system also has optical advantages. Because the lens moves with the eye there are none of the problems associated with looking through the edge of the lens experienced by the wearer of spectacles. In addition a more subtle effect is the more accurate representation of image size on the retina in subjects with high degrees of refractive error.

Although the original type of moulded scleral contact lenses are still occasionally used, they have been largely replaced by the modern rigid and soft lenses which are much smaller and thinner and hence causes less interference with corneal physiology. Rigid lenses are made from gas-permeable plastics and have generally replaced the early 'hard' lenses which were impermeable to oxygen. In 1960 the hydrophilic soft contact lens was introduced. This had the great advantage of being soft and malleable and hence more comfortable to wear, but optically it has never been quite as good as the rigid lens, especially when the patient has high degrees of astigmatism. Several different materials have now been used in the production of soft lenses although the basic material used is hydroxmethylmethacrylate (HEMA). The different types of soft lenses differ in their ability to take up water and transmit oxygen. Lenses are now being made which can be worn for long periods without needing to be removed and cleaned. Similarly disposable and 'planned-replacement' contact lenses are now widely available. Care should be taken that such lenses are used under professional care.

Soft contact lenses tend to absorb and adsorb material from the tear film. It is particularly important to ensure that a patient is not wearing a soft lens before fluorescein dye is instilled into the eye.

Side-Effects

In general soft contact lenses have more side effects than rigid lenses in the long-term. The commonest complication of wearing modern contact lenses is losing them. Patients are well advised to have a pair of glasses at hand in case they have contact-lens-wearing problems or a lens is lost. More serious trouble may result from clumsy handling of the lens or leaving a rigid lens in the eye for too long a period. Such patients quite often present with severe pain in the eye, and examination reveals a partially healed corneal abrasion. This must be treated in the usual manner and the patient advised against wearing the lens again for several weeks, depending on the extent of the abrasion. The contact lenses themselves should also be examined by the patient's fitter to make sure that they are not faulty. Bearing in mind the troubles, which may ensue when an abrasion becomes recurrent, the indications for wearing the lenses in the first place should be reconsidered.

The risk of infections by lens contamination or secondary to corneal abrasions is increased. Recently acanthamoeba keratitis has been described. This disease occurs more often in contact lens wearers. The widespread use of both daily and planned-replacement soft lenses does not appear to have completely solved the problem of serious complications resulting from lens wear.

Another sequel to wearing contact lenses, either rigid or soft, is the appearance of chronic inflammatory changes in the conjunctiva, often characterised by a papillary conjunctivitis. The resulting irritation and redness of the eyes may persist for some weeks after the wearing of the contact lenses ceases. Unfortunately these symptoms may appear after wearing lenses successfully for some years and they may tend to recur in spite of renewing or modifying the lenses. Some patients who tolerate contact lenses very well may develop corneal changes after some years. Peripheral vascularisation may become evident and in neglected cases there may be band degeneration of the cornea. Some contact-lens wearers complain of recurrent blurring of their vision and

Fig. 10.1 Hard contact lens with lipid deposits (With acknowledgement to Professor M. Rubinstein)

this may be due to an ill-fitting lens producing corneal epithelial oedema or simply to the excessive accumulation of mucus on the lens (Fig. 10.1).

Indications

These may be considered as either cosmetic or therapeutic.

Cosmetic

There are obvious cosmetic advantages for the wearer of contact lenses, especially the teenager. However, the potential wearer should realise the possible difficulties involved: the need to clean and sterilise the lenses and the need for some degree of finger dexterity when they are inserted and removed. There are numerous and varied cleaning and disinfection systems on the market. Contact lenses may be required for certain occupations and pursuits such as golf or athletics where the spectacle wearer is handicapped by misting up of the glasses in wet weather. Patients over the age of 45 or 50 will find that they require reading glasses as well and these, of course, must be worn over the contact lenses, thereby somewhat reducing the cosmetic value of the latter. Multifocal contact lenses are available but have limited success. Some patients tolerate being corrected in one eye for distance vision and in the other for reading, with contact lenses. Care should be taken in this situation when assessing the visual acuity as the eye corrected for near vision will be blurred for distance.

Therapeutic

There are instances when the contact lens may result in much better vision than spectacles, for example in patients with high degrees of corneal astigmatism which are not fully correctable with glasses. This accounts for the benefit of contact lenses in patients with keratoconus or conical cornea. Soft contact lenses are sometimes used as 'bandage lenses' to protect the cornea after corneal burns or in patients with bullous keratopathy. The contact lens has a special importance in the correction of unilateral aphakia where the biological lens has been removed without replacement with an implant for whatever reason (see Chap. 11) The contact lens has the effect of reducing the image size on the retina to such an extent that the two eyes can once again be used together. If eye drops are being regularly instilled into the eyes, soft contact lenses may absorb the drug being used or the preservative in the drops. In fact, attempts have been made to use soft contact lenses as a slow-release system by impregnating them with the drug before fitting.

When you have read this chapter you should be able to answer the following questions:

1. What are the advantages and disadvantages of wearing contact lenses?
2. What are the risks of wearing contact lenses?
3. What are the indications for wearing contact lenses?

Part III

Problems of the Eye Surgeon

Cataract

11

Abstract

In this chapter the anatomy and physiology of the lens are described. How cataracts develop, and their symptoms and signs, are then discussed. The current cataract surgery pathway is explained in detail.

Cataract means an opacity of the lens and it is the commonest potentially blinding condition, which confronts the eye surgeon. This is not to say that every person with cataract is liable to go blind. Many patients have relatively slight lens opacities that progress very slowly. Fortunately the results of surgery are very good, a satisfactory improvement of vision being obtained in over 90% of cases. It is usually possible to forewarn the patients when there is an extra element of doubt about the outcome. To the uninformed patient the word cataract strikes a note of fear and it may be necessary to explain that opacities in the lens are extremely common in elderly people. It is only when the opaque lens fibres begin to interfere with the vision that the term 'cataract' is used. Many patients have a slight degree of cataract, which advances so slowly that they die before any visual problems arise. Nobody need now go blind from cataract; however one still encounters elderly people who from ignorance or neglect, are left immobilised by this form of blindness, and it is especially important that the general practitioner is able to recognise the condition.

The Lens

The human lens is a surprising structure. It is avascular and yet it is actively growing throughout life, albeit extremely slowly. It receives its nourishment from the aqueous fluid that bathes it. The lens is enclosed in an elastic capsule and for this reason tends to assume a spherical shape, or would do if the moulding of the lens fibres allowed. In situ the shape of the lens is maintained by a series of taut fibres known as the zonule. The fibres exert radial tension on the lens but the tension is reduced when the circular part of the ciliary muscle contracts. The reduced tension of the zonule allows the lens to assume a more spherical shape and hence the antero-posterior diameter of the lens increases. As a result, the refracting power of the lens increases, that is to say, light rays are more bent and the eye becomes focused on near objects. This process of accommodation, which is produced by relaxation of the lens but contraction of the ciliary muscle, gradually becomes less effective as we grow older, probably because the lens becomes less malleable rather than because the ciliary muscle is becoming weaker. This reduction in the range of accommodation explains why the little child will present an object close to an adult's eyes and expect him or her to see it clearly. It also explains why, in the mid-forties it becomes necessary to hold a book further from ones eyes if it is to be read easily and also the subsequent inability to read without the assistance of a spectacle lens which provides additional converging power. The need for reading glasses occurs in people with normal eyes at about the age of 45 (presbyopia) but this is only a milestone in a slowly progressive path of deterioration that begins at birth.

Histological section of the lens reveals that beneath the capsule there is an anterior epithelium with a single layer of cells, but no such layer is evident beneath the posterior capsule. Furthermore, if one follows the single layered anterior epithelium to the equator of the lens, then the epithelial cells can be seen to elongate progressively and lose their nuclei as they are traced into the interior of the lens. Thus one can deduce from histological sections that the lens fibres are being continuously laid down from the epithelial cells at the equator. The actual arrangement of the lens fibres is quite complex; each fibre being made up of a prismatic six sided band bound to its fellow by an amorphous cement substance.

Slit lamp examination of the lens reveals the presence of the lens sutures, which mark the points of junction of the end of the lens fibres. Two such sutures are usually seen, both often taking the form of the letter 'Y', the posterior suture being inverted. The lens fibres contain proteins known as 'crystallins' and have the property of setting up an antigen-antibody reaction if they are released into the eye from the lens capsule. One other feature of the lens, which can usually be seen with the slit lamp microscope, is an object looking like a pig's tail which hangs from the posterior capsule. This is the remains of the hyaloid artery, a vessel that runs in the embryonic eye from the optic disc to the vascular tunic of the lens, which is present at that stage (Fig. 11.1).

Fig. 11.1 Cross-section of a child's lens: aqueous on left, vitreous on right. Note the hyaloid remnant and the "Y" sutures (With acknowledgement to M. L. Berliner, 1949)

Aetiology

Having learned of the complex structure of the lens, perhaps one should be more surprised that the lens retains its transparency throughout life than that some of the lens fibres may become opaque. There are a number of reasons why lens fibres become opaque but the commonest and most important is ageing. The various causes will now be considered.

Age

The majority of cataracts are associated with the ageing process, and some of the biochemical changes in the lens fibres are now being understood. We know that certain families are more susceptible to age related cataract, but a degree of opacification of the lens is commonplace in the elderly. Often the opacity is limited to the peripheral part of the lens and the patient may be unaware of any problem. It is usual to limit the term 'cataract' to the situation where the opacities are causing some degree of visual impairment. Elderly patients are often reassured to learn that their eye condition is part of the general ageing process and that only in certain instances does the opacification progress to the point where surgery is required.

Diabetes

The new trainee doctor working in an eye hospital must be impressed by the number of diabetics with cataracts who pass through his or her hands, and might be forgiven for deducing that diabetes is a common cause of cataract. To see the situation in perspective one must realise that both cataracts and diabetes are common diseases of the elderly and coincide quite often. Of course, the matter has been investigated from the statistical point of view and it has been shown that there is a somewhat higher incidence of cataract in diabetics, mainly because they tend to develop lens opacities at an earlier age. A special type of cataract is seen in young diabetics and in these cases the lens may become rapidly opaque in a few months. Fortunately this is not very common, usually occurring in insulin dependant patients who have had difficulty with the control of their diabetes. It is claimed that in its early stages this type of cataract can be reversible, but such an occurrence is so rare that it has not presented much opportunity for study.

Secondary

Cataract may be secondary to disease in the eye or disease elsewhere in the body.

Secondary to disease in the eye. More or less any terminal event in the eye tends to be associated with cataract. Advanced uncontrolled glaucoma is often associated with an opaque lens, as are chronic iridocyclitis and intraocular tumours. Certain specific eye diseases are accompanied by cataract; for example, patients who suffer from the inherited retinal degeneration, retinitis pigmentosa, sometimes develop a particular type of opacity in the posterior part of the lens. The removal of such a cataract may sometimes restore a considerable amount of vision, at least for a time.

Secondary to disease elsewhere. It may be recalled that the lens is ectodermal, being developed as an invagination of the overlying surface ectoderm. It is not surprising therefore, that some skin diseases are associated with cataract. In particular patients suffering from asthma and eczema may present to the eye surgeon in their late fifties. Dysfunction of the parathyroid glands is a very rare cause of cataract and Down's syndrome is a more common association.

Trauma

Contusion A direct blow on the eye, if it is severe enough, may cause the lens to become opaque. A squash ball injury is a typical example of the type of force required. Sometimes the appearance of the cataract may be delayed even for several years. The onset of unilateral cataract must always make one suspect the possibility of previous injury, but a cause and effect relationship may be difficult to prove in the absence of any other signs of previous contusion. It seems unlikely that a cataract would form unless there had been a direct blow on the eye itself, although occasionally medico-legal claims are made for compensation when a cataract has developed following a blow on the side of the head.

Perforation A perforating wound of the eye bears a much higher risk of cataract formation. If the perforating object (for example, a broken beer glass) passes through the cornea without touching the lens, then usually the lens is spared and, in the absence of significant contusion, a cataract does not form. This, of course, also depends on careful management of the corneal wound and the prevention of infection. Unfortunately such perforating injuries may also involve splitting of the lens capsule with spilling out of the lens fibres into the anterior chamber. The series of events, which follow such an injury, is dependent on the age of the individual. When the lens capsule of a child is ruptured, a vigorous inflammatory reaction is set up in the anterior chamber and the lens matter will usually gradually become absorbed, in the absence of treatment, over a period of about a month. This leaves behind the lens capsule and often a clear pupil. In spite of this the patient cannot see clearly because most of the refractive power of the eye is lost. This has serious optical consequences and the need for an artificial intraocular lens. When the lens capsule of an adult is ruptured, a similar inflammatory reaction ensues, but there tends to be more fibrosis, and a white plaque of fibrous tissue may remain to obstruct the pupil. Very rarely, it is possible for a lens to be perforated with subsequent opacity limited to the site of perforation—indeed, one occasionally sees a foreign body within the lens surrounded by opaque fibres but limited to a small part of the lens.

Radiation Visible light does not seem to cause cataract, although claims have been made that individuals from white races living for long periods in the tropics may show a higher incidence of cataract. In practice this is not easy to confirm. In spite of public misapprehension, ultraviolet light probably does not cause cataract either, since the shorter wavelengths fail to penetrate the globe. These shorter wavelengths beyond the blue end of the visible spectrum can produce a dramatic superficial burn of the cornea, which usually heals in about 48 h. This injury, which is typified by 'snow blindness' and 'welders flash', will be discussed in Chap. 15. Prolonged doses of infra red rays can produce cataract; this used to be seen occasionally in glassblowers and steel workers, but the wearing of goggles has now more or less eliminated this. X-rays and gamma rays may also produce cataracts, as was witnessed by the mass of reports, which followed the explosion of the atomic bombs at Nagasaki and Hiroshima. Radiation cataract is now seen following whole body radiation for leukaemia but the risk is only significant when therapeutic doses of x-rays are used.

Congenital Factors

Many of the cases of congenital cataract seen in ophthalmic practice are inherited. Sometimes there is a dominant family history and there are many other possible associated defects, some of which fit into named syndromes. Acquired congenital cataract may result from maternal rubella infection during the first trimester of pregnancy. The association of deafness, congenital heart lesions and cataract must always be born in mind. The ophthalmic house surgeon must take special care when examining the congenital cataract case preoperatively and likewise the paediatric house surgeon must bear in mind that congenital cataracts may be overlooked, especially if they are not very severe. Sometimes the cataracts may be slight at birth and gradually progress subsequently, or sometimes they may remain stationary until later years.

Toxicity

Toxic cataracts are probably rare, although several currently used drugs have been incriminated, the most notable being systemic steroids. Chlorpromazine has also been shown to cause lens opacities in large doses, and so has the use of certain meiotics, including Pilocarpine. Much of our knowledge of drug induced cataracts is based on former animal experiments. The potential danger of new drugs causing cataract was shown in the 1930s after the introduction of dinitrophenol as a slimming agent. This produced a large number of lens opacities before it was eventually withdrawn.

Symptoms

Many patients complain of blurred vision, which is usually worse when viewing distant objects. If the patient is unable to read small print, the surgeon may suspect that other pathology such as macular degeneration may be present. One must bear in mind that some elderly patients say that they cannot read when it is found that they *can* read small print when carefully tested. It is a curious fact that when the cataract is unilateral the patient may claim that the loss of vision has been quite sudden. Elucidation of the history in these cases sometimes reveals that the visual loss was noted when washing and observing the face in the mirror. When one hand is lowered before the other, the unilateral visual loss is noticed for the first time and interpreted as a sudden event. The history in cataract cases may be further confused by a natural tendency for patients to project their symptoms into the spectacles, and several pairs may be obtained before the true cause of the problem is found. In order to understand the symptoms of cataract it is essential to understand what is meant by index myopia. This simply refers to the change in refractive power of the lens, which occurs as a preliminary to cataract formation. Index myopia may also result from uncontrolled diabetes. If we imagine an elderly patient who requires reading glasses (for presbyopia) in the normal way but no glasses for viewing distant objects, then the onset of index myopia will produce blurring of distance vision, but also the patient will discover to his or her surprise that it is possible to read again without glasses. In the same way the hypermetropic patient will become less hypermetropic and find that it is possible to see again in the distance without glasses. The ageing fibres in the precataractous lens become more effective at converging light rays so that parallel rays of light are brought to a focus more anteriorly in the eye.

Apart from blurring of vision, the cataract patient often complains of monocular diplopia. Sometimes even a very slight and subtle opacity in the posterior part of the lens can cause the patient to notice, for example, that car rear lights appear doubled, and this may be reproduced with the ophthalmoscope light. Monocular diplopia is sometimes regarded as a rather suspect symptom, the suggestion being that if a patient continues to see double even when one eye is closed, then he or she may not be giving a very accurate history. In actual practice nothing could be further from the truth and this is quite a common presenting feature of cataract.

Glare is another common presenting symptom. The patient complains that he or she cannot see so well in bright light and may even be wearing a pair of dark glasses. Glare is a photographic term but here it refers to a significant reduction in visual acuity when an extraneous light source is introduced. Light shining from the side is scattered in the cataractous lens and reduces the quality of the image on the retina. Glare becomes an important consideration when advising an elderly cataractous patient on fitness to drive. The visual acuity may be within the requirements laid down by law (seeing a number plate at 20.5 m) but only when the patient is tested in the absence of glare.

A consideration of all these factors makes it relatively easy to diagnose cataract even before examining the patient. To summarise, a typical patient may complain that the glasses have been inaccurately prescribed, that the vision is much worse in bright sunlight, that sometimes things look double, and that there is difficulty in recognising peoples faces in the street rather than difficulty in reading. Patients with cataracts alone do not usually complain that things look distorted or that straight lines look bent, nor do they experience pain in the eye.

Very rarely, cataracts become hypermature; that is to say, the lens enlarges in the eye and this in turn may lead to secondary glaucoma and pain in the eye. Urgent surgery may be needed under these circumstances. In its late stages, a cataract matures and becomes white, so that exceptionally a patient may complain of a white spot in the middle of the pupil.

Signs

Reduced Visual Acuity

A reduction in visual acuity may, of course, be an early sign of cataract formation but this is not always the case. Some patients see surprisingly well through marked lens opacities, and the effect on visual acuity as measured by the Snellen test type depends as much on the position of the opacities in the lens as upon the density of the opacities.

Findings of Ophthalmoscopy

The best way of picking up a cataract in its early stages is to view the pupil through the

Fig. 11.2 Opaque areas in the lens can be seen clearly against the red refl ex

ophthalmoscope from a distance of about 50 cm. In this way the red reflex is clearly seen. The red reflex is simply the reflection of light from the fundus and it is viewed in exactly the same manner that one might view a cat's eyes in the headlamps of one's car or the eyes of one's friends in an ill judged flash photograph. In fact such a flash photo could well show up an early cataract if an elderly relative were included in the photograph. When using the ophthalmoscope, the opacities in the lens are often seen as black spokes against the red reflex (Fig. 11.2). It is important to focus one's eyes onto the plane of the patient's pupil if the cataract is to be well seen, and it is preferable to dilate the pupil beforehand or at least examine in a darkened room. Typical age related lens opacities are wedge shaped, pointing towards the centre of the pupil. At the same time the central nucleus of the lens may take on a yellowish-brown colour, the appearance being termed 'lens sclerosis', and ultimately the lens may become nearly black in some instances.

After inspecting a cataract with the ophthalmoscope held at a distance from the eye, one must then approach closer and attempt to examine the fundus. Further useful information about the density of the cataract can be obtained in this way. It is generally true that if the observer can see in, then the patient can see out. If there is an obvious discrepancy between the clarity of the fundus and the visual acuity of the patient, then some other pathology may be suspected. Sometimes the patient may not have performed too well on subjective testing and such an error should be apparent when the fundus is viewed. Some types of cataract can be misleading in this respect and this applies particularly to those seen in highly myopic patients. Here there is sometimes a preponderance of nuclear sclerosis, which simply causes distortion of the fundus while the disc and macula may be seen quite clearly.

Findings on Slit Lamp Microscopy

A really detailed view of any cataract can be obtained with the slit lamp. By adjusting the angle and size of the slit beam, various optical sections of the lens can be examined, revealing the exact morphology of the cataract. The presence of small vesicles under the anterior lens capsule may be seen as an early sign of age-related cataract. Cataracts secondary to uveitis or to drugs may first appear as an opacity in the posterior subcapsular region. For optical reasons, an opacity in this region tends to interfere with reading vision at an early stage. Opacities in the lens may appear in a wide range of curious shapes and sizes, and earlier in the last century there was a vogue for classifying them with Latin names which are now largely forgotten. Such a classification is of some help in deciding the cause of the cataract, although it may sometimes be misleading. Congenital cataracts are usually quite easily identified by their morphology, as also are some traumatic cataracts. When a unilateral cataract appears many years after a mild contusion injury, it may be difficult to distinguish this from an age related one.

Other Important Signs

Certain other important signs need to be carefully elicited in a patient with cataracts. The pupil reaction is a particularly useful index of retinal function and it is not impaired by the densest of cataracts. A poor reaction may lead one to suspect age related macular degeneration or chronic glaucoma, but a brisk pupil with a mature cataract might be described as a 'surgeon's delight' because it indicates the likelihood of restoring good vision to a blind eye. The function of the peripheral retina can be usefully assessed by performing the light projection test. This entails seating the patient in a darkened room, covering one eye, and asking him or her to indicate, by pointing, the source of light from a torch positioned at different points in the peripheral field. Checking the pupil and the light projection test take a brief moment to perform and are by far the most important tests of retinal function when the retina cannot be seen directly. A number of other more sophisticated tests are available; ultrasonography, electroretinography and measurement of the visually evoked potential to mention some. Sometimes at least an area of the peripheral retina may be seen when the pupils have been dilated, and all cataract patients should be examined in this way before one embarks on more complex tests. A search for the signs of cataract thus involves a full routine eye examination including a measurement of the best spectacle correction.

Fig. 11.3 A typical plastic intraocular implant. There are different designs to suit different surgical techniques

Management

At the present time there is no effective medical treatment for cataract in spite of a number of claims over the years. Some reports have suggested that oral aspirin may delay the progress of cataract in female diabetics. Although this might be expected to have some effect on theoretical grounds any benefit is probably marginal. Occasionally patients claim that their cataracts seem to have cleared, but such fluctuation in density of the lens opacities has not been demonstrated in a scientific manner. Cataracts associated with galactosaemia are thought to clear under the influence of prompt treatment of the underlying problem. More recent animal studies have shown that lanosterol reverses protein aggregation in cataracts with some increase in transparency of the lens, however at this stage no human studies are available.

Cataract is therefore essentially a surgical problem, and the management of a patient with cataract depends on deciding at what point the visual impairment of the patient justifies undergoing the risks of surgery. The cataract operation itself has been practised since pre-Christian times, and developments in recent years have made it safe and effective in a large proportion of cases. The operation entails removal of all the opaque lens fibres from within the lens capsule and replacing them with a clear plastic lens (Fig. 11.3).

In the early part of the last century the technical side of cataract surgery necessitated waiting for the cataract to become 'ripe'. Nowadays no such waiting is needed and it is theoretically possible to remove a clear lens. The decision to operate is based on whether the patient will see better afterwards. Modern cataract surgery can restore the vision in a remarkable way and patients often say that they have not seen so well for many years. Indeed many patients have quite reasonable vision without glasses but this cannot be guaranteed even with extended depth of focus or multifocal implants. Glasses may be necessary for some distances. Probably the worst thing that can happen after the operation is infection leading to endophthalmitis and loss of the sight of the eye. Although this only occurs in about one out of two thousand cases the patient contemplating cataract surgery needs to be aware of the possibility. Before the operation, it is essential to measure the length of the

Fig. 11.4 Instrument for measuring length of eye and curvature of cornea

eye and the corneal curvature (Fig. 11.4). Knowing these two measurements, one can assess the strength of lens implant that is needed. When deciding on the strength of implant it is necessary to consider the other eye. The aim is usually to, make the two eyes optically similar because patients find it difficult to tolerate two different eyes.

When to Operate

Even though the decision to operate on a cataract must be made by the ophthalmic surgeon, optometrists and the non specialist general practitioner need to understand the reasoning behind this decision. Elderly patients tend to forget what they have been told in the clinic and may not, for example, understand why cataract surgery is being delayed when macular degeneration is the main cause of visual loss. An operation is usually not required if the patient has not noticed any problem although sometimes the patient may deny the problem through some unexpressed fear. The requirements of the patient need to be considered; those of the chairbound arthritic 80 year old who can still read small print quite easily are different from the younger business person who needs to be able to see a car number plate at

20.5 m in order to drive. The visual acuity by itself is not always a reliable guide. Some patients who have marked glare may need surgery with a visual acuity of 6/9 whereas others with less visual demands may be quite happy with a vision of 6/12 or 6/18. Early surgery may be needed to keep a joiner or bus driver at work for which good binocular vision is needed.

Age of the Patient

By itself, the age of the patient need have little influence on the decision to operate. Many people over the age of 100 years have had their cataracts successfully removed. The general health of the patient must be taken into account and this may influence ones decision in unexpected ways. Occasionally one is presented with a patient who has difficulty with balancing perhaps as a result of Meniere's disease or some other cause. The patient asks for cataract surgery in the hope that this will cure the problem. Unless the cataracts are advanced the result may be disappointing. Sometimes cataract surgery is requested in a nearly blind demented patient on the grounds that the dementia will improve with improvement of the vision. Although this occasionally happens, often the patient's mental state is made worse even though the sight is better. This raises some interesting ethical problems for the surgeon and relatives.

In the case of the child with congenital cataracts, the indications for surgery depend largely on the degree of opacification of the lens. An incomplete cataract may permit a visual acuity of 6/12 or 6/18 and yet the child may be able to read small print by exercising the large amount of available focusing power. Such a child could undergo normal schooling, and cataract surgery may never be required. A complete cataract in both eyes demands early surgery and this may be undertaken during the first few months of life. There is a high risk that one eye may become amblyopic in these young patients, even after cataract surgery.

Traumatic Cataract

This is usually a unilateral problem in a younger patient and sometimes the nature of the damage to the eye prevents the insertion of an intraocular lens. The patient may be left with no lens in the eye, a situation known as aphakia. Vision can be restored by a very strong convex spectacle lens but the difference between the two eyes makes it impossible to wear glasses. This is partly because everything looks much bigger with the corrected aphakic eye; the image on the retina is abnormally large. By wearing a contact lens on the cornea the optical problems may be solved but it is an unfortunate fact that patients with traumatic cataracts usually have working conditions which are unsuited to the wearing of a contact lens. The problem of aphakia may also be solved by means of an artificial lens implant but only there is sufficient supporting tissue.

The Cataract Operation

Every medical student should witness at least one cataract operation during the period of training. It is an example of a classical procedure, which has been practised for 3000 years. The earliest method for dealing with cataract was known as couching. This entailed pushing the lens back into the vitreous where it was allowed to sink back into the fundus of the eye. Although this undoubtedly proved a simple and satisfactory procedure in some instances there is a tendency for the lens to set up a vigorous inflammatory reaction within the eye and subsequent loss of sight.

Modern cataract surgery was founded by the French surgeon Jacques Daviel in the eighteenth century. The operation that he devised involved seating the patient in a chair and making an incision around the lower half of the cornea. The lens was then removed through the opening. The results claimed were remarkable considering the technical difficulties that he must have encountered. Subsequently the procedure was facilitated by lying the patient down and making the incision around the upper part of the cornea where, in the postoperative period, it was protected by the upper eyelid. The use of local anaesthesia was introduced at the end of the nineteenth century and at the same time attempts were made to suture the cornea back into position. By the beginning of the twentieth century two methods had evolved for the actual removal of the lens. The safest way was to incise the anterior lens capsule and then wash out or express the opaque nucleus, preserving the posterior lens capsule as a protective wall against the bulging vitreous face. This is known as the extracapsular technique. The intracapsular cataract extraction became the standard operation of choice in most patients over the age of 50 years during the early part of the twentieth century. It involved removing the complete lens within its capsule and by this means avoided subsequent operations to open up residual opaque posterior capsule.

Perhaps the most dramatic change in cataract surgery has occurred in the latter half of the last century with the introduction of intraocular acrylic lens implants. Initially they were mostly employed with intracapsular surgery but a new technique for extracapsular surgery was then developed and found to be very successful with implants. Many different types and designs of intraocular lens have been used over the years. The illustration shows a commonly used type of lens implant (Fig. 11.3). The trend is now towards smaller incision surgery and the use of injectable implants, which unfold into position as they are being inserted into the eye. An important and universal technique in the UK is phaco-emulsification. Here the opaque lens nucleus is removed through a complex cannula, which breaks up the lens matter ultrasonically before sucking it from the eye (Figs. 11.5, 11.6 and 11.7). Additionally, femtosecond laser cataract surgery helps to speed up parts of surgery (such as lens fragmentation). This type of laser can also be used to perform the initial incisions into the cornea and the lens capsule.

Fig. 11.5 Type of probe used for phakoextraction of the opaque lens nucleus

Fig. 11.6 Injection of intraocular lens implant through small incision

Fig. 11.7 Intraocular lens implant within capsular bag

Time Spent in Hospital

Most cataract operations are now done under local anaesthesia as day cases. General anaesthesia is an option for younger patients or where there is a risk of the patient moving during the procedure, for example when the patient has a movement disorder or advanced dementia. An overnight stay is occasionally needed after a general anaesthetic. The elderly patient living alone with no relatives is also usually kept overnight in hospital but the trend is towards more and more day case work, dictated partly by economic reasons but also by safer surgery. Although surgery itself generally takes less than 15–20 min, typically patients having surgery will be in hospital for 2–3 h.

Convalescence

It is a fair generalisation to say that an eye requires about 4–6 weeks for full healing to take place following a cataract operation. On the other hand, most of the healing takes place in the first 2 weeks. It is usual for patients to return to work after 2 weeks; a prescription for glasses is usually issued beyond 3 weeks once the refraction becomes more stable. The visual recovery is undoubtedly quicker with smaller incision surgery (compared to when a larger incision is required) and with smaller wounds the ultimate visual result is typically improved with less chance of astigmatism. Hospitals invariably provide a 'hand out' of do's and don'ts for patients, detailing also how to put in eye drops, and with information about follow up arrangements (typically with an optometrist, rather than in the hospital). The important thing is for the patient to avoid rubbing the eye and to seek immediate medical advice if the eye becomes painful, because this may indicate infection which requires immediate treatment to prevent blindness. Following routine cataract surgery, it is usual to instil antibiotic drops combined with a steroid (often combined together in one bottle) four times daily for 3–4 weeks.

Infection is the rare but dreaded complication and this is usually heralded by pain, redness, discharge and deterioration of vision. The infection may be acquired from the patient's own commensal eyelid flora, or from contamination at the time of surgery. The commonest types of bacterial infection are streptococcal and staphylococcal species.

About 10–20% of patients develop opacification of the posterior lens capsule behind the implant after months or years. This is very simply cured by making an opening in the capsule with a special type of laser. This is a day case procedure, which requires only topical (eye drop) anaesthetic and takes 2 or 3 min. Rarely, when corneal sutures have been used these may sometimes need to be removed and this can also be done on a 'while you wait' basis in the outpatient department.

Figure 11.8 is a final reminder of the signs and symptoms of cataract. An elderly woman would not normally be able to read small print without glasses and this lady's eyes must be abnormal. She may have inherited myopia allowing her to see near objects without the need for a presbyopic lens, but the myopia may also be index myopia, which in turn may be due to early cataract formation. Another cause of index myopia could be uncontrolled diabetes.

Summary

At primary care level it is important to be able to diagnose cataract but also to understand the benefits and risks of cataract surgery in order to be able to give the patient advice as to when the cataract is bad enough to need an operation. An understanding of the meaning of aphakia and the optical consequences of an implant are also useful. Most patients who present with cataracts are diagnosed as having age related cataracts and investigations as to the cause are limited to tests to exclude diabetes and to confirm that the patient is fit for surgery. An understanding of the symptoms of cataract is helped by understanding the meaning of index myopia.

After reading this chapter you should be able to answer the following:

1. What are the commonest causes of cataract?
2. What are the symptoms of cataract?
3. What are the signs of cataract?
4. When is the best time to proceed with cataract surgery?
5. What are the main post-operative complications of cataract surgery?

Fig. 11.8 An elderly person cannot read without glasses unless he or she is myopic. Myopia in the elderly can be caused by cataract ("Rembrandt's mother", with acknowledgement to Rijksmuseum-Stichting)

Glaucoma

12

Abstract

In this chapter the basic physiology and measurement of eye pressure is discussed, and the various causes of glaucoma are described. The causes and treatments of the different types are then discussed in further detail.

The word 'glaucoma' refers to the apparent grey-green colour of the eye suffering from an attack of acute narrow angle glaucoma. Nowadays the term has come to include a group of eye diseases characterised by raised intraocular pressure. These diseases are quite distinct and the treatment in each case quite different. Glaucoma might be defined as a 'pathological level of intraocular pressure sufficient enough to damage vision'. This is to distinguish the normal elevation of intraocular pressure seen in otherwise normal individuals. Here we consider what is meant by the 'normal intraocular pressure'.

Normal Intraocular Pressure

Measurement of the intraocular pressure in a large number of normal subjects reveals a normal distribution extending from pressures of 10–12 mmHg to pressures of 25–28 mmHg. The pattern of distribution fits a Gaussian curve, so that the majority of subjects have a pressure of about 16 mmHg. For clinical purposes it is necessary to set an arbitrary upper limit of normal. By and large, the eye can stand very low pressures remarkably well, but when the pressure is abnormally high, the circulation of blood through the eye becomes jeopardised and serious damage may ensue. For clinical purposes, an upper level of 21 mmHg is often accepted. Above this level, suspicions are raised and further investigations undertaken.

Maintenance of Intraocular Pressure

If the eye is to function as an effective optical instrument, it is clear that the intraocular pressure must be maintained at a constant level. At the same time, an active circulation of fluid through the globe is essential if the structures within it are to receive adequate nourishment. The cornea and sclera form a tough fibrous and unyielding envelope and within this an even pressure is maintained by a balance between the production and drainage of aqueous fluid.

Aqueous is produced by the ciliary epithelium by active secretion and ultrafiltration. A continuous flow is maintained through the pupil, whence it reaches the angle of the anterior chamber.

On reaching the angle of the anterior chamber, aqueous passes through a grill known as the trabecular meshwork and then reaches a circular canal embedded in the sclera known as Schlemm's canal. This canal runs as a ring around the limbus (corneoscleral junction) and from it minute channels radiate outwards through the sclera to reach the episcleral circulation. These channels are known as aqueous veins and they transmit clear aqueous to the episcleral veins, which lie in the connective tissue underlying the conjunctiva. In actual fact, the proof of the route of drainage of aqueous can be verified by any medical student—it simply entails examining the white of the eye around the cornea with extreme care, using the high power of the slit-lamp microscope. After a time one can sometimes detect that some of the deeper veins convey parallel halves of blood and aqueous in the region beyond the junction of aqueous and episcleral vein.

The relative parts played by ciliary epithelium and trabecular meshwork in maintaining what is a remarkably constant intraocular pressure throughout life is not fully understood. It would appear that the production of aqueous is an active secretion whereas the drainage is more passive, although changing the tone of the ciliary muscle can alter the rate of drainage. In normal subjects the intraocular pressure does not differ in the two eyes by more than about 3 mmHg. Wider differences may lead one to suspect early glaucoma, especially if there is a family history of the disease. The normal intraocular pressure undergoes a diurnal variation, being highest in the early morning and gradually falling during the first half of the day. This diurnal change may become exaggerated as the first sign of glaucoma.

Measurement of Intraocular Pressure

The gold standard method of intraocular pressure measurement is Goldmann applanation tonometry. The Goldmann tonometer is supplied as an accessory to the slit-lamp microscope. The principle of applanation is as follows: when two balloons are pushed together so that the interface is a flat surface, then the pressure within the two balloons must be equal. By the same argument, when a fixed flat surface is pressed against a spherical surface such as the cornea, then at the

point at which the spherical surface is exactly flattened the intraocular pressure is equal to the pressure being applied. The applanation head is a small Perspex rod with a flattened end, which is fitted to a moveable arm. The tension applied to the moveable arm can be measured directly from a dial on the side of the instrument. The observer looks through the rod using the microscope of the slit lamp, and the point at which exact flattening occurs can thus be gauged. For applanation tonometry, the patient is seated at the slit lamp and not lying down but it is still necessary to instill a drop of local anaesthetic beforehand. Because the measurement of the intraocular pressure is such a basic requirement in any eye clinic, attempts have been made to introduce even more rapid and efficient devices. Perhaps the most ingenious to date is the tonometer which measures the indentation of the cornea in response to a puff of air by a photoelectric method. This air puff tonometer is less accurate than applanation, but it is useful for screening, although abnormal results should be confirmed by Goldmann tonometry.

Clinical Types of Glaucoma

It has been mentioned above that the word 'glaucoma' refers to a group of diseases. For clinical purposes these may be subdivided into five types:

1. Primary open angle glaucoma (POAG)
2. Normal pressure glaucoma
3. Acute angle closure glaucoma
4. Secondary glaucoma
5. Congenital glaucoma

Primary Open Angle Glaucoma

The first important point to note about this disease is that it is very common, occurring in about 5% of the population over the age of 65 years. The second point is that the disease is inherited, and whereas the practice of screening the whole population for the disease is problematic in terms of finance, it is well worth screening the families of patients with the disease if those over the age of 40 are selected. This leads to the third point, which is that the incidence increases with age, being very rare under the age of 40. This insidious, potentially blinding disease affects those who are least likely to notice its onset, and elderly patients with advanced chronic open angle glaucoma are still seen from time to time in eye clinics.

Primary open angle glaucoma occurs more commonly in high myopes and diabetics; patients with Fuchs' corneal endothelial dystrophy and retinitis pigmentosa also have a higher incidence. Glaucoma is commoner in different racial groups. For example, individuals of African descent, especially those from West Africa and the Caribbean, carry a significantly greater risk of glaucoma.

Pathogenesis and Natural History

Histologically there are remarkably few changes to account for the raised intraocular pressure, at least in the early stages of the disease. Subsequently, degenerative changes have been described in the juxta-canalicular trabecular meshwork, with endothelial thickening and oedema in the lining of Schlemm's canal. It has been shown that in the majority of cases the problem is one of inadequate drainage rather than excessive secretion of aqueous. In the untreated patient the chronically raised pressure leads to progressive damage to the eye and eventual blindness. The rate of progress of the disease varies greatly from individual to individual. It is possible for gross visual loss to occur within months, but the process may take 5 years. Younger eyes survive a raised pressure rather better than older eyes, which may already have circulatory problems. Very few eyes can withstand a pressure of 50 mmHg for more than a week or 2 or a pressure of 35 mmHg for more than a few months.

Primary open angle glaucoma is nearly always bilateral, but often the disease begins in one eye, the other eye not becoming involved immediately. It is important to realise that the progress of chronic glaucoma can be arrested by treatment, but unfortunately many ophthalmologists experience the natural history of the disease by seeing neglected cases.

Symptoms

Most patients with chronic glaucoma have no symptoms. That is to say, the disease is insidious and is only detected at a routine eye examination either by an optometrist or ophthalmologist before the patient notices any visual loss. Occasionally younger patients notice a defect in their visual field but this is unusual. Unfortunately, the peripheral loss of visual field my pass unnoticed until it has reached an advanced stage.

Signs

The three cardinal signs are:

1. Raised intraocular pressure
2. Cupping of the optic disc
3. Visual field loss

Without treatment, the intraocular pressure creeps up gradually to 30–35 mmHg, and it is this gradual rise which accounts for the lack of symptoms. Such a rise in intraocular pressure impairs the circulation of the optic disc, and the nerve fibres in this region become ischaemic. The combined effect of raised intraocular pressure and atrophy of nerve fibres results in gradual excavation of the physiological cup, and it is extremely useful to be able to identify this effect of raised intraocular pressure at an early stage (Fig. 12.1) shows an optic disc undergoing various stages of pathological cupping. In the first instance the central physiological cup becomes enlarged, with its long axis arranged vertically. Notching of the neuroretinal rim of the optic disc tissue especially in the inferotemoral and superotemporal region is common. The edge of the optic disc cup corresponds to the bend in the blood vessels as they cross the disc surface. In some eyes the area of pallor may correspond to the cup whilst in others the cup is larger than the area of pallor. It is particularly useful to observe the way in which the vessels enter and leave the nerve head (Fig. 12.2). A flame shaped haemorrhage at the disc margin may be seen. Localised loss of retinal nerve fibres may be observed especially with a red free light. Diagnostic instrumentation such as Ocular Coherence Tomography (OCT) scanning is capable of measuring the thickness of the retinal nerve fibre layer in microns, and offers an adjunctive objective measure for diagnosing and monitoring glaucoma (Fig. 12.3).

The changes in the visual field can be deduced from observing the disc and from considering the arrangement of the nerve fibres in the eye. If we gaze fixedly with one eye at a spot on the wall and then move a small piece of paper on the end of a paper clip, or even the end of our index finger, in such a manner as to explore our peripheral field, it is soon possible to locate the blind spot. In the case of the right eye, this is found slightly to the right of the point of fixation because it represents the projected position of the optic nerve head in the right eye. The blind spot is rounded and about 8°–12° lateral to and slightly below the level of fixation. It has already been mentioned that the glaucomatous disc is initially excavated above and below so that the patient with early glaucoma has a blank area in the visual field extending in an arcuate manner from the blind spot above and below fixation. This typical pattern of field loss is known as the arcuate scotoma (Fig. 12.4). If the glaucoma remains uncontrolled, this scotoma extends peripherally and centrally. It can be seen that even at this stage the central part of the field may be well preserved and the patient may still be able to read the smallest letters on the Snellen test chart. If the field loss is allowed to progress further, the patient develops severe visual impairment.

Treatment

Prostaglandin analogue medications are now the mainstay of treatment in most types of glaucoma. These are often effective enough when used in isolation, but can if necessary be combined with Betablockers (e.g. timolol) or other medications such as alpha agonists (e.g. brimonidine) or carbonic anhydrase inhibitors (e.g. brinzolamide). Tolerability to these medications varies and sometimes is affected by the preservatives in eye drop bottles. Preservatives e.g. benzalkonium chloride can cause dry eye symptoms, however if

Fig. 12.1 The effect of glaucoma on the optic disc

Fig. 12.2 (**a**) Glaucomatous cupping of the disc early cupping; (**b**) advanced cupping

Fig. 12.3 OCT nerve fibre layer scans from a left eye. (**a**) 3D topographical map of the optic nerve head. (**b**) 3D map of optic nerve (red pixels indicate nerve fibre layer loss)

this becomes problematic then preservative-free formulations are available.

Another medication less commonly used nowadays is pilocarpine. Pilocarpine is very effective in reducing intraocular pressure, however after about half an hour from the moment of instillation, the pupil becomes small and the patient experiences dimming of the vision, aching over the eyebrow and a spasm of accommodation which blurs the distance vision. After about 4 h the intraocular pressure begins to rise again and the side effects wear off. This, of course, means that a further drop of pilocarpine must be instilled if good control is to be continued. It is here that we find the most difficult problem of treatment. Human nature is such that drops are rarely instilled four times daily on a regular basis, although patients are genuinely anxious to preserve their eyesight. Poor compliance with glaucoma medication is a major problem when medications are taken more than once daily, and is a relatively common reason for disease progression.

Timolol and other betablockers are effective over a 12 h period and are most often instilled twice daily. As an ocular hypotensive agent these are probably not quite as effective as pilocarpine, but many cases of chronic glaucoma are now satisfactorily controlled by them and furthermore the drug may be used in combination with pilocarpine. Betablockers have the further advantage that they do not cause any miosis. The main side

Fig. 12.4 Superior arcuate visual field defect, right eye

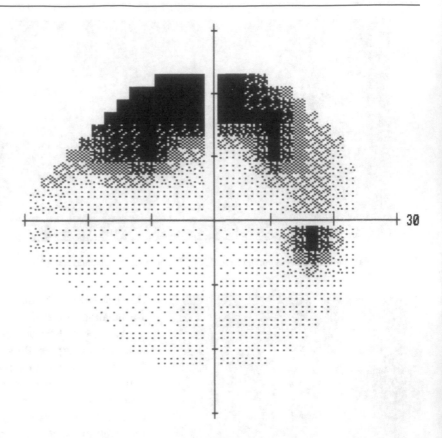

effects of betablockers are bronchospasm, reduced cardiac contractility and bradycardia. They are therefore contraindicated in patients with chronic obstructive airway disease, heart block, hypotension and bradycardia.

The cholinergic drugs such as pilocarpine act by increasing the rate of outflow of aqueous, whereas timolol is thought to inhibit the production of aqueous. Adrenaline drops also have the effect of reducing aqueous production and they were in use for some years as a supplement to pilocarpine. However, their limited effectiveness and the numerous side-effects (chronic dilatation of the conjunctival vessels, deposition of pigment in the conjunctiva and subconjunctival fibrosis) has curtailed their use nowadays.

Oral acetazolamide is only occasionally used in chronic glaucoma because of its long-term side effects. Acetazolomide (e.g. Diamox) is a carbonic anhydrase inhibitor, which was introduced many years ago as a diuretic. Its diuretic action is not very well sustained, but it is a potent drug for reducing intraocular pressure. If a normal subject takes a 250–500 mg tablet of the drug, the eye becomes soft after about an hour. Most patients taking Acetazolomide experience paraesthesiae of the hands and feet and some complain of gastric symptoms. Occasionally patients become lethargic or even confused. Young patients, particularly young males, may suffer renal colic. It should be pointed out that these more serious side-effects are rare, and long-term acetazolamide is still sometimes used when no other means of controlling the intraocular pressure is available.

More modern glaucoma medications include Latanoprost, Dorzolamide and Brimonidine. Latanoprost is a prostaglandin analogue, which produces its intraocular pressure lowering effect through increased uveoscleral outflow. The main side effects are slight conjunctival congestion (hyperaemia) and increased iris pigmentation in some patients with mixed coloured irides. Prostaglandin analogues are licenced as first-line

Table 12.1 Topical glaucoma medication

Drug type	Examples	Mechanism of action
Prostglandins	Latanoprost	Increased uveo-scleral outflow
	Travoprost	
	Bimatoprost (prostaglandin-2-a)	
β-Blockers	Timolol	Reduce aqueous production
	Betaxolol	
	Levubunolol	
	Carteolol	
Cholinergics	Parasympathomimetics: Pilocarpine	Increase aqueous outflow through trabecular meshwork
Adrenergic agonists	Adrenaline and prodrug (Dipivefrine)	Decrease aqueous production and increase uveo-scleral outflow
α2-agonist	Brimonidine, apraclonidine	Reduce aqueous production
Carbonic anhydrase inhibitors	Dorzolamide	Reduce aqueous production
	Brinzolamide	

medication for glaucoma and have superceded Betablockers in effectiveness and tolerability. Other prostaglandin-related medications include Bimatoprost (Lumigan) and Travaprost (Travatan) which have similar mechanisms of action to Latanoprost.

Dorzolamide (Trusopt) and Brinzolamide (Azopt) are topically administered carbonic anhydrase inhibitors. Their pressure lowering effect is inferior to that of Timolol, but they are useful adjunctive medications.

Brimonidine (Alphagan) is an alpha-2 adrenergic agonist, which decreases aqueous production and also increases the uveoscleral outflow. It has a pressure lowering effect comparable to that of Timolol. It has the advantage of not having any effect on the respiratory system. It can therefore be used in patients with obstructive airway disease (Table 12.1).

If the intraocular pressure remains uncontrolled by safe medical treatment and there is evidence of continued loss of visual field, then surgical treatment is indicated. A large number of operations have been devised for the management of primary open angle glaucoma and most of these entail allowing the aqueous to drain subconjunctivally through an artificial opening made in the sclera. One of the commonest operations performed currently is known as a "trabeculectomy". In this operation a superficial 'trapdoor' of sclera is raised and the deeper layer, including the trabecular mesh-

Fig. 12.5 Trabeculectomy bleb

work, is removed. The trapdoor is then sutured back into position. Aqueous drains out around the edge of this scleral flap into the subconjunctiva (Fig. 12.5). Although most of these operations may reduce the intraocular pressure very effectively and often for many years, they all tend to increase the rate of formation of cataract. This and the risk of postoperative endophthalmitis are the main reasons why surgery is usually not considered the first line of treatment in chronic open angle glaucoma by most ophthalmologists. Often such surgery is augmented by the use of anti-fibrotic agents per-operatively, such as mitomycin C or 5-fluorouracil. These agents inhibit fibroblast activity, and increase the success rate of surgery, but carry potential side-effect and need to be used cautiously. Newer, less invasive surgeries known as

MIGS (micro-invasive glaucoma surgery) hold great promise in simplifying surgery, and these include various types of miniature tubes/stents. Variants of trabeculectomy avoid a full thickness cut into the eye however are more time-consuming to perform. Additionally, selective laser trabeculoplasty (SLT) is a less invasive laser procedure that is effective in many patients with open angle glaucoma, and in view of its safety is often a preferred option for patients, ahead of any more formal surgical procedure. SLT is suitable for use first line for many patients and is known to be a cost-effective option by delaying the need for more complex, riskier surgery.

In some patients laser treatment known as 'cyclodiode' is applied externally to the eye to lower intraocular pressure by ablating part of the ciliary body (this area produces the aqueous humour). Such treatment however is irreversible, and although easier to perform than conventional glaucoma surgery, is mostly reserved for patients with advanced uncontrolled glaucoma. A gentler version of this treatment known as "ECP laser" can be performed at the time of cataract surgery, endoscopically, without the same risk of hypotony (eye pressure that is too low) that occurs after standard diode laser.

Normal Pressure Glaucoma (NPG)

This condition is similar to POAG except that the intraocular pressure is within normal limits i.e. 21 mmHg or less at the initial and subsequent visits. The condition is probably due to low perfusion pressure at the optic nerve head so that the nerve head is susceptible to damage at normal intraocular pressure. Patients with NPG may often have associated cardiovascular disease such as hypertension.

Certain conditions that may mimic NPG include compressive lesions of the optic nerve and chiasma, carotid ischaemia and congenital optic disc anomalies.

Treatment of NPG aims to reduce intraocular pressure to 12 mmHg or less.

Management

Most eye units now run special clinics for dealing with glaucoma patients. From what has been said, it should be clear that patients with glaucoma require much time and attention. Initially the nature of the disease must be explained and patients must realise that the treatment is to arrest the progress of the condition and not to cure it. Furthermore, any visual loss that occurs is irretrievable, so that regular follow-up visits are essential for checking the intraocular pressure and carefully assessing the visual fields.

The initial treatment is a single topical agent— usually a prostaglandin analogue. The second line treatments of choice are most often alpha agonists, or carbonic anhydrase inhibitors. Commonly, patients with glaucoma require several different medications to control intraocular pressure effectively.

Increasingly, monitoring units now use technical staff to assist in collecting the large about of data required to help inform decisions on treatment. A team approach is required however, with nursing staff and optometrists often working alongside hospital consultant-led teams. Additionally, many staff work in the community to 'refine referrals' and reduce the number of false-positive referrals to a specialist glaucoma clinic.

Acute Angle Closure Glaucoma

This condition is less common than chronic open angle glaucoma, comprising about 5% of all cases of primary glaucoma. It is a much more dramatic condition than the chronic disease and fits in more closely with the popular lay idea of 'glaucoma'. It tends to affect a slightly younger age group than chronic glaucoma and only occurs in predisposed individuals. There is a particular type of eye, which is liable to develop acute glaucoma: this is a small hypermetropic eye with a shallow anterior chamber. One rarely meets a myope with acute glaucoma in Caucasians (in Asian populations, however, angle-closure and myopia more often coexist).

Pathogenesis and Natural History

Eyes that are predisposed to develop closed angle glaucoma generally have a shallow anterior chamber and are very often hypermetropic. These characteristics may be heritable, and genome-wide association studies have identified a clear association with increased angle closure risk. In susceptible individuals, there is forward bowing of the iris and the corneal diameter may be slightly smaller than in normal eyes. Another factor is the gradual but slight increase in size of the lens, which takes place with ageing. Raised intra-ocular pressure in angle closure is due to occlusion of the angle by the iris root and it may be precipitated by dilating the pupil and causing "pupillary block". Medications such as topiramate can induce an ciliary effusion, pushing the lens and iris forward, therefore causing angle closure by a different mechanism. An uncontrolled acute attack of glaucoma can lead to rapid and permanent loss of the sight of the affected eye. Although it is known that occasionally patients recover spontaneously from such an attack, they may be left with chronic angle closure and a picture similar to that of chronic open angle glaucoma. About half the patients with closed angle glaucoma will develop a similar problem in the other eye if steps are not taken to prevent this, and prophylactic treatment for the other eye *at the initial visit* is now strongly recommended.

Symptoms

The subacute attack. Here it might be helpful to consider a typical patient, who might be a male or female, aged about 50. Such a patient would have a moderate degree of hypermetropia and rather a narrow gap between iris and cornea as shown by the shallow anterior chamber. During the autumn months, this patient's pupil might be noted to be slightly wider, as one might expect with the dimmer illumination and one evening the pupil dilates sufficiently to allow the iris root to nudge across the angle and obstruct the flow of aqueous. Immediately the intraocular pressure rises acutely, perhaps to 30 or 40 mmHg and pain is felt over the eye. At the same time the acute rise of pressure causes the cornea to become oedematous. Since it is evening, the patient observes that streetlights when viewed through the oedematous cornea appear to have coloured rings around them, as if they were being viewed through frosted glass. At this point the patient retires to bed and on sleeping the pupil becomes small and the intraocular pressure rise is relieved. After several of these attacks, the patient may seek attention from the family doctor. Patients present as healthy people with evening headaches associated with blurring of the vision and they are wearing moderately thick convex lenses in their spectacles. Subacute glaucoma is easily missed, partly because it is rare amongst the large number of sufferers from headache. If attention is not sought at this stage or if the diagnosis is missed, then one evening the acute attack develops.

The Acute Attack. After a number of subacute attacks an irreversible turn of events may occur. The iris root becomes congested, raising the intraocular pressure further and producing further congestion. The headache becomes much worse and the vision becomes seriously impaired. The doctor, who may be called in the following morning, is confronted with a patient who is nauseated and vomiting and at first sight an acute abdominal problem may be suspected until the painful red eye should make the diagnosis obvious. Sometimes acute glaucoma does not cause much pain or nausea and in these cases the physical signs in the eye become especially important (Fig. 12.6).

Fig. 12.6 Acute angle-closure glaucoma

Signs

The most obvious physical sign is the semi-dilated fixed pupil. The iris and the constricting sphincter muscle of the pupil are damaged by the raised intraocular pressure. The pupil is not able to constrict and after a day or two the iris becomes depigmented, taking on the grey atrophic colour, which gave glaucoma its name. Prompt and effective treatment should prevent any damage to the iris. The eye is red and a pink frill of engorged deeper capillaries is seen around the corneal margin; this important sign, as opposed to conjunctival inflammation is known as ciliary injection. Corneal oedema can usually be detected without optical aids by observing the lack of lustre in the eye and any attempts to assess the hardness of the eye by palpating it through the eyelids will elicit another sign, that of tenderness of the globe. The visual acuity may be reduced to 'hand movements' in a severe attack. There are two rather subtle signs that often persist permanently after the acute attack has been resolved. The first is the presence of a white irregular microscopic deposit just deep to the anterior surface of the lens, and the second is the presence of whorl atrophy in the iris. The pattern of the iris becomes twisted as if the sphincter has been rotated slightly. Both these signs may provide useful evidence of a previous attack, which has resolved spontaneously.

Measurement of the intraocular pressure at this point may reveal a reading of 70 mmHg or more. Very gentle palpation of the globe is usually enough to confirm that the eye has the consistency of a brick, especially when the pressures of the two eyes are compared. It should be realised that digital palpation of the globe can be very misleading and the method cannot be used to detect smaller rises in intraocular pressure with any degree of reliability (Table 12.2).

Table 12.2 Signs of acute glaucoma

1. Corneal oedema with resulting poor visual acuity
2. Shallow anterior chamber
3. Ciliary injection
4. Semi-dilated oval pupil (due to iris ischaemia)
5. Tenderness of globe
6. Hard eye

Examination of the other eye will reveal a shallow anterior chamber. Shining a focused beam of light obliquely through the cornea and noting the width of the gap between where the light strikes the cornea and where it strikes the iris can assess the depth of the anterior chamber. After inspecting a few normal eyes in this way, the observer can soon learn when an anterior chamber is abnormally shallow. This facility is important to anyone who intends to instill mydriatic drops into an eye A shallow anterior chamber does not contraindicate mydriatic drops but it does indicate the need for extreme caution and care that the pupil is afterwards restored to its normal size. The angle of the anterior chamber itself is not exposed to direct inspection and it can only be seen through a gonioscope (Fig. 12.7). This instrument is a contact lens with a mirror mounted on it and through it the width of the angle can be estimated. If the angle is open, the various structures adjacent to the iris root and inner surface of the peripheral cornea can be identified. Gonioscopy forms a routine part of the examination of any patient with glaucoma although in acute narrow angle glaucoma the presence of a closed angle can often be presumed by the presence of the other physical signs. Where there is any doubt, it may be necessary to apply a drop of hypertonic glycerol to the cornea to clear the oedema before applying the gonioscope.

The sooner closed angle glaucoma is diagnosed and treated then, the better are the results of treatment. Unfortunately, it is in the early sub-acute stage of the disease that the diagnosis may be difficult. A number of provocative tests have been devised for the patient who presents with suspicious symptoms but a normal intraocular pressure. The simplest test is the 'dark room test': The patient's intraocular pressure is measured before he or she is seated in a darkened room for half an hour. The intraocular pressure is again measured immediately after this, and a rise in pressure of more than 5 mmHg may be taken to be significant. Certain drugs can have a similar effect by having a mildly mydriatic action when taken by mouth. The phenothiazines have been incriminated in this respect. Of course, such

Fig. 12.7 Preparing for gonioscopy

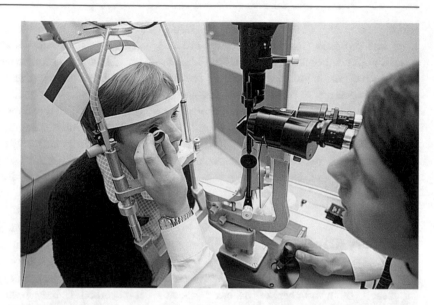

drugs will have no adverse effect on patients who have already been treated and identified as cases of narrow or closed angle glaucoma. Only in unsuspected cases of subacute narrow angle glaucoma is there a real risk of precipitating an acute attack.

Treatment

Acute narrow angle glaucoma may present as a surgical problem and any patient suffering from the condition requires urgent assessment in a hospital setting. To do less than this is to undertreat the condition and run the risk of developing uncontrolled chronic narrow angle glaucoma. On admission, the affected eye is treated with combination therapy including miotic drops. A typical regime would be the application of pilocarpine 2%, dorzolamide 2%/timolol 0.5%, and apraclonidine 0.5%. This treatment is supported by an injection of acetazolamide. If the renal function is unimpaired, acetazolamide may be given intravenously (250 mg) followed by an oral dose of 250 mg q.i.d. Additionally, reduction of inflammation and iris congestion with topical steroids may help achieve a quicker lowering of intraocular pressure. In many cases these measures relieve the acute attack within hours. However, some patients may require an intravenous infusion of mannitol. During this period the

patient is kept under closer nursing observation, and analgesics are given if required. It is important that the other eye is also treated with pilocarpine 2% q.i.d. in order to prevent a second disaster.

Once the intraocular pressure has been controlled, the cure is maintained by performing a peripheral iridotomy or iridectomy. This allows the bulging iris bombe to sink backwards like a punctured ship's sail and is a sure means of preventing further acute attacks. Usually, the fellow eye is at risk of a similar problem and is lasered at the same time. In some patients the angle of the anterior chamber remains partially occluded by peripheral adhesions from the iris. In these cases a simple peripheral iridectomy may not be adequate and it may be necessary to carry out a drainage operation such as a trabeculectomy. Most patients with acute narrow angle glaucoma are cured by surgery, although a small proportion develop significant cataract in later years. The prognosis in adequately treated narrow angle glaucoma is therefore very good, but in the absence of treatment the result is disastrous.

The treatment of narrow angle glaucoma has undergone a small revolution over the last few decades, with the advent of specific lasers; it is relatively simple now to create the small necessary iris aperture with just a few laser applications. The YAG (Yttrium-Aluminium-Garnet) laser has replaced surgical iridectomy in most cases. A special contact lens is used to focus the laser on the peripheral iris, and one or two full thickness openings in the peripheral iris are created. Following such laser treatment, topical steroids and pupil dilatation are given to minimize the effects of uveitis. Occasionally, trabeculectomy surgery is performed if intraocular pressures remain persistently high despite other treatments.

Secondary Glaucoma

The intraocular pressure may become raised as the result of a number of different disease processes in the eye quite apart from the causes of primary glaucoma, which have just been described.

Secondary to Vascular Disease in the Eye

Central Retinal Vein Occlusion This is a common cause of sudden blurring of the vision of one eye in the elderly. The retinal veins can be seen to be dilated and surrounded by haemorrhages. In some cases, recovery is marred by a rise in intraocular pressure, which typically appears approximately 3 months after the onset of the condition. The prompt appearance of this very painful complication has given it the name of 'hundred day glaucoma'. This type of glaucoma is usually difficult to control and even surgical measures may prove ineffective. A typical feature is the appearance of a vascular network over the anterior surface of the iris and sometimes in the angle of the anterior chamber. This vascularised tissue lends a pinkish hue to the iris and is termed rubeosis iridis. Patients with a central retinal vein occlusion followed by secondary glaucoma have another problem because there is a recognised association between chronic open angle glaucoma and central retinal vein occlusion. This means that some patients who present with an occluded vein may be found to have chronic glaucoma in the other eye.

Diabetes Patients with severe diabetic retinopathy may also develop rubeosis iridis and secondary glaucoma. The vascular occlusive features of diabetic eye disease give it many resemblances to central retinal vein occlusion and the secondary glaucoma which develops is also very resistant to medical treatment. Panretinal laser photocoagulation when applied early causes regression of the rubeosis. The ultimate outcome is sometimes a blind and painful eye, which has to be removed.

Secondary to Uveitis

During an attack of acute iridocyclitis the intraocular pressure is often below normal because the production of aqueous by the ciliary body is reduced. When the normal production of aqueous is resumed it may induce a rise in pressure because the outflow channels have been obstructed by inflammatory exudate. This type of secondary glaucoma responds to vigorous treatment of the iridocyclitis, and here it is essential to dilate and not constrict the pupil and to apply steroid treatment. Acetazolamide and topical beta-blockers for example Timolol and Betagan may also be required. The type of secondary glaucoma, which develops after the iridocyclitis of herpes zoster infections, can be particularly insidious. The intraocular pressure may remain high without obvious pain and with relatively slight inflammatory changes in the eye. Secondary glaucoma usually responds well to treatment and once the underlying inflammation has subsided the eye returns to normal.

In iridocyclitis glaucoma may also be due to pupil block (inability of aqueous to pass from the posterior to anterior chamber) because of posterior synechiae (adhesions between the iris and lens). Treatment is YAG laser iridotomy.

Secondary to Tumours

Malignant melanoma of the choroid and retinoblastoma may cause glaucoma. The raised intraocular pressure can be an important diagnostic feature when a suspected lesion is seen in the fundus. When a patient presents with a blind glaucomatous eye the possibility of malignancy must always be in the back of one's mind.

Secondary to Trauma

Trauma may precipitate a rise in intraocular pressure in a number of different ways. Sometimes, especially in children, bleeding may occur into the anterior chamber after a contusion injury. This can seriously obstruct the flow of aqueous both through the pupil and into the angle. Such an episode of bleeding may occur on the second or third day after the injury, turning a slight event into a very serious problem. On other occasions a contusion injury may cause splitting or recession of the angle which is associated with glaucoma. The iridocyclitis, which follows perforating injuries, tends to be complicated by glaucoma and the ophthalmologist must be constantly aware of such a complication.

Drug-Induced Glaucoma

Local and systemic steroids can cause a rise in intraocular pressure and this is more likely to occur in patients with a family history of glaucoma. Steroid-induced glaucoma is a well recognised phenomenon and 'steroid responders' can be identified by measuring the intraocular pressure before and after instilling a drop of steroid. The less potent steroids, hydrocortisone and prednisolone, are less likely to cause this problem and other steroids have been manufactured which have less effect on intraocular pressure, but the anti-inflammatory strength is significantly weaker. The use of systemic steroids may be associated with glaucoma: and asthmatics who use steroid inhalers very frequently are at a significantly greater risk of developing glaucoma.

The possibility of inducing an attack of acute glaucoma by drugs has already been mentioned.

Secondary to Abnormalities in the Lens

A cataractous lens may become hypermature and swell up, pushing the iris diaphragm forwards and obstructing the angle of the anterior chamber. This is referred to as phacomorphic glaucoma. Removing the lens relieves the situation. Phacolytic glaucoma occurs when a mature cataract causes a type of uveitis. This is thought to result from leakage of lens proteins through the lens capsule. A dislocated or subluxated lens, either the result of trauma or as a congenital abnormality, can be associated with a rise in intraocular pressure.

Congenital or Developmental Glaucoma

These glaucomas occur in eyes in which an anomaly present at birth produces an intraocular pressure rise.

This type of glaucoma is extremely rare and it is often, though not always, inherited. This means that the affected child may be brought to the ophthalmologist by the parents because they are aware of the condition in the family. Children may be born with raised intraocular pressure and for these cases the prognosis is not so good as in those where the pressure rise does not occur until after the first few months of life.

In primary developmental glaucoma the glaucoma is due to defective development of the angle of the anterior chamber, and gonioscopy shows that the normal features of the angle are obscured by a pinkish membrane. Raised intraocular pressure in infancy has a dramatic effect because it causes enlargement of the globe. This can best be observed by noting an increase in the corneal diameter. The enlarged eye has given the condition the name of buphthalmos or 'bull's eye' (Fig. 12.8). Other important signs are photophobia and corneal oedema. The diagnosis is confirmed by an examination under anaesthesia, which includes measuring the corneal diameters

Fig. 12.8 Congenital glaucoma: note the enlarged left cornea (With acknowledgement to Mr R. Gregson)

and the intraocular pressure. Surgical treatment is nearly always required and this involves passing a fine knife through the peripheral cornea so that the point reaches the opposite angle of the anterior chamber. Once in the angle, it is moved gently to and fro to open up the embryonic tissue which covers the trabecular meshwork (goniotomy). The other (or secondary) developmental glaucomas include the rubella syndrome, Aniridia, mesodermal dysgenesis, Peter's anomaly and the phacomatoses where the intraocular pressure rise is associated with other ocular and systemic developmental anomalies.

After reading this chapter you should be able to answer the following:

1. Compile a list of the different types of glaucoma.
2. List several examples of secondary glaucoma.
3. What are the symptoms of acute angle closure?
4. What are the treatments for angle closure episodes?
5. What are the signs of congenital glaucoma?
6. Which drugs can cause glaucoma?

Retinal Detachment

13

Abstract

Detachment of the retina signifies an inward separation of the sensory part of the retina from the retinal pigment epithelium (RPE). There is an accumulation of fluid in the space between the neural retina and the retinal pigment epithelium known as subretinal fluid (Fig. 13.1). The retina bulges inwards like the collapsed bladder of a football. Once detached, the retina can no longer function and in humans it tends to remain detached, unless treatment is available.

Fig. 13.1 Histology of retinal detachment showing the location of subretinal fluid. This eye has an underlying choroidal melanoma

Although the condition is relatively rare in the general population, it is important for several reasons. First it is a blinding condition which can be treated very effectively and often dramatically by surgery. Second, retinal detachment may on occasions be the first sign of malignant disease in the eye. Finally, nowadays the condition may often be prevented by prophylaxis in predisposed eyes.

Incidence

Retinal detachment is rare in the general population but an eye unit serving a population of 500,000 might expect to be looking after three or four cases a week. It can be seen, therefore, that a doctor in general practice might see a case once in every 2 or 3 years, especially if we consider that some retinal detachment patients go directly to eye casualty departments without seeking non-specialist advice. Although children are sometimes affected, the incidence increases with age and reaches a maximum in the 50–60 age group. There is a smaller peak in the mid-twenties to thirties due to traumatic detachments in young males.

Certain groups of people are especially liable to develop detachment of the retina: severely shortsighted patients have been shown to have an incidence as high as 3.5% and about 1% of patients who have had cataract surgery without the insertion of an implant (see the Chap. 11) have detachments.

In just under a quarter of cases, if there is no intervention, the other eye becomes affected at a later date. This means that the sound eye must be examined with great care in every instance.

Pathogenesis

There is an embryological explanation for retinal detachment in that the separating layers open up a potential space which existed during the early development of the eye as described previously (Chap. 2). The inner lining of the eye develops as two layers. In its earliest stages of development, the eye is seen as an outgrowth of the forebrain, the optic vesicle, the cavity of which is continuous with that of the forebrain. The vesicle becomes invaginated to form the optic cup, and the two-layered cup becomes the two layered lining of the adult eye. Anteriorly in the eye the two layers line the inner surface of the iris and ciliary body. Posterior to the ciliary body the outer of the two layers remains as a single layer of pigmented cells, known as the pigment epithelium. The inner of the two layers becomes many cells thick and develops into the sensory retina. In the adult the sensory retina is closely linked, both physically and metabolically, with the pigment epithelium and, in particular the production of visual pigment relies on this juxtaposition. When the retina becomes detached and the sensory retina is separated from the pigment epithelium, the retina can no longer function and the sight is lost in the detached area. Both pigment epithelium and sensory retina are included in the term 'retina' and in this sense 'retinal detachment' is a misnomer.

The retina receives its nourishment from two sources: the inner half deriving its blood supply from the central retinal artery, and the outer half from the choroid. The important foveal region is supplied mainly by the choroid. When the retina is detached, the central retinal artery remains intact and continues to supply it since it is also detached with it. The outer half of the retina is deprived of nourishment, being separated from pigment epithelium and choroid. Eventually degenerative changes appear, the fovea being affected at an early stage. It is interesting that after surgical replacement the retina regains much of its function during the first few days but further recovery may occur over as long a period as 1 or even 2 years.

Classification

Detachment of the retina can be classified as follows:

Rhegmatogenous Retinal Detachment

This is the most common form of retinal detachment, caused by the recruitment of fluid from the vitreous cavity to the subretinal space via a full-thickness discontinuity (a retinal 'break') in the sensory retina.

Retinal 'breaks' can be further subdivided into 'tears', which are secondary to dynamic vitreo-retinal traction, and 'holes', which are the result of focal retinal degeneration (see below).

Tractional Retinal Detachment

This form of retinal detachment develops as a result of tractional forces within the vitreous gel pulling on the retina, causing the retina to be tented up from the retinal pigment epithelium. The pure form of tractional retinal detachment is different from rhegmatogenous retinal detachment in that there are no retinal breaks. Examples of tractional retinal detachment include proliferative diabetic retinopathy, and vitreo-macular traction syndrome.

Exudative Retinal Detachment

This group of retinal detachments also occurs in the absence of retinal breaks. The fluid gains access to the subretinal space through an abnormal choroidal circulation, e.g. from a choroidal malignant melanoma (Fig. 13.1), or rarely secondary to inflammation of the retinal pigment epithelium or deeper layers of the eye (e.g. scleritis).

Rhegmatogenous Retinal Detachment

The Presence of Breaks in Retinal Detachment

It was noticed as long ago as 1853, only a short time after the invention of the ophthalmoscope, that many detached retinae have minute full-thickness discontinuities (breaks) in them, but it was not until the 1920s that the full significance of these breaks as the basic cause of the detachment became realised. The break may be single or multiple and are more commonly situated in the anterior or more peripheral part of the retina. In order to understand how these breaks occur, it is necessary to understand something of retinal degeneration and vitreous changes.

Retinal Degeneration

When examining the peripheral retina of otherwise normal subjects, it is surprising to find that from time to time there are quite striking degenerative changes. Perhaps this is not so surprising when one considers that the retinal arteries are end arteries and these changes occur in the peripheral parts of the retina supplied by the distal part of the circulation. Peripheral retinal degenerations are more commonly seen in myopic eyes, especially in association with Marfan's and Ehlers-Danlos Syndromes and Stickler's disease (see reading list).

Different types of degeneration have been described and named and certain types are recognized as being the precursors to retinal breaks formation. The most important degenerations are lattice degeneration and retinal tufts. Lattice degenerations consist of localized areas of thinning in the peripheral retina. Progressive thinning of the retina within areas of lattice degeneration can eventually lead to formation of retinal 'holes'.

In addition, both lattice degenerations and retinal tufts also represent areas with abnormally strong adhesions between the vitreous and the retina. The presence of exaggerated vitreoretinal adhesions can result in the formation of retinal 'tears' within areas of lattice degeneration and retinal tufts during posterior vitreous detachment (see below).

The Vitreous

The normal vitreous is a clear gel, which occupies most of the inside of the eye. Its consistency is similar to that of raw white of egg and, being a gel, it takes up water and salts. It is made up of a meshwork of collagen fibres whose interspaces are filled with molecules of hyaluronic acid. The vitreous is adherent to the retina at the ora serrata (junction of ciliary body and retina) and around the optic disc and macula. If we move our eyes, the vitreous moves, and, being restrained by its attachment, swings back to its original position again. The vitreous is usually perfectly transparent but most people become aware of small particles of cellular debris, which can be observed against a clear background such as a blue sky or an x-ray screen (vitreous floaters). These particles can be seen to move slowly with eye movement and appear to have momentum, just as one would expect if one considers the way the vitreous moves.

Posterior Vitreous Detachment

Vitreous floaters are commonplace and tend to increase in number as the years pass. But the vitreous undergoes a more dramatic change with age. Often in the late fifties, it becomes more fluid and collapses from above, separating from its normal position against the retina and eventually lying as a contracted mobile gel in the inferior and anterior part of the cavity of the globe. The rest of the globe is occupied by clear fluid. This then is the process known as posterior vitreous detachment (PVD).

When this happens the patient may complain of something floating in front of the vision and also the appearance of flashing lights. This is because the mobile shrunken vitreous sometimes causes slight traction on the retina. As a rule, the same symptoms are then experienced subsequently in the other eye. On the other hand, it is also very common to find a detached vitreous in an elderly person's eye in the absence of any symptoms.

Retinal Breaks Formation

In the majority of eyes the vitreous separates 'cleanly' from the retina during PVD. Such 'uncomplicated' PVD is common and is usually of no pathological significance. Unfortunately on rare occasions, the collapsing vitreous causes a retinal 'tear' to form at a point of abnormally strong adhesion between vitreous to retina, for example within an area of lattice degeneration or retinal tufts. There may even be an associated vitreous haemorrhage, when the PVD cause the avulsion of a peripheral retinal blood vessel.

Mechanism of Rhegmatogenous Retinal Detachment

Once a retinal tear forms as a result of abnormal vitreous traction following PVD, the fluid from within the vitreous cavity can gain access to the subretinal space through the retinal tear. The progressive accumulation of fluid in the subretinal space eventually causes the retina to separate from the underlying retinal pigment epithelium, similar to wallpaper being stripped off a wall. This inward separation of the retina from the retinal pigment epithelium through the recruitment of fluid via a retinal break is the basis for 'rheg-matogenous' retinal detachment, which is the most common form of retinal detachment.

Rhegmatogenous Retinal Detachment Associated with Trauma

Most rhegmatogenous retinal detachments occur as a result of spontaneous PVD-induced retinal breaks. However, retinal tears can also occur as a result of trauma. A perforating injury of the eye can produce a tear at any point in the retina, but contusion injuries commonly produce tears in the extreme retinal periphery and in the lower temporal quadrant or the superior nasal quadrant. This is because the lower temporal quadrant of the globe is most exposed to injury from a flying missile such as squash ball. The threatened eye makes an upward movement as the lids attempt to close. Tears of this kind often take the form of a dialysis, the retina being torn away in an arc from the ora serrata. Warning symptoms in these patients are usually masked by the symptoms of the original injury and they tend to present some months, or occasionally years, after the original injury with the symptoms of a retinal detachment. This is unfortunate because the tear can be treated if it is located before the detachment occurs.

Signs and Symptoms of Retinal Tear and Retinal Detachment

Let us now consider a typical patient, possibly a myope in the middle fifties either male or female, who suddenly experiences the symptoms of 'flashes and floaters', sometimes spontaneously or sometimes after making a sudden head movement. Proper interpretation of such symptoms can save sight and they will therefore be considered in more detail.

Flashes ('Photopsiae')

When questioned, the patient usually says that these are probably present all the time but are only noticeable in the dark. They seem to be especially apparent before going to sleep at night. The flashes are usually seen in the peripheral part of the visual field. They must be distinguished from the flashes seen in migraine, which are quite different and are usually followed by headache. The migrainous subject tends to see zigzag lines, which spread out from the centre of the field and last for about 10 m. Elderly patients with a defective vertebrobasilar circulation may describe another type of photopsia in which the flashing lights tend to occur only with neck movements or after bending.

Floaters

It has already been explained that black spots floating in front of the vision are commonplace but often called to our attention by anxious patients. When the spots are large and appear suddenly, they may be of pathological significance. For some reason patients often refer to them as tadpoles or frogspawn or even a spider's web. It is the combination of these symptoms with flashing lights that makes it important.

Flashes and floaters appear because the vitreous has tugged on the retina producing the sensation of light and often when the tear appears there is a slight bleeding into the vitreous, causing the black spots. When clear-cut symptoms of this kind appear, they must not be overlooked. The eyes must be examined fully until the tear in the retina is found. Sometimes a small tear in the retina is accompanied by a large vitreous haemorrhage and thus sudden loss of vision.

Shadow

Once a retinal tear has appeared, the patient may seek medical attention, and effective treatment of the tear may ensue. Unfortunately some patients do not seek attention, or, if they do, the symptoms may be disregarded. Indeed, in time the symptoms may become less, but after a variable period between days and years, a black shadow is seen encroaching from the peripheral field. This may appear to wobble. If the detachment is above, the shadow encroaches from below and it may seem to improve spontaneously with bedrest, being at first better in the morning. Loss of central vision or visual blurring occurs when the fovea is involved by the detachment, or the visual axis is obstructed by a bullous detachment. Inspection of the fundus at this stage shows that fluid seeps through the retinal break, raising up the surrounding retina like a blister in the paintwork of a car. A shallow detachment of the retina may be difficult to detect but the affected area tends to look slightly grey and, most importantly, the choroidal pattern can no longer be seen. The analogy is with a piece of wet tissue stuck against grained wood. If the tissue paper is raised slightly away from the wood, the grain is no longer visible. As the detachment increases, the affected area looks dark grey and corrugated and the retinal vessels look darker than in flat retina. The tear in the retina shines out red as one views the pigment epithelium and choroid through it.

Once a black shadow of this kind appears in front of the vision, the patient usually becomes alarmed and seeks immediate medical attention. Urgent admission to hospital and retina surgery are needed.

Traction Retinal Detachment

In tractional retinal detachment, the retina may be pulled away by the contraction of fibrous bands in the vitreous. Photopsia and floaters are usually absent but a slowly progressive visual field defect is noticeable. The detached retina is usually concave and immobile.

Advanced proliferative diabetic retinopathy may be complicated by tractional retinal detachment of the retina when a contracting band tents up the retina by direct traction. Not infrequently such a diabetic patient experiences further sudden loss of vision in the eye, when the traction exerted by the contracting vitreous pulls a hole in the area of tractional retinal detachment, resulting in a combined rhegmatogenous and tractional retinal detachment.

Exudative Retinal Detachment

In such detachments there are no photopsiae but floaters may occur from associated vitritis or vitreous haemorrhage. A visual field defect is usual. Exudative detachments are usually convex shaped and associated with shifting fluid.

A malignant melanoma of the choroid may present as a retinal detachment. Often the melanoma is evident as a black lump with an adjacent area of detached retina. If the retina is extensively detached over the tumour, the diagnosis may become difficult. It is important to avoid performing retinal surgery on such a case because of the risk of disseminating the tumour. Suspicion should be raised by a balloon detachment without any visible tears, and the diagnosis may be confirmed by transilluminating the eye to reveal the tumour.

Retinal detachments secondary to inflammatory exudates are not common. One example is Harada's disease, which is the constellation of exudative uveitis with retinal detachment, patchy depigmentation of the skin, meningitis and deafness. Its cause is unknown. Exudative detachments do not require surgery but treatment of the underlying cause.

Management of Rhegmatogenous Retinal Detachment

Prophylaxis

Retinal tears without significant subretinal fluid can be sealed by means of light coagulation. A powerful light beam from a laser is directed at the surrounds of the tear (Fig. 13.2). This produces blanching of the retina around the edges of the hole and, after some days, migration and proliferation of pigment cells occurs from the pigment epithelium into the neuroretina and the blanched area becomes pigmented. A bond is formed

Fig. 13.2 Laser photocoagulation of retinal tear (With acknowledgement to Mr R. Gregson)

across the potential space and a retinal detachment is prevented. This procedure can be carried out, with the aid of a contact lens, in a few minutes.

A wider and more diffuse area of chorioretinal bonding can be achieved by cryopexy, which entails freezing from the outside. Cryopexy is occasionally necessary if the retinal hole is very peripheral, or when there is limited blanching of the retina from laser photocoagulation due to the presence of vitreous haemorrhage. A cold probe is placed on the sclera over the site of the tear and an ice ball is allowed to form over the tear. A similar type of reaction (as occurs after photocoagulation) develops following this treatment, but it tends to be uncomfortable for the patient and local or general anaesthesia is required.

Retinal Surgery

In the early part of the twentieth century it was generally accepted that there was no known effective treatment for retinal detachment. It was realised that a period of bedrest resulted in flattening of the retina in many instances. This

Fig. 13.3 Retinal detachment (**a**) before and (**b**) after treatment (After Gonin)

entailed a prolonged period of complete immobilisation with the patient lying flat with both eyes padded. This treatment can restore the sight but only temporarily because the retina redetaches when the patient is mobilised. It was also very dangerous for the patient in view of the risk of venous thrombosis and pulmonary embolism. In the 1920s it began to be realised that effective treatment of retinal detachment depends on sealing the small holes in the retina (Fig. 13.3). It was already known by then that the fluid under the retina could be drained off externally simply by puncturing the globe, but up till then no serious attempt had been made to associate this with some form of cautery to the site of the tear. Once it became apparent that cautery to the site of the tear combined with the release of subretinal fluid was effective, it also became evident that not all cases responded to this kind of treatment. It was almost as if the retina was too small for the eye in some cases, an idea, which led to the design of volume-reducing operations, which effectively made the volume of the globe smaller. This in turn led to the concept of mounting the tear on an inward protrusion of the sclera to prevent subsequent redetachment.

Modern retinal reattachment surgery is carried out by one of the following techniques:

Cryobuckle

This involves the sewing of small inert pieces of material, usually silicone rubber onto the outside of the sclera in such a way as to make a suitable indent at the site of the tear (Fig. 13.4). This is combined with cryopexy to the break. It is often necessary to drain off the subretinal fluid and inject air or gas into the vitreous. In more difficult cases the eye may be encircled with a silicone strap to provide all-round support to a retina with extensive degenerative changes.

Vitrectomy

The detached retina can also be reattached from within the vitreous cavity. This involves the use of fine calibre instruments inserted through the pars plana into the vitreous cavity. A light probe is used to illuminate the operative field, whilst a 'vitrectomy cutter' is used to remove the vitreous and hence relieving the abnormal vitreous adhesions that produced the retinal tear in the first instance (Fig. 13.5). The detached retina is 'pushed-back' into place from within and temporarily supported by an internal tamponade agent (air, gas or silicone oil) while the retina heals. The retinal breaks are identified and treated by either laser photocoagulation or cryo-

Fig. 13.4 (a) Retinal detachment surgery: retinal tear surrounded by cryopexy and covered by indent. (b) A–C show positioning of an encircling silicone band (With acknowledgement to Professor D. Archer)

Fig. 13.5 Vitrectomy

pexy at the same time. Vitrectomy may also be combined with a silicone strap encirclement if further support of the peripheral retina is needed.

Historically, vitrectomy is reserved for the more difficult and complex cases of rhegmatogenous retinal detachment where multiple tears and posteriorly located tears are present, or as a 'salvage' operation following failed cryobuckle. With advances in instruments, vitrectomy is increasingly being used as the primary operation for the repair of most acute PVD related rhegmatogenous retinal detachments, regardless of the complexity of the detachment.

Prognosis

The retina can now be successfully reattached by one operation in about 85% of cases. Of the successful cases, those in which the macular region was affected by the retinal detachment do not achieve a full restoration of their central vision, although usually the peripheral field recovers. The degree of recovery of central vision in such macula-detached cases depends largely on the duration of the macular detachment prior to surgery. Even when the retina has been detached for 2 years, it is still possible to restore useful navigational vision.

The main cause of failure of modern retinal reattachment surgery is proliferative vitreoretinopathy (PVR). This is characterized by excessive 'scarring' following initial retinal reattachment surgery, with the formation of fibrous tractional membrane within the eye, resulting in recurrent detachment of the retina.

When retinal surgery has failed, further surgery may be required and for a few patients a series of operations is necessary. If it is thought that more than one operation is going to be needed, then it is important that this is fully discussed in the preliminary interview.

Squint

14

Abstract

The word 'squint' refers to a failure of the visual axes to meet at the point of regard. For normal vision each eye must be focused on and lined up with the object of regard. The fact that we have two eyes positioned some 60 mm apart means that we can accumulate considerably more data about our environment than would be possible with one eye alone. This can best be exemplified by considering what happens when one eye is suddenly lost as the result of injury or disease. Apart from the obvious loss of visual field which necessitates turning the head to the blind side, the patient experiences impaired distance judgement. The skilled worker notices a deterioration in the ability to perform fine tasks and the elderly notice that they pour tea into the saucer rather than the cup. In time, depth perception may improve and the patient adapts to the defect to some extent; children may adapt to one eyed vision in a remarkable way. But it seems that modern civilised living does not have such great demands for binocular vision now that many tasks are carried out by machines. It is no coincidence that those animals whose survival depends on catching their food by means of accurate distance judgement have their eyes placed in front of their head, enabling the two eyes to be focused together on their prey.

The word 'squint' refers to a failure of the visual axes to meet at the point of regard. For normal vision each eye must be focused on and lined up with the object of regard. The fact that we have two eyes positioned some 60 mm apart means that we can accumulate considerably more data about our environment than would be possible with one eye alone. This can best be exemplified by considering what happens when one eye is suddenly lost as the result of injury or disease. Apart from the obvious loss of visual field which necessitates turning the head to the blind side, the patient experiences impaired distance judgement. The skilled worker notices a deterioration in the ability to perform fine tasks and the elderly notice that they pour tea into the saucer rather than the cup. In time, depth perception may improve and the patient adapts to the defect to some extent; children may adapt to one eyed vision in a remarkable way. But it seems that modern civilised living does not have such great demands for binocular vision now that many tasks are carried out by machines. It is no coincidence that those animals whose survival depends on catching their food by means of accurate distance judgement have their eyes placed in front of their head, enabling the two eyes to be focused together on their prey.

Investigation of a normal human population reveals that although the eyes may be situated on

Fig. 14.1 The synoptophore. An instrument for measuring the angle of deviation of a squint and the ability of the eyes to work together

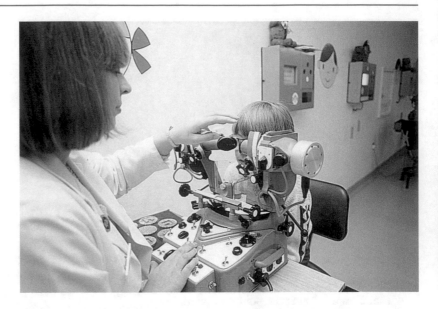

the front of the face, they do not always work together, and it will be seen that there are a number of reasons why the mechanism may fail. The ability to use the eyes together is called binocular vision. It can be measured and graded by presenting each eye separately but simultaneously with a series of images. The instrument used to do this is called a synoptophore (Fig. 14.1).

1. *Simultaneous macular perception* is said to be present if the subject can see two dissimilar images which are presented simultaneously to each eye, e.g. a triangle to one eye, a circle to the other.
2. *Fusion* is present if the subject can see two parts of a whole image as one whole when each half is presented to a separate eye. E.g. a picture of a house to one eye, a picture of a chimney to the other, and the whole picture is maintained as one as the eyes converge. The range of fusion can be measured in degrees.
3. *Stereopsis*, the third grade of binocular vision, is present if, when slightly dissimilar views of an object are presented to each eye separately, a single three dimensional view of the whole is seen. Stereopsis itself can also be graded if very fine degrees of impairment of binocular function need to be measured.

This ability of ours to put together the images from each eye and make a single picture in our minds seems to develop during the early years of life and furthermore its development seems to depend on visual input. Below the age of 8 years any misalignment of the eyes which disturbs binocular vision may permanently damage this function.

If the alignment of the eyes is disturbed for any reason during childhood, the child may at first, as one might expect, notice double vision but very quickly learns to suppress the image from one eye, thereby eliminating the annoyance of diplopia at the expense of binocular vision. In fact most, but not all, children learn to suppress when using monocular instruments, switching the other eye on again when the instrument is not being used. Prolonged suppression seems to lead to a more permanent state of visual loss called amblyopia of disuse. The word 'amblyopia' simply means blindness. Suppression is a temporary switching off of one eye when the other is in use, whereas amblyopia of disuse is a permanent impairment of vision, which could affect the career prospects of the patient. Amblyopia of disuse can also occur if the sight of one eye is defective as the result of opacities in the media, even though the alignment of the eyes has not been disturbed. Again this only occurs in children under the age of 8 years. Covering one eye of a baby could lead to permanent impairment of the vision of that eye as well as impairment of the ability to use the eyes together. An adult may have one eye covered for many months or even years without suffering visual loss.

Before considering the causes and effects of squint in children and adults, it is necessary to know something of the different kinds of squint.

Types of Squint

In lay terms the word squint can just mean screwing up the eyes but here we are referring to a deviation of one eye from the line of sight. This may be present all the time or just when the patient is tired. It is important to notice whether the eye movements are normal. For example, if there is weakness of one lateral rectus muscle, the affected eye will not turn outwards and the angle of the squint will be much greater when looking to that side. Most childhood squints are not associated with weakness of one or more extraocular muscles so that the angle of the squint is the same in all directions of gaze. The deviation of the squint may be horizontal or sometimes vertical or the eyes may be convergent or divergent.

Squint in Childhood

During the first few weeks of life the eyes may seem to wander about aimlessly with limited ability to fix. Between the ages of 2 and 6 months, fixation becomes steadier even though the fovea is not fully developed, and by the age of 6 months convergence on a near object may be maintained for several seconds. Even at birth some degree of following movement of the eyes can be seen in response to a flashing light, but only the most gross squints can be diagnosed during these very early months of life. If the eyes are definitely squinting at the age of 6 months then urgent referral to an ophthalmologist is indicated. Prior to this or when there is some doubt, referral to an orthoptic screening service may be considered. These have been set up in many parts of the country. Orthoptists might be regarded as 'physiotherapists of the eyes' and they are trained to examine the eye movements in great detail. We need to detect squints early in children for the following reasons:

1. The squint may be caused by serious underlying intracranial or intraocular disease.
2. The squint may result in amblyopia which is more effectively treated, the younger the child.
3. The cosmetic effect of a squint is an important consideration.

Amblyopia of Disuse

A special word is needed about this curious condition, which accounts for unilateral impairment of vision in over 2% of the population. Any eye casualty officer is familiar with the patient with a foreign body on the cornea of one eye and the other eye being amblyopic. (how can I drive home with this patch on doctor?). The words 'lazy eye' are sometimes used but in lay terms this can also mean squint.

The eye suffering from amblyopia of disuse shows certain features:

1. Impaired Snellen visual acuity but usually able to decipher vertical lines of letters better than horizontal ones.
2. Normal fundus
3. Small residual squint or, if not, the affected eye relatively hypermetropic.
4. A vague central scotoma, which is difficult to assess by routine visual field testing.
5. History of poor vision in one eye since childhood.

The diagnosis of amblyopia may be by exclusion but it must never be reached without a careful examination of the eyes. In recent years there has been a considerable research interest in this subject and there appear to be nerve conduction anomalies in the occipital cortex, which can be induced by visual deprivation.

Causes of Squint in Childhood

1. Refractive error—hypermetropia (most common) and myopia.
2. Opaque media—corneal opacities, cataract, uveitis.
3. Disease of retina or optic nerve—retinoblastoma, optic atrophy.
4. Congenital or acquired weakness of extraocular muscles.
5. Abnormalities of facial skeleton leading to displacement of extraocular muscles.

Refractive Error

In order to understand how refractive error can cause squint, one must first understand how the act of accommodation is linked to the act of convergence. That is to say, we must realise that when we focus upon an object, not only is each individual eye separately focused on it, but the eyes swivel together by the requisite amount to allow them both to view the object at once (convergence). A given amount of accommodation must therefore be associated with an equivalent amount of convergence. In hypermetropic subjects this relationship is disturbed. In order to overcome hypermetropia, the eyes must accommodate and sometimes this excessive focusing induces an excess of convergence hence causing a squint. This type of accommodative squint may be fully corrected by wearing spectacles; when the glasses are on the eyes are straight, when they are off one eye turns in. More often the squint is only partially accommodative and the squint is improved but not eliminated by wearing glasses. The convergent squint associated with hypermetropia is the commonest type of childhood squint.

Opaque Media

Congenital cataract can occasionally present as a squint. In a similar manner, a corneal opacity, as might result from herpes simplex keratitis or injury, may cause a squint to appear. A completely blind eye from whatever cause tends to converge if the blindness occurs in early childhood. Blindness of one eye in an adult tends to result in a divergent squint. This is sometimes a useful indicator of the age of onset of blindness.

Disease of the Retina or Optic Nerve

Such a possibility provides an important reason for the careful examination of the fundus in every case.

Congenital or Acquired Muscle Weakness

6th, 3rd or 4th cranial nerve palsies are sometimes seen after head injuries and the surgeon must always bear in mind the possibility of a 6th or other cranial nerve palsy being associated with raised intracranial pressure. Myasthenia gravis is extremely rare in children but it may present as a squint. In some cases of squint there is a degree of facial asymmetry. These patients may also have 'asymmetrical eyes', one being myopic or hypermetropic relative to the other. Sometimes there is no refractive error but there may be an asymmetry of the insertions of the extraocular muscles as a possible cause of squint. There is a group of conditions known as musculofascial anomalies in which there is marked limitation of the eye movements from birth in certain directions. They are accompanied by abnormal eye movements such as retraction of the globe and narrowing of the palpebral fissures on lateral gaze.

Overaction of muscles can cause a squint. This is seen in schoolchildren sometimes with a background of domestic or other stress. The eyes tend to overconverge and overaccommodate especially when being examined.

Abnormalities of Facial Skeleton

This is not a very common cause but it should be kept in mind

Diagnosis

History When faced with a case of suspected squint there are certain aspects of the history, which may be very helpful in assisting with the diagnosis. It is often useful to ask who first noticed the squint. Sometimes a parent has been made anxious by a well wishing neighbour or relative, and in these cases there may be no true squint but merely the appearance of one. The parent themself is usually the best witness. Unfortunately some children have a facial con-

Fig. 14.2 Pseudosquint. The configuration of the eyelids gives the appearance of a squint but the corneal reflexes show that this is not the case

figuration which makes the eyes look as though they are deviating when they are not and it is essential that the student or general practitioner should be able to make this distinction in order to avoid sending unnecessary referrals to the local eye unit. (Fig. 14.2). Childhood squints often show a dominant pattern of inheritance and the family history provides a useful diagnostic indicator. From the point of view of prognosis it is useful to find out whether the squint is constant or intermittent and also the age of onset. A full ophthalmic history must be taken which should include the birth history and any illness which might have caused or initiated the problem.

Examination While the history is being taken from the parents, one should be making an assessment of the child. If the child is obviously shy or nervous, a useful technique is to introduce some-

thing of interest to the child in the conversation with the parents. At this point it is important not to approach the child directly but to allow him or her to make an assessment of the doctor. It is quite impossible to examine an infant's eyes in a noisy room, thus the number of people present should be minimal and they should not be moving about. The room lighting should be dim enough to enable the light of a torch to be seen easily. The first important part of the examination is to shine a torch at the patient so that the reflection of the light can be seen on each cornea. The position of these corneal reflections is then noted carefully. The more mobile the child the less time there is to observe this. If there is a squint the reflections will be positioned asymmetrically in the pupil. If the patient has a left convergent squint, the reflection from the left cornea is displaced outwards towards the pupil margin. A rough assessment of the angle of the squint can be made at this stage by noting the abnormal position of the reflection. One of the difficulties experienced at this point is due to the continuous movement of the child's eyes, which make it difficult at first to know whether the light is being accurately fixated. By gently moving the torch slightly from side to side, it is usually possible to confirm that the child is looking, albeit momentarily, at the light.

Once the light reflections have been examined, the *cover test* can be performed. Once again the reflection of light from each eye is noted but this time one of the eyes is smartly covered, either with the back of the hand or a card. If the fixating eye is covered, a movement of the non-fixing eye to take up fixation may then be observed (Fig. 14.3). After some practice it is possible to detect even very slight movements of this kind. The result of the test may be misleading if the non-fixing eye is too weak to take up fixation, and quite often, an assessment of the vision of the non-fixing eye can be made at this stage.

If, having performed this first stage of the cover test, no deviation can be detected then the cover can be quickly swapped from one eye to the other and any movement of the covered eye can be noted. That is to say, the latent deviation

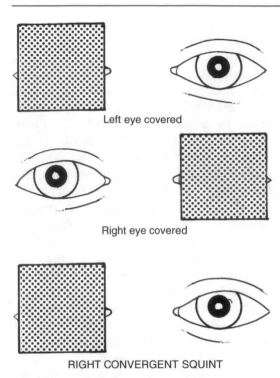

Left eye covered

Right eye covered

RIGHT CONVERGENT SQUINT

Fig. 14.3 The cover test

produced by covering one eye is spotted by noting the small recovery movement made by the previously covered eye. Finally the cover test must be repeated with the patient looking at a distant object. One type of squint in particular can be missed unless this is done. This is the divergent squint seen in young children, which is often only present when viewing distant objects. The parents may have noticed an obvious squint and yet testing by the doctor in the confines of a small room reveals nothing abnormal, with ensuing consternation all round.

After the cover test has been performed it is necessary to test the ocular movements to determine whether there is any muscle weakness. At this stage it is usual to instil a mydriatic and cycloplegic drop (e.g. cyclopentolate 1% or 0.5%) in order to obtain a measure of the refractive error, by retinoscopy, when the eyes are completely at rest. Next the optic fundi are examined.

In most instances the nature of the squint becomes apparent by this stage and further test-

ing of the binocular function and more accurate measurement of the angle of the squint are carried out using the synoptophore.

Management of Squint in Childhood

Glasses Any significant refractive error is corrected by the prescription of glasses. Sometimes the squint is completely straightened when glasses are worn but more often the control is partial, the glasses simply acting to reduce the angle of the squint. Glasses may be prescribed in a child as young as 6–9 months if really necessary. It is important that the parents have a full understanding of the need to wear glasses if adequate supervision is to be expected. When the spectacles are removed at bedtime, a previous squint may appear to become even worse and the parents should be warned about this possible rebound effect.

Orthoptic Follow-Up The orthoptic department forms an integral and important part of the modern eye unit. It is run by orthoptists who carry out the careful measurement of visual acuity with and without glasses and the measurement of eye movements and binocular function. Once the patient has been seen for the initial visit, follow up in the orthoptic department is arranged and the question of treatment by occlusion of the good eye has to be considered. By covering the good eye for a limited period, the sight of the amblyopic eye can be improved. The younger the child, the better are the chances of success. In older children beyond the age of 7 or 8 years, not only is amblyopia more resistant to treatment, but the treatment itself can interfere seriously with schoolwork. The type and amount of occlusive treatment have to be planned and discussed with the parents. Sometimes atropine eye drops are used as an alternative to patching one eye. Orthoptic exercises may also be used in an attempt to strengthen binocular function.

Surgery If the squint is not controlled by glasses, surgery should be considered. Some parents ask if an operation can be carried out as a substitute for wearing glasses. Unfortunately surgery to correct refractive error is not yet at a stage where it can be applied to children with squints. Squint surgery involves moving the muscle insertions or shortening the muscles and from the cosmetic point of view is highly effective. The adjustment of the muscles is measured in millimetres to correspond with the angle of the squint in degrees. Sometimes two or more operations are needed due to occasionally unpredictable results, but from the cosmetic point of view, nobody need suffer the indignity of a squint even though a series of operations may be needed. Once the eyes have been put straight or nearly straight by surgery, the functional result depends on the previous presence of good binocular vision and good vision in each eye.

Squint occurs in about 2% of the population and so it is a very common problem, but it is only a small proportion of these cases that eventually require surgery. The commonest type of squint in childhood is the accommodative convergent squint associated with hypermetropia and here surgery is indicated only when spectacles prove inadequate. Divergent squints are less common but more often require early surgery.

The aim of treatment for a child with squint is to make the eyes look straight, to make each eye see normally and to achieve good binocular vision. Unfortunately, all too often, the first one of these aims alone is achieved in spite of modern methods of treatment. The fault may lie partly in late referral or difficulty with patient co-operation but better methods of treatment are needed.

Squint in Adults

Adults who present with a squint have usually suffered defective action of one or more of the extraocular muscles. It is important to have a basic understanding of these muscles.

Anatomy of the Extraocular Muscles
These can be divided into three groups.

The Horizontal Recti The medial and lateral recti act as yoke muscles, like the reins of a horse.

They rotate the eye about a vertical axis. The lateral rectus abducts the eye (turns it out) and the medial rectus adducts the eye (turns it in).

The Vertical Recti These act as vertical yoke muscles but they run diagonally from their origin at the apex of the orbit to be inserted 7 or 8 mm behind the limbus above and below the globe. The action of these muscles depends on the initial position of the eye. For example the primary action of the superior rectus is to elevate the abducted eye and the inferior rectus depresses the abducted eye. The secondary action of the superior rectus is to adduct and intort the adducted eye; the inferior rectus adducts and extorts the adducted eye. Intorsion and extorsion refer to rotation about an antero-posterior axis through the globe. The important thing to realise is that the action of these muscles depends on the position of the eye (Fig. 14.4).

The Obliques These are also vertical yoke muscles but they run on a different line to the vertical recti. The superior oblique depresses the adducted eye (makes the eye go down when it is turned in) and the inferior oblique elevates the adducted eye.

Needs a diagram of muscles and actions

When a patient has a fourth cranial nerve palsy on the right side, the right eye can no longer look down when it is turned in due to the defective action of the superior oblique muscle. Double vision is experienced which is maximal (i.e. widest displacement of images) when looking down to the left.

When a patient has a sixth cranial nerve palsy on the right side, the right eye can no longer abduct or turn outwards. A right convergent squint is seen and the patient experiences double vision worse when looking to the right. There may be a head turn to the right.

When a patient has a third cranial nerve palsy on the right side, the right eye is turned down and to the right and, if the palsy is complete, the upper lid droops and the pupil is dilated. Movement of the eye is very limited.

Fig. 14.4 Primary and secondary actions of the superior rectus muscle

Intorts the adducted eye   Elevates the abducted eye

Causes of Adult Squint

Adults who *present* with a squint usually have a well defined ocular muscle palsy. This may be due to a pathological process at any point from the brain, through the nerve to the muscle. These will be discussed elsewhere but two important causes are demyelination in the younger age groups and hypertensive vascular disease in older patients. Diabetes is another important cause that must be excluded in all age groups.

Some adult squints prove to be concomitant squints neglected from childhood. Sometimes a latent squint, which has been well controlled throughout childhood, breaks down in adult life.

In adult life a blind eye tends to turn outwards and a divergent squint may be due solely to impaired vision in one eye.

Diagnosis

In contrast to the situation with children, who usually present with concomitant squint (same magnitude regardless of gaze position) associated with hypermetropia, the sudden onset of a squint in adult life is extremely disabling because of intractable double vision. The double vision is less apparent when the lesion is more central, involving the level of the cranial nerve nucleus or above. In the latter case, the patient tends to complain more of blurred vision and confusion.

A carefully taken history may reveal the diagnosis. First it is necessary to ensure that the double vision is only present with both eyes open and then the patient can be questioned about the posi-

tion of the second image and whether the separation of the images is maximal in any particular direction of gaze. The duration and constant or intermittent nature of the squint must be determined as must the history of any associated disease, past or present.

Once the history has been obtained, the nature of the squint can be investigated by the cover test and measured by use of prisms. In addition, an accurate record of the impaired muscle action can be recorded on the Hess screen.

Hess Screen

Here the eyes are dissociated by using either coloured filters or a mirror. The system is arranged so that a screen is viewed with one eye and the end of a pointer with the other. The patient is told to place the pointer on various points on the screen. If the eyes are not straight the pointer is placed away from the correct position. A map of the incorrect positions is made (Fig. 14.5). The shape of the map is diagnostic of particular ocular muscle problems and serial records can be very helpful in assessing progress.

Causes of a squint in an adult

Demyelination
Raised intracranial pressure
Microvascular occlusion secondary to diabetes
    and hypertension
Giant cell arteritis
Thyroid eye disease
Myesthenia gravis
Orbital fracture

Fig. 14.5 Hess chart depicting a right lateral rectus palsy

Treatment

Many cases of adult squint recover spontaneously within a period of 3-6 months. Once the cause of the squint has been investigated the immediate treatment entails eliminating the diplopia by occluding one or other eye. This may be conveniently achieved by applying adhesive tape to the spectacle lens. If the angle of the squint is sufficiently small, it may be possible to regain binocular vision by means of a prism. Fresnel prisms are thin and flexible and can be simply stuck onto the spectacle lens as a temporary measure during the recovery period. When the squint shows no sign of recovery over a period of 9 months or more, then surgery is usually required to restore binocular vision. Before applying these principles of management it is essential to treat the underlying cause of the squint. It would be a serious error to treat diplopia due to raised intracranial pressure by means of prisms without instituting a full neurological investigation, just as it would not help the patient with myasthenia gravis to undergo squint surgery before medical treatment has been started.

Ocular Muscle Imbalance

Mild latent squints may sometimes go undetected until a period of stress or perhaps excessive reading precipitates symptoms of eyestrain and headache. The effort to maintain both eyes in line causes the symptoms. The latent deviation may be inwards or outwards but because most people's eyes tend to assume a slightly divergent position when completely at rest, a degree of latent divergence (exophoria) is almost the rule and of no significance. Vertical muscle imbalance is less well tolerated and even a slight deviation may cause symptoms. Small but significant degrees of vertical muscle imbalance are seen in otherwise normal individuals who show a marked difference in refractive error between the two eyes or in those with facial asymmetry. The provision of a small prism incorporated into the spectacle lenses of such patients may produce dramatic relief, but we must always remember that the appearance of an ocular muscle imbalance may be the first indication of more serious disease. A small vertical deviation may be the first sign of a tumour of the lacrimal gland or thyrotoxic eye disease and a wide range of investigations may be needed before one can be satisfied with the excellent but sometimes deceptive results of symptomatic treatment.

Summary

Squint is a relatively common condition that can affect both children and adults. It implies a misalignment of the eyes so that they fail to look at the object of regard simultaneously. In children, the most common cause is refractive error (hypermetropia). This can often be treated with glasses. Sometimes the cause in children is central and surgery is required to realign the eyes if glasses do not correct the deviation. In adults, the cause is usually poor function of one or more of the extraocular muscles. Causes include hypertension, diabetes and stroke, and in all cases the patient should undergo a thorough ocular and systemic evaluation as the squint may be due to more serious problems.

Tumours of the Eye and Adnexae

15

Abstract

In this chapter the more important ocular tumours will be considered. There are a considerable number of other rare tumours and the interested student should refer to one of the more specialised and comprehensive textbooks of ophthalmology for further reading.

The Globe

Expanding tumours in the eye present diagnostic problems because it is not usually possible to biopsy them without significant risk to the eye.

Choroidal Melanoma

The most common primary intraocular tumour is the malignant melanoma of the choroid. In Caucasians, the tumour has an incidence of 1 in 2500 and the average age at presentation is 50 years. The incidence rises with age with a peak at 70 years, however, it is important to appreciate that no age is exempt since choroidal melanomas have been reported in children as young as three years old. It is extremely rare in Afro-Caribbeans. It differs from melanoma of the skin in that it grows more slowly and metas-tasises late. Most choroidal melanomas are thought to originate from choroidal naevi which are present in up to 10% of the population At first it is seen as a raised pigmented oval area which may be anywhere in the fundus (Fig. 15.1a, b). It is usually brown in colour although it may be amelanotic (or greyish). As the tumour enlarges there may be associated lipofuscin accumulation, giving it an orange hue, exudative retinal detachment or, less often, secondary glaucoma if the lesion originates in the ciliary body. Other associated features may include choroidal haemorrhage and serial photography may be needed to confirm the growth. The usual presentation is with decreased vision or a visual field defect. Diagnosis is confirmed with careful clinical examination including indirect ophthalmoscopy and slit lamp biomicroscopy, fundus autofluorescence, OCT scans, ultrasonography, occasionally fluorescein angiography and transvitreal fine needle aspiration in equivocal cases. The most common site for metastases is the liver, so regular abdominal ultrasound examination is recommended. The appearance of liver metastases may be delayed for several years and may occur even if the eye has been removed signifying micrometastases at the time of presentation. Approximately 50% of patients develop metastases within 10 years while the estimated five-year mortality rate for treated medium size melanomas is between 15 and 23%. A poor

Fig. 15.1   Choroidal melanoma poorly pigmented (amelanotic) melanoma (**a**) Fundus photograph. (**b**) Bisected eye showing pigmented and nonpigmented portions of melanoma in same eye (With acknowledgement to Mr A. Foss)

prognosis is associated with age, large size, origin in the cilairay body and loss of 1 copy of chromosome 3 on fine needle aspiration. The differential diagnosis of choroidal melanoma includes retinal detachment, metastatic choroidal tumours, wet macular degeneration, large choroidal naevi, choroidal haemangioma or choroidal effusion. Historically treatment involved enucleation (removal of the globe) however today many alternative eye sparing treatments are available, partly dependant on the size and local spread of the tumour. Options include radiotherapy (most commonly external plaque and proton beam), laser photocoagulation for small lesions and local resection by both internal and external approaches. Untreated, the tumour may extend into the orbit.

Choroidal Metastases

These make up the most common intraocular tumour in adults. Although lesions can be demonstrated in at least 1–2.5% of patients with carcinomas, many cases remain asymtomatic unless the macula is involved. In males the most common primary tumour is found in the lung and in females it is the breast. The metastatic tumours are usually treated with external beam radiotherapy or by systemic chemotherapy

Retinoblastoma

This is a rare tumour of childhood which arises not from the choroid but, as its name suggests, from the retina. It is, however, the commonest primary intraocular tumour in children with an incidence of 1 in 15000 live births. It shows certain rather strange and unusual features. It is not usually present from birth, but occurs most frequently in infancy to three years (although it can occur in older patients); it is either be inherited as an autosomal dominant trait or may be sporadic in nature. Approximately 40% of cases are considered to be inherited. In a third of inherited cases it appears in both eyes. A change in the RB1 gene on chromosome 13 is found in the inherited cases. Initially it may be seen in an individual, suspected on account of the family history, as a small white, raised mass. Examination under anaesthesia is essential in such cases because the tumour may be in the extreme periphery of the fundus. A larger tumour may present as a white mass in the pupil ('leucocoria') and such an appearance in infancy demands immediate referral to an ophthalmologist (Fig. 15.2). Other presenting features include strabismus, secondary glaucoma, proptosis or intra ocular inflammatory signs. CT scanning and ultrasound may show a calcified intraocular mass. Extension tends to occur locally along the

Fig. 15.2 Retinoblastoma: leucocoria

optic nerve and enucleation is often life saving. Until recently, enucleation was the treatment of choice and cure rates of 90–95% were achieved. Nowadays, eye sparing therapy is preferred, in an attempt at avoiding the physical and psychological trauma involved in enucleating a young child. Alternative treatment options include initial systemic or local tumour chemoreduction with carboplatin based regimes followed by external beam radiotherapy, plaque radiotherapy, cryotherapy or laser photocoagulation. Genetic counselling is essential for these patients in order to prevent the increasing incidence of the tumours, which will result from effective medical treatment.

Melanoma of the Iris

This rare iris tumour usually presents as a solitary nodule, usually on the inferior iris, which may or may not be pigmented. It may cause distortion of the pupil, which may be an early warning sign. Other features which may point to the diagnosis are localised lens opacity, iris neovascularisation and elevation of intraocular pressure. It is extremely slow growing and probably much less malignant than choroidal melanomas with a survival rate of at least 95% at 5 years. Treatment is usually in the form of a sector or total iridectomy.

The Eyelids

Benign Tumours

Meibomian Cysts (Chalazion) This is the commonest eyelid lump in all ages. It is due to blockage of the meibomian gland orifice such that the secretions accumulate. A granulomatous inflammation is set up which results in a painless, round, firm slowly growing lump in the tarsal plate (Fig. 15.3). The cyst may become infected when it becomes red hot and painful. Treatment is usually conservative with warm compresses and lid hygiene however incision and curettage may occasionally be required.

Molluscum Contagiosum This is caused by a viral infection and is most commonly seen in children. The lesions consist of several pale, waxy, umbilicated nodules on the eyelids and face. Similar lesions may be located on the trunk. The eyelid lesions shed viral particles, which produce a chronic conjunctivitis and less often superficial keratitis. The lesions may disappear in about six months, but may need curettage or cautery.

Papilloma This is the name used to describe a rather common virus induced nodule or filiform wart often seen on the lid margin.

Fig. 15.3 Chalazion

Seborrhoeic Keratosis This is common in the elderly and consists of slow growing sessile, greasy lesions of the eyelid. They are usually brown and friable.

Senile Keratosis Senile keratosis consists of multiple, flat, scaly lesions, which may occasionally undergo transformation into a squamous cell carcinoma.

Xanthelasma These are slightly elevated lesions consisting of lipid deposits usually on the medial aspect of the eyelids. They may be associated with hyperlipidemia especially in the younger patient.

Keratoacanthoma This is an example of a lesion, which grows rapidly, too rapidly for a neoplasm, over a period of a few weeks and then resolves spontaneously (Fig. 15.4). It usually starts as a red papule, which grows quickly into a nodule with a keratin filled crater. The lesion may resemble a basal cell carcinoma. Small lumps on the eyelids should be removed and biopsied. Larger lumps may be biopsied by taking a small segment from them prior to total excision if this proves necessary. Special care should be taken with the excision of any lesion on the eyelid in view of the risk of causing distortion of the lid margin or exposure keratitis.

Kaposi Sarcoma This is a well known association with AIDS. The lesions consist of purple nodules on the eyelid and similar lesions in the lower conjunctival fornix composed of proliferating endothelial and spindle shape cells. Inflammatory cells may also be present with vascular channels without endothelial cell lining. Human Herpes virus 8 is thought to be important in the pathogenesis of these lesions.

Benign vascular tumours of the eyelids fall into three types:

Capillary Haemangioma of the Newborn (Strawberry Naevus) This is usually seen before the age of six months, and nearly all examples regress spontaneously between 3 months and 5 years. Tumours appear as red, slightly raised marks on the skin. Even very extensive tumours of this kind can show a dramatic improvement over several years and conservative management is usually indicated unless the tumour is associated with a fold of skin, which occludes the eye, causing amblyopia. Larger tumours may produce orbital enlargement. If treatment is required, intralesional steroid injections or systemic propanalol have proved beneficial.

Cavernous Haemangioma These tumours lie more deeply in the skin and appear as a bluish swelling in the lid which expands when the child cries. These lesions may also disappear spontaneously or, if persistent, they may be treated by freezing.

Telangiectatic Haemangioma Also known as the port wine stain or naevus flammeus, this tumour tends to be distributed over the area supplied by one or more of the branches of the fifth cranial nerve and usually remains throughout life as a dark red discolouration in the skin (Fig. 15.5). The importance of this particular appearance is its association with secondary glaucoma and haemangioma of the meninges. The latter produces calcification and a characteristic x-ray appearance. The combination of lesions is known as the Sturge-Weber syndrome. There may be hypertrophy of the affected area of the face leading to asymmetry.

Fig. 15.4 Keratoacanthoma (With acknowledgement to Mr A. Sadiq)

Fig. 15.6 Early basal cell carcinoma of medial canthus

Fig. 15.5 Port wine stain (naevus flammeus)

Malignant Tumours of the Eyelids

Basal Cell Carcinoma This is the most common malignant tumour of the eyelid in adults (80–90% of cases). Pathogenesis is related to exposure to UV light hence it most frequently involves the lower lid and medial canthus. The tumour begins as a small insignificant nodule, which turns into a small crater-like lesion with a slightly raised pearly colored edge with fine dilated blood vessels on its surface (Fig. 15.6). Although the tumour rarely metastasizes, it is locally invasive, therefore early diagnosis and treatment is important. In the early stages it is a simple matter to remove the lesion and confirm the diagnosis by biopsy, but if left the tumour tends to spread into surrounding structures and into the underlying bone and orbit (Fig. 15.7).

Treatment depends on the size, extent and location of the tumour. Usually surgical excision with wide margins is the technique of choice either by a simple excisional biopsy or by the more complex Mohs' procedure. The more extensive, neglected basal cell carcinomata are treated by radical surgery, cryotherapy or palliative radiotherapy.

Squamous Cell Carcinoma It is the second most common malignant eyelid lesion and constitutes 5–10% of cases. It occurs most commonly in the elderly and is related to sun light exposure. The tumour may initially resemble a basal cell carcinoma although the edges are usually not rolled. Spread tends to occur to the local lymph nodes, (preauricular for the upper lid and submandibular for the lower lid). Treatment is similar to a basal cell carcinoma

Sebaceous Gland Carcinoma This uncommon tumour constitutes 1–3% of malignant eyelid tumours (higher in Asians). It arises from the meibomian glands in the tarsal plate. It appears as a discrete, firm nodule, which often presents as a 'recurrent chalazion' thereby delaying diagnosis. Treatment involves wide excision ± radiotherapy. Mortality ranges from 6% to 30%, depending on site, size, symptom duration and histological classification.

Melanoma of the Eyelid Malignant melanoma of the eyelids is similar to malignant melanoma

Fig. 15.7 Extensive basal cell carcinoma involving the orbit and extending across the nose to the opposite side. (**a**) Clinical photograph; (**b**) Computerised tomography scan

elsewhere, appearing as a raised often shiny black lump. It metastasises at a very early stage and the prognosis does not seem to be altered by excision

The Conjunctiva

Benign Lesions

Benign Pigmented Lesions of the Conjunctiva

Conjunctival epithelial melanosis occurs in approximately 90% of Afro-Caribeans and 10% of Caucasians and is noticeable in early life. The lesions are flat, brownish patches scattered throughout the conjunctiva, but may be more noticeable at the limbus (Fig. 15.8). They do not grow usually. Other pigmented lesions, for example the benign naevus, require closer attention and specialist evaluation.

Non-Pigmented Lesions

Pingueculum is a common mass lesion of the conjunctiva. It is seen as a yellowish nodule usually on the medial interpalpebral fissure. It is a fibrovascular degeneration and is seen in all climates.

  Pterygium is a growth of abnormal fibrovascular tissue usually extending from the nasal conjunctiva over the cornea (Fig. 15.9). It is thought to be due to chronic irritation from dust and solar radiation. It is commoner in hot cli-

Fig. 15.8 Conjunctival melanosis

Fig. 15.9 Pterygium

mates and individuals that work out of doors. Recurrent inflammation of the pterygium is often self-limiting but responds to a short course of topical steroids. If it extends over the visual axis of the cornea it may cause visual impairment,

Fig. 15.10 Melanoma of conjunctiva

Table 15.1 Primary orbital tumours

Vascular	Capillary haemangioma
	Cavernous haemangioma
	Lymphangioma
Neural	Optic nerve glioma
	Meningioma
	Neurofi bromatoma
Lacrimal gland	
Lymphoproliferative	
Rhabdomyosarcoma	
Histiocytosis	

therefore surgical excision may be required although regrowth occurs in a large proportion of patients.

Malignant Lesions

Melanoma of the Conjunctiva Malignant mela-nomata may occur on the conjunctiva (Fig. 15.10) but they should not be confused with the rela-tively common benign conjunctival naevus. The latter is a slightly raised pigment-stippled lesion often seen at the limbus on the temporal side. Closer examination with the hand lens or micro-scope may reveal one or two minute cysts. It is generally accepted that these benign lesions should be excised and biopsied if they become irritable or sometimes simply on cosmetic grounds, but thcy rarely bccome malignant. The treatment of conjunctival malignant melanoma involves wide surgical excision with adjuvant cryotherapy, radiotherapy or topical mitomycin C or interferon. The five year survival rate is approximately 85%.

The Orbit (see Table 15.1)

Lacrimal Gland and sac Tumours Lacrimal gland tumours may either be inflammatory, mixed cell tumours or adenocarcinomas. They present with proptosis or mass in the outer part of the eyelid superotemporal orbit. Lacrimal sac tumours are less common and present with sac swelling. Benign lesions and infections need to be excluded.

Dermoid Cyst Dermoid cysts are congenital and are the most common orbital mases seen in chil-dren. The cystic swelling is usually seen at the level of the eyebrow in the upper outer part of the orbit. It is smooth and fluctuant and often fixed to bone. Sometimes a deeper part of the cyst may occupy a cavity in the bone and a CT scan is advisable when this is suspected. Rupture of the cyst can lead to profound orbital inflammation. Excision on cosmetic grounds and for diagnosis is usually indicated.

Cavernous Haemangioma This is the common-est primary neoplasm of the orbit in adults. It is benign. It is unusual for surgery to be necessary in such cases. It is usually located within the muscle cone, and gives rise to axial proptosis. If treatment is required, surgical removal is recommended.

Glioma of the Optic Nerve This rare tumour causes progressive proptosis and optic atrophy but it may be very slow growing. There is an association with Von Recklinghausen's disease (Neurofibromatosis type 1) and the presence of pigmented patches in the skin should make one suspect this. Treatment by surgical resection and/ or radiotherapy is indicated if intracranial spread is documented

Rhabdomyosarcoma This rare but highly malig-nant orbital tumour is seen in children. Its growth is so rapid that it may be misdiagnosed as orbital cellulitis. If a correct diagnosis is made at an early stage, there is some hope of reaching a cure by combining radiotherapy and chemotherapy. The tumour is thought to arise from striated muscle and the histological diagnosis is confirmed by finding striation in the tumour cells. It is usually located in the superonasal orbit.

Metastatic Tumours and Tumours from Neighbouring Sites A wide variety of tumours may invade the orbit and produce proptosis and often diplopia. Lymphoma is one example. It may present as an isolated lesion or in association with Hodgkin's disease or leukaemia. Examples of local spread from adjacent structures include carcinoma of the nasopharynx, carcinoma of the lacrimal gland and meningioma. In children orbital metastases arise most commonly from neuroblastoma and Ewing's sarcoma. In the adult the commonest primary sites are bronchus, breast, prostate and kidneys.

Idiopathic Orbital Inflammatory Disease (Pseudotumour) This is a non—infectious, inflammatory swelling in the orbit of unknown cause, which may present with pain, proptosis and diplopia. A mass may be palpable in the orbit and biopsy reveals non-specific inflammatory tissue consisting mainly of lymphocytes. Diagnosis may eventually be made by exclusion of other causes of proptosis. In severe cases a course of systemic steroids and or radiotherapy is usually very effective.

Exophthalmos and Proptosis

Both these terms mean forward protrusion of the eyes but traditionally exophthalmos refers to the bilateral globe protrusion in thyroid disease. Proptosis refers to unilateral forward displacement of the globe from whatever cause. In practice the terms tend to be used rather loosely and are now almost synonymous.

Causes of Proptosis (see Table 15.2)

When one eye seems to bulge forward the doctor may have a serious problem on his hands and he should be able to consider the likely causes.

Table 15.2 Causes of proptosis

Endocrine
Vascular abnormalities
Inflammatory disorders
Primary orbital tumours
Metastases

Pseudoproptosis An apparent bulging forward of the eye occurs if the eye is too big, as in unilateral high myopia and unilateral congenital glaucoma or if the other eye is sunken following a blow-out fracture of the maxilla (orbital floor). These need to be distinguished from a true proptosis.

Thyrotoxicosis This is the commonest cause of unilateral or bilateral proptosis; diagnosis is achieved from the history, examination and tests of thyroid function (Fig. 15.11). At presentation, assessment of corneal health and optic nerve function should be carried out as dysfunction is an ophthalmic emergency and may require urgent treatment. MRI is often used to assess the state of

Fig. 15.11 Proptosis: dysthyroid disease

the extra ocular muscles and any optic nerve compression

Infection Orbital cellulitis, usually from neighbouring sinuses, requires urgent otorhinological (ENT) opinion.

Trauma Proptosis can occur as a result of retroorbital haemorrhage. Diagnosis should be possible from the patient's history. In severe cases, compression of the optic nerve may occur and require urgent decompression by a lateral canthotomy

Haemangioma This may expand after bending down or crying. Ultrasound and CT scanning may confirm the diagnosis. Occasionally angiography, may be required

Idiopathic Orbital Inflammatory Disease (Pseudotumour) Biopsy should be carried out if possible, and other causes excluded.

Mucocele of Sinuses Diagnose by x-ray or CT scan.

Lymphoproliferative Disease A biopsy, full blood count and sternal marrow puncture should be carried out.

Assessment of Proptosis

In the clinic, proptosis is best assessed by standing behind the seated patient and asking them to look down. The position of each globe in relation to the lids and face can be best seen by this means. Proptosis can be measured by means of an exophthalmometer. A number of such instruments are on the market and they depend on measuring the distance from the rim of the outer margin of the orbit to the level of the anterior part of the cornea. These measurements are not always very accurate (especially for the novice) but best results are achieved by ensuring that they are made by the same person, using the same instrument on each occasion for a given patient.

Once thyroid disease and trauma have been excluded, the patient would require further investigations including systemic examination, full blood picture, orbital ultrasound, CT scan, MRI scan, possibly carotid angiography and sometimes orbital biopsy.

Summary

Ocular tumours are rare. However it is important to diagnose them as early as possible because they can have life threatening consequences. Even after choroidal melanomas have been diagnosed and treated, patients need follow up for many years due to the risk of metastatic disease. Far more common are adnexal tumours such as basal cell carcinoma and squamous cell carcinoma. Although these have a much lower life threatening potential, it is still important to diagnose them early so as to reduce the requirement for major disfiguring oculoplastic surgery and radiotherapy.

Abstract

The fact that injuries to the eye and its surrounding region demand special attention and create great concern for patient and doctor is self evident when the eye alone is involved, but when other life threatening injuries are present the eye injury, seeming slight at the time, may be overlooked. Sometimes the eyelids may be so swollen that it is difficult to examine the eyes and a serious perforating injury may be obscured. When other injuries are present and an anaesthetic is needed, it is essential that the eyes are examined carefully, if possible under the same anaesthetic. As in the case of injuries elsewhere, those to the eye demand urgent and immediate treatment, and neglect can result in tragedy even though the problem may have at first seemed very slight.

The fact that injuries to the eye and its surrounding region demand special attention and create great concern for patient and doctor is self evident when the eye alone is involved, but when other life threatening injuries are present the eye injury, seeming slight at the time, may be overlooked. Sometimes the eyelids may be so swollen that it is difficult to examine the eyes and a serious perforating injury may be obscured. When other injuries are present and an anaesthetic is needed, it is essential that the eyes are examined carefully, if possible under the same anaesthetic. As in the case of injuries elsewhere, those to the eye demand urgent and immediate treatment, and neglect can result in tragedy even though the problem may have at first seemed very slight.

Injuries to the Globe

Contusion

The eye casualty officer comes to recognise a familiar pattern of contusion, the effect of squash ball injuries and blows from flying objects in industry or after criminal assault. Injuries from industrial causes have now become quite uncommon thanks to better control by means of protective clothing and proper guarding of machinery. Sporting injuries have as a result become more evident although here also increasing public concern has led to some improvement. Notable instances of good control are the use of protective guards in ice hockey and cricket and the use of protective goggles in squash. The surrounding orbital margin provides good protection to the eyes from footballs and even tennis and cricket balls but the rare golf ball contusion injury usually leads to loss of the sight of the eye. Squash balls and especially shuttle cocks have earned a bad reputation for inflicting contusion injuries and, from the economic point of view, leading to loss of time at work and hospital expenses.

The extent of damage to the eye from contusion depends on whether it has been possible to close the eyelids in time before the moment of impact. If the lids have been closed, bruising and swelling of the eyelids is marked and the injury to the eye may be minimal. It must be remembered though that this is not an infallible rule and the eyes themselves must always be carefully examined, even when there is extreme swelling of the lids. It is always possible to examine an eye, if necessary using an eye speculum under general anaesthesia. In the primary care situation one must be very careful not to apply more than gentle pressure to the eyelids in case the globe of the eye has been perforated and when there is doubt referral to the eye department is advisable. The important clinical features of contusion injury are best considered by looking at the anatomical parts of the eye.

Cornea The commonest injury to the cornea is from the corneal foreign body and this has already been described in Chap. 6. Almost as common is the corneal abrasion. It is odd how this is so often caused by the edge of a newspaper, a comb or a child's finger nail. Abrasions from the leaves of plants or twigs need special attention because of the type of infection that can occur (fungal), but any abrasion can lead to the condition known as recurrent erosion. Here the patient experiences a sharp pain in the eye in the early morning usually on waking, sometimes many months after the initial injury. It is thought that the lid margin adheres to the area of weakened healed corneal epithelium during sleep. The diagnosis is easily missed if the patient has forgotten about the original injury and if the cornea is not examined carefully with the slit lamp biomicroscope. This problem of recurrence is a reason to treat these abrasions with some care and to provide the patient with a lubricating ointment to be used at night for some time after the original injury has healed. Sometimes recurrent erosion is due to a rare inherited disorder of the corneal epithelium.

When a patient presents with a corneal abrasion, the eyelids are often swollen perhaps from rubbing and the distress and agitation can be con-

Fig. 16.1 Hyphaema showing anterior chamber half filled with blood

siderable. Examination may be impossible without first instilling a drop of local anaesthetic . These drops should never be continued as treatment because they could seriously delay the healing of the cornea.

Anterior Chamber A small bleed into the anterior chamber of the eye is seen as a fluid level of blood inferiorly ('hyphaema') (Fig. 16.1). This is a sign of potential problems because of the risk of secondary bleeding after 2 or 3 days. This risk is especially serious in children and the complication can lead to secondary glaucoma and at worst the loss of the eye. The parents need to be warned about this if there is a hyphaema. Treatment is by strict rest with little or no head movement to avoid further bleeding and regular measurement of the intraocular pressure.

Iris When confronted by a flying missile, the normal reaction is to attempt to close the eyelids and to rotate the eyes upwards. This is the reason why the commonest point of impact is the lower temporal part of the eye and it is in this region of the iris that one is most likely to see peripheral iris tears ('iridodialysis').

When the eye is compressed the iris periphery is torn at its root, leaving a crescentic gap which looks black, but through which the fundus and red reflex can be observed. Such an injury also provides an excellent view of the peripheral part of the lens and the lens zonules (Fig. 16.2).

Fig. 16.2 Iridodialysis or splitting of the iris root in lower temporal quadrant. A sure sign of previous contusion

Contusion may result not in a tear of the iris root, but in a tangential splitting of the iris and ciliary body from the sclera producing recession of the angle of the anterior chamber; the appearance is often associated with secondary glaucoma, sometimes many years after the injury and is identified using the special contact lens known as the gonioscope.

A sudden impact on the eye may also produce microscopic radial tears in the pupillary sphincter of the iris. This may be a subtle microscopic sign of previous injury when no other signs are present, or the damage may be more severe resulting in persistent dilatation of the pupil (traumatic mydriasis). Unless the eye is examined this widening of the pupil after injury can be mistaken for a third cranial nerve palsy.

Lens Any severe contusion of the eye is liable to cause cataract, but the lens may not become opaque for many years after the injury. The lens may also become subluxated (slightly displaced due to partial rupture of the zonular ligament) or even dislocated either anteriorly into the anterior chamber or posteriorly into the vitreous.

Vitreous The vitreous may become displaced from its attachments around the processes of the ciliary body or around the optic disc after a contusion injury if it has not already undergone this change as part of the normal ageing process. The patient may be aware of something floating in front of the vision. More extensive floating black spots can indicate a vitreous haemorrhage caused by excessive vitreous traction on a retinal blood vessel. Although such haemorrhages usually clear completely in time they tend to accompany more serious damage to the retina which may only be fully revealed once clearing has taken place.

Retina Bruising and oedema of the retina are seen as grey areas with scattered haemorrhages. The macular region is susceptible to oedema after contusion injuries causing permanent damage to the reading vision. Just as tears can occur to the peripheral iris, so a similar problem is seen in the peripheral retina. These crescentic retinal dialyses are also most common in the lower temporal quadrant and their importance lies in the fact that they may lead to a detachment of the retina unless the tear is sealed by laser treatment. Any significant contusion injury of the eye requires a careful inspection of the peripheral retina.

Choroid Tears in the choroid following contusion have a characteristic appearance. They are concentric with the disc and are seen as white crescents where the sclera is exposed. When near the macula, there is usually permanent damage to the central vision. (Fig. 16.3). They are also potential sites for choroidal neovascularisation.

Fig. 16.3 Healed choroidal tear. Another sign of previous injury

Optic Nerve A variable degree of optic atrophy may become apparent a few weeks after a contusion injury. Blunt injuries to the eye may cause bleeding into the optic nerve sheath or tearing of the tiny pial blood vessels that supply the nerve, both resulting in complete, irreversible loss of vision on the affected side. Attempts have been made to relieve the situation by emergency decompression of the optic nerve, nerve sheath fenestration, use of hyperbaric oxygen and high dose steroids. No treatment has shown a clear benefit except optic nerve decommpression in specific circumstances

Perforation

As soon as the globe of the eye is penetrated there is a serious risk of infection. The vitreous is an excellent culture medium and in the pre-antibiotic era eyes were totally lost within 2 or 3 days as a result of this. *A perforating wound of the eye must therefore be considered a surgical emergency.* Perforating injuries are seen in children from scissor blades, screwdrivers, darts and other more bizarre objects. In adults there has been a dramatic fall in the incidence of such injuries since the introduction of compulsory seat belts but 'DIY' accidents and assaults still take their toll. Following such an injury it is important to consider the possibility of an intraocular foreign body especially when there is a history of using a hammer and chisel.

The outcome of a perforating injury is dependent on the depth of penetration and the care with which the wound is cleaned and sutured. If the cornea alone is damaged, excellent results may be obtained by careful suturing under general anaesthesia using the operating microscope. If the lens has been damaged, early cataract surgery may be needed and deeper penetration may result in the need for retinal detachment surgery.

On admission or in the casualty department, the patient is given tetanus prophylaxis and both systemic and local antibiotics. If early surgery under general anaesthesia is likely to be needed then it is better for the patient not to eat or drink to avoid delays in hospital. If it becomes clear that the injury is a serious one, it is better to warn the patient at an early stage about the possible risk of losing the sight of the eye or even the need to replace it with an artificial one.

Intraocular Foreign Body

Metallic foreign bodies tend to enter the eyes of those who operate high speed grinders without goggles or those using a hammer and chisel on metal without eye protection. These injuries may seem slight at first and sometimes the patient does not attach much importance to it. *Any such eye injury with this occupational history warrants an X-ray of the eye.* When ferrous metals remain in the eye they may cause immediate infection, or at a later date the deposition of ferrous salts in a process known as siderosis. This may eventually lead to blindness of the eye. Other metals also tend to give reactions, particularly copper and for this reason the metallic fragment should be removed (Fig. 16.4). This is achieved either by using intravitreous forceps under microscopic control or using a magnet. The exact surgical technique is planned beforehand once the foreign body has been accurately localised in the eye. Airgun pellets cause particu-

Fig. 16.4 A small metallic foreign body lying on the retina

larly severe eye injuries and the eye is often lost because of the extensive disruption at the time of the injury. Some intraocular foreign bodies such as glass particles or some alloys may be tolerated quite well and a decision may have to be made as to whether observation is preferable in the first instance. This especially applies when the sight of the eye remains good. When a foreign body is not to be removed immediately, many ophthalmologists would insert intravitreal antibiotics as a prophylactic measure against endophthalmitis. When a foreign body is found lying deeply in the cornea, its removal may result in loss of aqueous and collapse of the anterior chamber. It is prudent to arrange that removal should be done under full sterile conditions in the operating theatre where the corneal wound can be sutured if necessary.

Sympathetic Ophthalmia

This rare complication of perforation occurs in the previously unaffected fellow eye and is more common in children. Over a period of two weeks to several months or even years, a granulomatous inflammatory response begins in the uvea of the traumatised eye. Subsequently, a similar reaction occurs in the "normal" eye. The inflammation in both eyes can be so severe as to cause blindness. The condition does however respond well to steroid treatment and it is extremely rare. Occasionally one sees patients who have an artificial eye complaining of transient blurring of the vision of their remaining eye. They need to be examined carefully for signs of uveitis.

Injuries to the Eyelids

Loss or destruction of eyelid tissue should always be treated as a threat to vision. The upper lid especially is important in this respect. The immediate concern is to ensure that the cornea is properly covered when the eyelids are closed. If more than one third of the margin of the upper lid is lost, this must be replaced by grafting from the lower lid. When less than one third is missing, the gaping wound can usually be closed directly. Up to one third of the lower lid can also be closed by direct suturing. When more than this is lost or when it has been transferred to the upper lid, a slide of tissue from the lateral canthus can be effected, combined if necessary with a rotating cheek flap.

One of the most important features of the repair of lid injuries is the method of suturing. If the lid margin is involved, the repair should be made using the operating microscope and the fine suture material available in an eye department (Fig. 16.5). An untidy repair can result in a permanently watering eye due to kinking of the eyelid. This interferes with the proper moistening of the cornea during blinking or when asleep. Special attention must be paid when the medial part of the eyelid has been torn as this contains the lacrimal canaliculus. Again unless repair is carried out using an accurate technique under general anaesthesia in theatre then the risk of a permanently watering eye is increased.

Contusion of the eyelids, otherwise known as a black eye, is of course a common problem especially on Saturday nights in a general casualty department. Usually the presence of a black eye is an indication that the afflicted was smart enough to close his eye in time to avoid injury to the globe. It is unusual to find damage to the eyes after Saturday night fistfights, unless a weapon was involved. Broken beer glasses produce devastating injuries to the eyes as well as to the eyelids.

Fig. 16.5 Full thickness lower lid laceration

Injuries to the Orbit

Blows on the side of the cheek and across one or other eye occur in fights, industrial accidents and road traffic accidents. The most common type is the ' blow out fracture'. Here the globe and contents of the orbit are forced backward causing fracture of the orbital floor and displacement of bone downwards into the antrum of the maxillary sinus. The inferior rectus muscle becomes tethered in the wound so that there is mechanical limitation of upward movement. The infraorbital nerve which traverses the orbital floor may also be injured producing anaesthesia of the skin of the cheek. Once the surrounding swelling has subsided, the posterior displacement of the globe becomes obvious and the globe of the eye itself often shows evidence of contusion. A considerable improvement from the functional and cosmetic point of view can be obtained by positioning a plastic or Teflon implant in the floor of the orbit after freeing the prolapsed tissue.

Fractures of the skull, which extend into the orbit, may be accompanied by retro-orbital haemorrhage and proptosis. Cranial nerve palsies affecting the ocular movements are also commonly seen in this type of injury and the vision may be affected by optic nerve damage. A blow on the eye may result in sudden blindness with at first no other evidence of injury (apart from an afferent pupillary defect), but subsequently the optic disc becomes pale and atrophic after 2 or 3 weeks.

Radiational Injuries

The eyes may be exposed to a wide range of electromagnetic radiation from the shorter wavelength ultraviolet rays through the wavelengths of visible light to the longer infra-red waves, X-rays and microwaves. X-rays pass straight through the eye without being focused by the optical media and, in large enough doses may cause generalised damage. It is important to realise that therapeutic but not diagnostic doses of X-rays tend to cause cataracts and the eye must be suitably screened during treatment. Excessive doses of X-rays also cause stenosis of the lacrimal canaliculi, destruction of the secretary cells within the lacrimal glands and retinal neovascularisation. As one might expect, visible light does not normally damage the eyes, although an intense light source may be absorbed by the pigment epithelium behind the retina and converted to heat, producing a macula burn. After eclipses of the sun there are usually a number of patients who arrive in the casualty departments of eye hospitals with macular oedema and sometimes serious permanent impairment of visual acuity. Sun gazing with consequent retinal damage has been reported after taking LSD. The laser beam provides a source of intense light, which is used widely in ophthalmology as a deliberate means of producing gentle burns in the retina or making holes in the lens capsule after cataract surgery. However uncontrolled use of lasers can cause blinding foveal burns as the subject tends to look directly at the beam momentarily, until they realise what it is. Ultraviolet rays, which are shorter than visible light, do not normally penetrate the eye but in large enough doses produce burns of the eyelids and cornea. On the skin this is seen as erythema and later pigmentation, and on the cornea a punctate keratitis is seen with the slit lamp. Ultraviolet damage of this kind is seen after gazing with unprotected eyes at welder's arcs, after exposure of the eyes to sunray lamps, and after exposure to the sun under certain conditions such as in snow on mountain tops. All these types of ultraviolet injury show a delayed effect, the symptoms appearing 2 or 3 h after exposure and lasting for about 48 h. There is usually severe pain and photophobia so that it may not be possible to open the eyes, hence the term 'snow blindness'. The use of locally applied steroid and antibiotic drops hastens recovery.

Unlike ultraviolet light, infrared rays penetrate the eye and can cause cataract. A specific kind of thermal cataract has been well described in glassblowers and furnace workers but this is now rarely seen due to the use of protective goggles. Microwaves, in the form of diathermy, can cause cataract but the eye must be in the path of the beam if damage is to occur, and microwave ovens would not be expected to be dangerous in this respect. Concern is quite often expressed in the press or elsewhere about the possibility of radiation damage to the eyes from visual display units. Such damage has never been demonstrated any more than it has from the face of a television set. Someone not used to working with a VDU who is suddenly made to spend several hours a day in front of one may experience eyestrain especially if incorrect spectacles are worn.

Chemical Injuries

These are quite common but usually not severe enough to warrant hospital attention. In industrial premises there is now nearly always a first aid post with facilities to wash out the eyes. Plain water or a salt solution is the best fluid to use and valuable time may be lost if washing is delayed in order to search for a specific antidote. More severe burns can result from the catalysts used in the manufacture of plastics or from alkalis such as caustic soda. Alkalis penetrate the eye rapidly as they saponify lipids within cell membranes aiding passage, and can quickly reach the posterior segment. Acid burns as from exploding car batteries are quite commonly seen in large casualty departments but are usually less severe as acids tend to coagulate corneal proteins thereby slowing penetration.

Summary

Trauma to the eyes and orbit, although relatively uncommon, can lead to devastating visual loss. Tissue can be damaged such as by a corneal laceration from a sharp insrtrument or indirectly such as the optic nerve damage in traumatic optic neuropathy. Correct management and diagnosis requires a careful and systemic examination technique so as not to miss potentially damaging sympathetic ophthalmia.

Part IV

Problems of the Medical Ophthalmologist

Testing Visual Acuity

17

Abstract

This chapter describes how visual acuity is tested clinically. It outlines the basic principles involved in the design and clinical recording and interpretation of these different tests, as well as indicates the tests that are available for children and illiterate persons. A basic introduction to refraction and auto-refraction is given.

Keywords

Visual acuity Snellen chart LogMAR chart Optokinetic drum 'E' test Preferential looking Refraction

Introduction

Measurement of visual acuity is the most important, quantifiable part of the ocular assessment performed by the doctor and yet it is surprising how often the non-specialist omits it in examination. It has already been shown that the differential diagnosis of the red eye can be simplified by noting the vision in the affected eye. After injuries of the eye it is just as important to note the vision in the uninjured eye as it is to note that in the injured eye. Simple measurement of visual acuity is of course, of limited value without knowledge of the spectacle correction or whether the patient is wearing the appropriate spectacles or not. The best corrected visual acuity (i.e. with lenses in place) therefore needs to be recorded for each eye. This corrected visual acuity can also be estimated with a pinhole held in front of the eye. The effect of the pinhole is to eliminate the effect of refraction by the cornea and the lens on the extremely thin beam of light produced by the pinhole.

Measuring the visual acuity means measuring the function of the macula, which is of course only a small part of the whole retina. A patient may have grossly impaired visual acuity and yet have a normal visual field enabling him to walk about and lead a normal life apart from being able to read. This state of affairs is seen in patients with age-related macular degeneration or macular dystrophies, and can be compared with the situation in which a patient has grossly constricted visual fields but normal macular function, as is sometimes seen in retinitis pigmentosa or advanced primary open angle glaucoma. Here the patient appears to be blind, being unable to find his way about, but he may surprise the ophthalmologist by reading the visual acuity chart from top to bottom once he has found it.

The simplest way to measure visual acuity might be to determine the ability to distinguish two points when placed very close together (resolution). Such a method was supposed to have been used by the Arabs when choosing their horsemen. They chose only those who were able to resolve the two stars which form the second 'star' in the tail of the Great Bear constellation. A point source of light such as a star, although it is infinitely small, forms an image with a diameter of about 11 μm on the retina. This is because the optical media are not perfect and allow some scattering of the light. In practice it is possible for a person with normal vision to distinguish two points apart if they are separated by 1 mm when placed 10 m away. Two such points would be separated by 2 μm on the retina. This might be surprising considering that a spot of light casts a minimum size of image of 11 μm due to scatter, but such an image is not uniform, being brighter in the centre than at the periphery. In fact, the resolving power of the eye is limited by the size of the cones, which have a diameter of 1.5 μm.

The principles and different ways of testing visual acuity in different persons are summarized in Tables 17.1 and 17.2.

Table 17.1 Testing visual acuity

Methods	• Tests used dependent on age/ability/cooperation of patient • For adults adopt Snellen type or LogMAR charts • Younger pre-verbal children = Orthoptist judges whether the child has seen the stimulus or not • Many qualitative assessments of whether a child can see or not • Fixing and following a light • Reaching for small toys
Why necessary?	• Need quantitative assessments • Monitor visual development in children • Quantify any increase/decrease in visual acuity • Determine and monitor treatment efficacy • Disease progression
Principles	• Need to test visual acuity UNIOCULARLY (one eye at a time), otherwise you will NEVER detect amblyopia—a visual acuity test with both eyes open only represents the visual acuity in the good eye • Importance of crowded vision tests Crowded tests = letters or pictures in a line • On a chart with other lines of letters/pictures above & below • One row of letters/pictures with a surrounding box Harder to detect crowded letters/pictures More accurate visual acuity test Patients with amblyopia often have 'crowding': Able to identify single letters well, but will struggle to identify letters in a line

Table 17.2 Visual Acuity Tests in children

1. Preferential Looking	• Used for young babies • 40 cm test distance • Uses black and white square wave gratings against a grey background • Gratings of decreasing width = higher spatial frequency (harder to see the gratings against the grey background) • Child looks towards the gratings if seen
2. Kay pictures (now in crowded form, measured in LogMAR units)	• Used for young verbal children • 3 m test distance • Four pictures in a line, surrounded by a box = crowded • Child names the pictures (can match pictures)
3. Cardiff acuity chart	• Gross test based on preferential looking, and that child will look at picture rather than plain background • Used mainly for screening in paediatric patients (12–36 months) • Consists of single picture objects: House, fish, boat etc. • Pictures are in black and white against a grey background • Test done at 1 m or 50 cm • Examiner watches the child's eye movements, up or down to estimate gaze direction: In direction of picture • Results may be recorded in Snellen, LogMAR or decimal notation

Table 17.2 (continued)

4. Stycar test	• Similar to Kay • Done at 3–6 m with different sized pictures • Based on Snellen principle • Chart consists of pictures of food items or toys
5. Sheridan Gardiner test	• Used in children 2–6 years old • Test done at 6 meters (or 3, if the VA is worse than 6/60) • Consists of letters HOTV at different sizes • Child given a card with the letters arranged to give correct orientation, and asked to match them against those on the main chart
6. LogMAR crowded/ uncrowded (measured in LogMAR units)	• Used to test distance vision in school going children and adults • Crowded: Four letters in a line, surrounded by a box • Uncrowded: Single letters (no crowding) • Used for young children more familiar with letters/shapes • 3 m test distance • Child can name/match letters

In the clinic, the distance visual acuity is measured by asking the patient to read a standard set of letters (called 'optotypes'), traditionally the Snellen chart. This is placed at a distance of 6 m from the eye. The single large letter at the top of this chart is designed to be just discernible to a normally sighted person at a range of 60 m. If the patient's vision is so poor that only this and no smaller letter can be seen at 6 m, then the vision is recorded as the fraction '6/60'. The normal-sighted person who can read the chart down to the smaller letters designed to be discerned at 6 m is recorded as having a visual acuity of 6/6. The normal range of vision extends between 6/4 and 6/9 depending on the patient's age. In some European countries, the visual acuity is expressed as a decimal instead of a fraction. Therefore 6/60 would be expressed as 0.1. In the USA, metres are replaced by feet, therefore 6/6 becomes 20/20. This is where the term "twenty twenty" vision originates from, meaning clear or near perfect vision.

The Snellen VA chart (Fig. 3.1), although the most commonly used measure of VA to date, exhibits well recognised design flaws. Such flaws include the non-geometric progression of letter sizes and the variable number of letters on each line which reduces test-retest variability, lack of systematic approach to letter legibility and crowding. The Snellen unequal visual demand at each level of visual acuity, i.e. one letter at 6/60 level, two letters at 6/36 level, seven or eight letters at 6/6 level (referred to as the "pyramid" shape of the Snellen chart). The

Fig. 17.1 LogMAR visual acuity chart

unequal distance between the letters, and between the lines of letters. Furthermore, the Snellen fraction notation is not easily subjected to statistical analysis, compared to a logarithmic system.

The LogMAR chart (also called the Bailey-Lovie chart, after Ian Bailey and Jan E. Lovie-Kitchin who co-designed it) was recently introduced into clinical practice (Fig. 17.1). The Early Treatment Diabetic Retinopathy Study

(ETDRS) chart is a specific type of logMAR chart developed for the ETDRS studies. It initially started as mainly a research tool, and was designed to provide more accurate estimates of visual acuity compared to traditional vision charts (including Snellen). It is more standardised and scientifically accurate measurement of visual acuity. The test is normally performed at 4 m, although it can be done at 1, 2, and 3 m, with appropriate allowance for the test distance in the test score.

The logMAR chart comprises rows of five letters (optotypes) whose size is scored with reference to the Logarithm of the Minimum Angle of Resolution (logMAR). There is a logarithmic progression of letter size and the distances between each letter and each line. This ensures an equal visual demand at each level of visual acuity, i.e. five letters on each line. Each letter has a score value of 0.02 log units. The total score for a line (of five letters) on the LogMAR chart represents a change of 0.1 log units. An eye which can resolve details as small as 1 min of visual angle scores LogMAR 0 (the base-10 logarithm of 1 is 0).

LogMAR VA is also available in 'reduced forms'.

Examples of Snellen and logMAR VA correlations are listed below:

- 6/6 Snellen or 0.0 LogMAR = 'normal' visual acuity.
- 6/12 Snellen or 0.3 LogMAR = UK minimum driving test VA requirement.
- 6/60 Snellen or 1.0 LogMAR = defective visual acuity (significantly reduced).
- 6/5 Snellen or—0.1 LogMAR = better than 'normal' visual acuity.

There are also smaller differences in type size between lines. The spacing between 2 lines is equal to the size of letters in the previous line. LogMAR vision is measured at 4 m usually, but can be measured at any distance, as long as this distance is recorded appropriately. Some of the advantages of using this new chart are that the measurement of poor visual acuity is more accurate as more larger letters are included and small

Fig. 17.2 Near reading type chart

changes in acuity are easier to detect (easier to detect disease progression or treatment success).

The near visual acuity is also measured using a standard range of reading types in the style of newsprint (Fig. 17.2). Here care must be taken to ensure that the correct spectacles for near work (reading glasses) are used if the patient is over the age of 45. (Fig. 17.3). LogMAR VA is also available for near vision measurements. Normally the results of testing the near visual acuity are in agreement with those for measuring distance vision providing the correct spectacles (for distance ['driving glasses'] or near ['reading glasses'] are worn if needed.

The visual acuity of each eye must always be measured by placing a card carefully over one eye and then transferring this to the other eye when the first eye has been tested. The visual acuity of both eyes together is usually the same or fractionally better than the vision of the better of the two eyes tested individually. In certain special circumstances the binocular vision may be worse than the vision of each eye tested sepa-

The news print these days isn't what
it used to be. . . .

Fig 17.3 Need for reading glasses in presbyopia

rately (e.g. in cases of macular disease causing
distortion).

A number of other tests have been developed
to measure visual acuity in the non-literate
patient. Infants below the reading age can be
measured with surprising accuracy using the
Stycar test. Here, letters of differing size are
shown to the child, who is asked to point to the
same letter on the card, which is given to him. Up
to the age of 18 months or 2 years, the optokinetic drum may be used. This makes use of the
phenomenon of optokinetic nystagmus produced
by moving a set of vertically arranged stripes
across the line of sight. When the stripes are sufficiently narrow, they are no longer visible and
fail to produce any nystagmus. The eyes are
examined using a graded series of stripes. This
kind of test can be used to measure visual acuity
in animals other than man. Other tests used in

pre-school children include the Sheridan-
Gardiner, Kay, or Cardiff Acuity cards which are
summarized in Table 17.2. The 'E' test is a way
of measuring the visual acuity of illiterate
patients. This is based on the Snellen type but the
patient is presented with a series of letter 'E's of
different sizes and orientations and is given a
wooden letter 'E' to hold in the hands. He is then
instructed to turn the wooden letter to correspond
with the letter indicated on the chart. Similar
optotypes with breaks in a ring called Landolt's
ring are available for non-literate persons.

The visual acuity charts have the great advantage of being widely used and well standardised,
but it must be realised that such measurement is a
measure of something more complex than simply
the function of the macula area of the retina. It
involves a degree of literacy and also speech, and
testing shy children or elderly patients may
sometimes be misleading.

Other ways of measuring visual acuity other
than letters have been developed. Another way is
to assess the patient's the ability to resolve a grating. Here, the word 'grating' refers to a row of
black and white stripes where the black merges
gradually into the white. Such a grating can be
varied by altering either the contrast of black and
white or the width of the stripes (the 'frequency').
Thus for a given individual, the threshold for
contrast and frequency (contrast sensitivity) can
be measured. This type of test has certain theoretical advantages over standard methods but it is
not widely used clinically as a routine. Finally,
the electrical potentials generated by the retina
and optic nerve (visual evoked potentials) may be
measured to give an estimate of visual acuity
when the eye is presented with targets of varying
size and contrast. This method is useful in infants
and in the assessment of adults with non-organic
visual loss.

Measuring for Spectacles

If a patient has not been recently tested for spectacles, then not only may the measurement of
visual acuity be inaccurate, but the presenting
symptoms may be due to the need for a correct

pair of glasses. The measurement, which deter-
mines the type of spectacles needed, requires skill
developed by practice and the use of the right
equipment. The most obvious way to measure
someone for a pair of glasses is to try the effect of
different lenses and ask the patient whether the
letters are seen better with one lens or another.
This is known as subjective testing and by itself it
is not a very accurate method because some
patients' observations as to the clarity of letters
may be unreliable. Furthermore, a healthy young
person may see quite clearly with a wide range of
lenses simply be exercising the ciliary muscle (i.e.
accommodation). Fortunately the refractive error
of the eye can be measured by an objective method
and an answer can be reached without consulting
the patient. The method entails observing the rate
of movement of the shadow of the iris against the
red reflex from the fundus of the eye after interposing different strengths of lenses (retinoscopy).
In order to make an accurate measurement of the
spectacle requirement, both objective and subjective refractions are performed and the results
compared.

Objective Refraction

The patient is fitted with a spectacle trial frame
into which different lenses can be slotted. In the
case of young children it is usually advisable to
instill a mydriatic and cycloplegic drop beforehand to eliminate focusing (accommodation).
The adult patient is asked to look at the topmost
letter on the distance vision chart e.g. Snellen) or
a light spot on the chart. The ophthalmologist
then views the eye to be examined through an
instrument known as a retinoscope, from a distance of about one arm's length. The red reflex
can be seen and the instrument is then moved
slightly so that the light projected from the retinoscope moves to and fro across the pupil. The
shadow of the iris on the red reflex is then seen to
move, and the direction and speed of movement
depend on the refractive error of the patient. By
interposing different lenses in the trial frame, the
movement of the iris shadow can be 'neutralised'
and the exact refractive error determined. The

trial frame can accommodate both spherical and
cylindrical lenses so that the amount of astigmatism can be measured.

Subjective Refraction

Here, considerable skill is also needed because
many patients become quite tense when being
tested in this way and may not initially give accurate answers. Lenses, both stronger and weaker
than the expected requirement, are placed in the
trial frames and the patient is asked to read the
letters of the distance (e.g. Snellen) chart and to
say whether they are more or less clear. A number
of supplementary tests are available which enable
one to check the patients' answers. It can be seen
that the word 'refraction' refers to the total test
for glasses, although the same word refers to the
bending of the rays of light as they pass from one
medium to another. Accurate refraction takes 10
or 15 min to perform, or longer in difficult cases
and it is an essential preliminary to an examination of the eye itself.

Automated Refraction

In recent years attempts have been made to develop
an automated system of refraction, and instruments are now commercially available. They are,
however, still expensive and not always accurate
when there are opacities in the optical media, or
when the patient over-accommodates. One further
way of assessing the refractive error without asking the patient any questions is by making use of
the visually evoked response. This is the name
given to the minute electrical changes detectable
over the back of the scalp when the eyes are
exposed to a repeated stimulus, usually a flashing
chequerboard. When fine checks are viewed, interposing different lenses can modify the response.
This method is of great interest but it is still not
very reliable and takes time to perform.

Considering the importance of the measurement of visual acuity, it is not surprising that a
number of tests have been developed for this, but
the simple Snellen chart remains an essential part

of any doctors' surgery (especially the general practitioner). It must be remembered that this is a measure of function in the centre of the visual field only, and it is possible to have advanced loss of peripheral vision with normal visual acuity as is seen sometimes in patients with chronic glaucoma or retinitis pigmentosa. The assessment of the rest of the visual field has also been standardised and a number of instruments have been developed to measure it. These have already been described in Chap. 3 together with various other measurements of different aspects of visual function.

Summary

After completing this chapter, the reader should appreciate the importance of measuring visual acuity, and the different methods that are used in clinical practice. The salient points are:

• Measuring visual acuity is the most important part of the ocular assessment performed in an ophthalmic examination by the specialist and non-specialist practitioner. It indicates to the ophthalmologist how good the resolving power of the eye is, and is compared to the normal for the patient's age.

• The visual acuity is dependent on the resolving power of the fovea, but is influenced by medial opacities and refractive errors.

• The traditional Snellen chart has been complemented with logMAR chart which is more standardised and scientifically accurate measurement of visual acuity.

• Appropriate tests for non-literate persons, including children, and illiterate adults are available.

• Appropriate correction at distance and near vision should therefore be worn before this resolving power (visual acuity) of the eye is determined.

• The power of spectacles can be measured by a trained person.

• The refraction can be determined objectively, and subjectively.

• Auto-refractors are available.

The Inflamed Eye

18

Abstract

This chapter deals with inflammatory conditions that affect the different parts of the eye, from different aetiologies, including trauma, allergy, infections and non-infectious ('auto-immune') conditions. It highlights uveitis, but in addition, the sclera and the episclera i.e. the more superficial coats of the eye may also be affected by similar inflammatory changes. Causes, clinical features of the different types of inflammation, their investigation and treatment are described.

In an earlier chapter we have already seen that 'the red eye' is an important sign in ophthalmology, and there are a number of reasons why the eye may become inflamed. When the exposed parts of the eye such as the conjunctiva and the cornea are the primary sites of inflammation, the cause is usually infection, allergy or trauma. Common examples are chronic conjunctivitis or a corneal foreign body. Here we will consider a type of inflammation, which arises, deeper in the eye and primarily from the uvea. The uvea has a tendency to become inflamed for no apparent external reason and in this respect can be compared to a joint; indeed, there is a recognised association between uveitis and arthritis. In spite of the fact that the eye is open to microscopic examination, the exact cause of uveitis is usually obscure, although there is evidence to indicate a relationship with other kinds of auto-immune disease. Uveitis can be divided into anterior, intermediate or posterior uveitis depending on which part of the uvea is predominantly involved. Anterior uveitis is the same entity as iritis or iridocyclitis, and is when the inflammation predominantly affects the anterior chamber and iris; intermediate uveitis, the same as pars planitis is where the vitreous and ciliary body are predominantly affected; posterior uveitis is the same as choroiditis, and refers to inflammation predominantly involving the choroid (and retina).

Apart from the uvea, the sclera and the episclera (that is, the connective tissue deep to the conjunctiva and overlying the sclera) i.e. the more superficial coats of the eye may also be affected by similar inflammatory changes.

The Role of Autoimmunity in Uveitis

Although it has been long recognised that bacterial and viral infection may account for some cases of uveitis, it is also recognised that the majority of cases fail to show any evidence of this. Furthermore, in many instances the eye disease may be associated with known autoimmune disease elsewhere in the body. There are several different ways in which the uvea might be expected to become the focus of an antigen-antibody reaction. A foreign agent such as a virus might reside in the uvea and cause an antibody response, which coincidentally involves uveal tissue, or, on the other hand, a foreign agent might react with specific marker on the cell membrane to produce a new active antigen. It is now recognised that patients who inherit certain of the human leucocyte antigens (HLA) are more susceptible to particular types of uveitis, for example the uveitis seen in ankylosing spondylitis and Reiter's disease (HLA B27), and birdshot choriodoretinopathy (HLA A29). It has been suggested that HLA may act as the specific marker in these cases. A further way in which the uvea might become the centre of an immune response concerns the question of self-recognition. It now appears that there is a mechanism in the body, which normally prevents antibodies in the serum from acting against our own tissues. This active suppression is maintained by a population of thymus-derived lymphocytes (T lymphocytes) known as T-suppressor cells. There is evidence to suggest that sympathetic ophthalmitis might arise from inhibition of the T-suppressor cells after uveal antigens have been introduced into the bloodstream. Patients with juvenile rheumatoid arthritis may develop uveitis, whereas rheumatoid disease in adults is more commonly associated with the dry eye syndrome and episcleritis. The causes of uveitis can be infectious or non-infectious (Table 18.1). A significant proportion (up to 70–80% of anterior uveitis, and 60% of posterior uveitis) of non-infectious uveitis is idiopathic. However, this conclusion should be arrived at only after excluding all known potential associations.

Anterior Uveitis

Anterior uveitis refers to inflammation affecting the iris (anterior uvea). When the ciliary body is inflamed at the same time, the condition is referred to as iridocyclitis (as described above).

Table 18.1 Common causes of anterior and posterior uveitis

Non –infectious uveitis	Infectious uveitis
• Idiopathic	• Parasitic
• Sarcoidosis	– Toxoplasmosis
• Bechets' disease	– Toxocariasis
• HLA B27 Associated disease (Reiter's, Ankylosing Spondylitis, Psoriasis)	– Onchocerchiasis
	• Fungal
	– Candida
	– Cryptococcus
• Juvenile Idiopathic Arthritis	– Histoplasmosis
• Birdshot Choroidoretinopathy (HLA A29 associated)	• Bacterial
	– Syphilis
	– Tuberculosis
	– Lyme disease
• Bowel diseases (ulcerative colitis, Crohn's and Whipple's' Diseases)'	– Cat-scratch
	– Leprosy
	• Viral
• Sympathetic ophthalmitis	– HSV
	– HZV
• Specific entities (MEWDS, PIC, MF)	– CMV
	– Ebola
• Others	• Others

Symptoms

The patient suffering from acute anterior uveitis is usually aware that there is something seriously amiss with the eye. The vision is blurred and the eye aches and often, may be extremely painful. Photophobia is usual and often the pain may worsen on focusing on near objects. The age incidence is wide but anterior uveitis is commonly seen in the third and fourth decades of life, and every eye casualty officer becomes very familiar with this particular form. When the disease presents for the first time in the elderly, the underlying cause is likely to be different and age provides an important diagnostic feature. In children, anterior uveitis may occur as a complication of juvenile rheumatoid arthritis, especially the pauci-articular type. Occasionally, it can complicate an acute viral illness or sarcoidosis in children. Acute anterior uveitis usually appears quite suddenly over a period of about 24 h and then resolves on treatment in 2 or 3 weeks; however, it may last as long as 6 weeks in some cases. A further exacerbation may occur during this period and there is a strong tendency towards recurrence after a few months or several years in the same or the other eye, depending on the cause.

Signs

The eye is red, but of especial importance is the presence of a pink flush around the cornea (the ciliary flush) which indicates an inflammatory process either in the cornea or within the anterior chamber of the eye itself. The pupil is small because the iris sphincter goes into spasm. Thus the pupil of iritis is small and treatment is aimed at making it larger, whereas the pupil of acute glaucoma is large and treatment is aimed at making it smaller. Unless there is secondary glaucoma, the cornea remains bright and clear, but with a pen torch it may be possible to see that the aqueous looks turbid. That is to say, a beam of light shone through the aqueous resembles a beam of sunlight shining through a dusty room. (Fig. 18.1). Normally, of course, the aqueous is crystal clear even when examined with the slit lamp biomicroscope or pen torch.

The presence of an occasional cell in the aqueous may be normal, especially if the pupil has

Fig 18.2 Keratic precipitates

been dilated with mydriatic eye drops, but suspicion should be raised if more than three or four cells are seen. In fact the early diagnosis of anterior uveitis can entail very careful slit-lamp examination. It is usual to discriminate between the presence of cells in the aqueous and the presence of flare. The latter reflects a high protein content and is a feature of more long-standing disease. Because there are convection currents in the aqueous, inflammatory cells are swept down the centre of the posterior surface of the cornea and become adherent to it, often forming a triangular-shaped spread of deposits known as keratic precipitates, or 'KP's. (Fig. 18.2) The microscopic appearance of the KP is determined by the type of cells. If a granulomatous type of inflammatory reaction is taking place involving epithelioid cells and macrophages, then the KP may be large, resembling oil droplets ('mutton fat KP'). This form of KP is seen in uveitis associated with sarcoidosis and also tuberculosis and leprosy. When the inflammation is non-granulomatous, a fine dusting of the posterior surface of the cornea may be evident. KPs tend to become absorbed over time but they may remain more permanently as pigmented spots on the endothelium.

Anterior uveitis is often associated with the formation of adhesions between the posterior surface of the iris and the anterior capsule of the lens. These adhesions are called posterior synechiae and become evident when attempts are made to dilate the pupil since parts of the iris

Fig 18.1 Flare

Fig 18.3 (**a**) Hypopyon. In addition, there are red blood cells and fi brinous exudate in the anterior chamber (with acknowledgement to Professor HS Dua). (**b**) 360° of posterior synechiae

remain stuck to the pupil giving it an irregular appearance. In severe cases of anterior uveitis, pus may collect in the anterior chamber to the extent that a fluid level may be seen where the layer of pus has formed inferiorly. This is known as hypopyon—literally, 'pus below'. (Fig. 18.3a). A hypopyon is an indication of severe disease in the eye and the patient should be, preferably, treated in hospital as an in-patient. Hypopyon tends to occur in certain specific types of anterior uveitis. It is occasionally seen in elderly diabetics with inadequately treated corneal ulcers, particularly those with vascular occlusive disease. It is also seen in Behcet's disease, which is a rare disorder characterized by hypopyon uveitis, and ulceration of the mouth and genitalia. A hypopyon is occasionally seen following cataract surgery and in such cases may often be infective in origin, although it could be non-infective. It is fortunately a rare complication of modern cataract surgery, with the use of intraocular lenses, strict asepsis, and prophylactic and post-operative use of antibiotics.

Complications

The visual prognosis of acute anterior uveitis as commonly seen in young people is usually good unless recurrences are frequent. Chronic uveitis is more prone to complications. Secondary glaucoma may cause serious problems and a careful

check on the intraocular pressure must be maintained. The rise in intraocular pressure may be due to direct obstruction of the aqueous outflow by inflammatory cells or by the presence of adhesions between the peripheral part of the iris and the posterior surface of the cornea (peripheral anterior synechiae). Sometimes, especially when treatment has been inadequate, the pupil margins adhere to the anterior surface of the lens (posterior synechiae). Posterior synechiae can become extensive enough to obstruct the passage of aqueous through the pupil (Fig. 18.3b). The iris bulges forwards (due to pressure of the trapped aqueous humor behind the iris) giving the appearance known as iris bombe. Secondary glaucoma may also result from the use of topical steroids in predisposed individuals. Cataract is a further serious complication, which may appear after repeated attacks of anterior uveitis. It nearly always first affects the posterior subcapsular zone of the lens and unfortunately interferes with the vision at an early stage. Cataracts may also result from long term use of topical or systemic steroids.

Causes

For the majority of patients who present to eye out-patient departments with this condition, no specific cause is found. However, there are many known causative agents. The ophthalmologist is obliged to exclude at least some of these although he/she knows that more often than not a negative result will be obtained. It is necessary to explain this to patients otherwise considerable anxiety may be created by the fact that 'no cause can be found' for their complaint. When we say no cause can be found we really mean that there is no evidence of any associated systemic disease and this should be of some reassurance to the patient.

As has already been mentioned, it is helpful to consider the age of the patient when trying to eliminate the possibility of underlying systemic disease. Uveitis is very rare in young children, but when seen, the possibility of juvenile rheumatoid arthritis or an antecedent must be borne in mind. In young adults sarcoidosis, gonorrhoea, Reiter's disease and ankylosing spondylitis are all recognised associations. In former years tuberculosis was very high on the list of suspected causes but this would appear to be a less common cause nowadays (although not eradicated). Herpes Simplex and Zoster may also cause anterior uveitis. Septic foci in adjacent structures, such as dental sepsis or sinusitis, have also been under suspicion but these are now thought to be relatively unimportant. In the case of the elderly, the onset of anterior uveitis may prove to be a recurrence of previous attacks and the same underlying causes must be suspected, but here there is also the possibility of lens-induced uveitis associated with by hypermature cataract.

Management

Once the diagnosis has been made, it is usual to embark on a number of investigations, guided in part by the history and taking into account especially any previous chest or joint disease (Table 18.2). It is mandatory to dilate the pupil in all eyes with presumed anterior uveitis. Such dilatation allows adequate examination of the posterior segment in order to exclude involvement of the posterior segment. An x-ray of chest, and a blood count including measurement of the ESR are routine in most clinics, but the expense of further investigations is now often spared if the patient appears completely fit and well in other respects. The history and background of the patient may lead one to suspect the possibility of sexually transmitted disease. In the case of some infective types of anterior uveitis, the diagnosis is usually made before the uveitis appears because the condition occurs as a secondary event. This is the case following herpes simplex keratitis and also in patients with herpes zoster affecting the upper division of the fifth cranial nerve. By contrast, anterior uveitis may be an important clue to the diagnosis of a sexually transmitted disease.

The treatment involves the administration of local steroids and mydriatic drops. When the condition is severe, a subconjunctival injection of steroid should be given and relief of symptoms may be further achieved by local heat in the form of a warm compress. Atropine is the mydriatic of first choice except in the mildest cases when homatropine or cyclopentolate drops may be used. Steroid drops should be administered every hour during the acute stage and then gradually tailed off over a period of a few weeks. Systemic steroids are not usually indicated and should be reserved for those cases in which the sight becomes seriously jeopardised. If any underlying systemic disease is identified, then of course, this should also be treated where effective treatment is available. The proper management of anterior uveitis demands the expertise of an ophthalmologist and, when the condition is severe and affecting both eyes, it may occasionally become necessary to admit the patient to hospital (Table 18.3).

Table 18.2 Investigations in uveitis

- Ocular Examination
- Fundus Examination of both eyes, with pupillary dilatation—mandatory even for presumed isolated anterior uveitis
- Laboratory investigations based on clinical findings and presumed clinical diagnosis

Table 18.3 Management of non-infectious uveitis

Treatment choice dependent on
- Anatomic location of inflammation: anterior/intermediate/posterior uveitis
- Laterality
- Age/Sex
- General health
- Patient wishes and compliance
- Potential benefit

A special word of warning is needed for those patients who have undergone previous intraocular surgery, including glaucoma draining surgery. For these patients what is normally a mild infective conjunctivitis may lead to intraocular infection through a compromised drainage site. The development of anterior uveitis, weeks, and occasionally even years, after the operation, can indicate disastrous consequences if urgent and intensive antibiotic treatment is not applied.

One specific type of anterior uveitis (called heterochromic iridocyclitis) must be mentioned at this stage.

Heterochromic Iridocyclitis (Fuch's)

This type of anterior uveitis presents commonly in 20–40 year olds and is usually unilateral. The vision becomes blurred and the iris becomes depigmented. Sometimes it may take several years for the diagnosis to be made. The eye usually remains white, the inflammatory reaction is low grade and chronic; posterior synechiae do not develop. As such mydriasis is not required. However, the inflammation may respond to topical treatment with steroids as the spillover of cells into the anterior chamber is curtailed. Intravitreal steroid therapy may be useful if the inflammation is complicated by cystoid macular oedema. Cataracts and chronic glaucoma occur very commonly. The condition has been mimicked by denervating the sympathetic supply of the eyes in experimental animals and it seems possible that there may be a neurological cause, unrelated and distinct from other types of uveitis.

Intermediate Uveitis (Pars Planitis)

Intermediate uveitis refers to an inflammatory response, predominantly affecting the intermediate uvea (ciliary body) usually seen in young adults, which may vary from low grade to severe. It affects both eyes in up to 80% of cases, although the severity may be asymmetrical. There may be minimal to moderate evidence of anterior uveitis, where there is significant spillover of inflammatory cells. The patient usually complains of floating spots in front of the vision, and in the later stages blurring of vision. Fundus examination reveals vitreous opacities (including inflammatory cells), and careful inspection of the peripheral retina shows whitish exudates in the overlying vitreous base (described as 'snow banking'), or in the vitreous ('snow balls') especially inferiorly. A mild to moderate peripheral retinal phlebitis may occur. The condition runs a chronic course and occasionally may be complicated by cataract, cystoid macular oedema and tractional retinal detachment. The cause of intermediate uveitis is unknown in the majority of cases although there is a known association with sarcoidosis and multiple sclerosis.

Treatment and Management

The investigations recommended here are similar to those for anterior uveitis.

In the mild forms of intermediate uveitis, management is observation. However, when the condition is complicated by cystoid macular oedema, or optic disc swelling, or the vitreous debris is significantly symptomatic, treatment is recommended with systemic steroids or intravitreal steroids. Steroid sparing systemic immunosuppression may be helpful. Associated systemic disease, including sarcoidosis and multiple sclerosis, where present, should be appropriately treated.

Posterior Uveitis

Inflammation of the choroid is referred to as choroiditis or posterior uveitis. Often the inflammation spreads from choroid to overlying retina and then to the vitreous. Alternatively the inflammation may originate from the retina and spread to involve the choroid and vitreous subsequently.

Symptoms

When the choroid, as opposed to the ciliary body and iris, becomes inflamed, the eye is not usually painful or red and the patient complains of blurring or loss of vision, which may vary. If the focus of choroiditis remains peripheral, then the disease may remain unnoticed, as is witnessed by the relatively frequent observation of isolated healed foci in the fundi of asymptomatic patients. Spread of inflammation from choroid and retina to the vitreous, results in vitreous floaters (from cells and debris). When this happens the vision becomes markedly blurred, even when the original focus is remote from the macula region. Choroiditis (or chorioretinitis) at the macula itself usually leads to permanent loss of central vision as damage to the cone photoreceptors is usually irreversible.

Signs

In its early stages, choroiditis may be seen as a grey or yellowish raised area which may be discrete or multiple and anywhere in the fundus. In the mild or early stages of the disease the vitreous may be fairly clear to allow a good view of the fundus. As the disease progresses, a cellular reac-

tion may appear in the overlying vitreous, seen as localised misting with the ophthalmoscope, and eventually the whole vitreous may become clouded, obscuring any view of the fundus and the original site of inflammation. The patient usually presents at this stage so that the origin of the problem only becomes apparent after the inflammation has subsided. Retinitis manifests as an indistinct white cloudy area. When a patch of choroiditis heals, the margins become pigmented and a white patch of bare sclera remains (Fig. 18.4a). This is the result of atrophy of the pigment epithelium and choroid. Sometimes larger choroidal vessels survive as a clearly seen network overlying the white sclera surrounded by a pigment halo. During the active stage, inspection of the vitreous with the slit lamp reveals the presence of cells and very often the anterior chamber also contains cells. Posterior uveitis comes into the differential diagnosis of a white eye with failing vision. When the vitreous becomes cloudy the condition must be distinguished from vitreous haemorrhage. The latter nearly always occurs acutely over a period of hours, whereas the cloudiness following uveitis takes a few days to develop. Examination of the vitreous with the slit lamp can reveal whether the vitreous is filled with inflammatory cells or red cells. Retinal vasculitis may occur. A predomi-

Fig. 18.4 Chorioretinitis. (**a**) active inflammation with hazy vitreous; (**b**) inactive scar

nantly retinal arteriolar inflammation indicates a viral cause whereas venous involvement is more common with other aetiologies. Macular oedema, or optic nerve inflammation and/or oedema may also occur.

Causes

As in the case of anterior uveitis, it is often impossible to pinpoint any systemic cause and the condition seems to be confined to the eye. However, a number of systemic associations have been recognised and often are related to specific types of posterior uveitis (Table 18.1). The fundus appearance may provide a clue to the cause of the inflammation.

Management

The fundus appearance may give a clue to the diagnosis, although this is not always possible and laboratory investigations may be necessary refine the diagnosis, and guide treatment.

Non-infectious posterior uveitis is treated when the condition is complicated by cystoid macular oedema, optic disc swelling, or the vitreous debris is significantly symptomatic enough to aggravate the patient or impair the visual acuity, or if the lesion is close to and threatens the fovea. Systemic steroids are the usual first line therapy, and may be supplemented with intravitreal steroids. Large doses of systemic steroids are best administered, sometimes, on admission to hospital. This has the added advantage of allowing a more detailed pre-treatment examination and investigations, and often the opinion of a general physician or immunologist (as part of a multidisciplinary team [MDT]) may be valuable at this stage. Secondary glaucoma may also need to be treated as necessary.

Increased interest in immunological diseases in recent years, which has accompanied advances in tissue grafting and cancer research, has led to attempts to treat uveitis with means other than steroids. Immunosuppressive agents, given systemically, e.g. cyclosporin A, tacrolimus, azathioprine, cyclophosphamide, methotrexate, mycophenolate mofetil and biologics including anti-TNF drugs (including adalimumab) are now sometimes used to supplement or replace systemic steroids in difficult cases.

The infectious causes of uveitis have specific therapies directed at the pathologic agent, and are described below with each specific entity.

Specific Uveitis Entities

Toxoplasmosis

Toxoplasma gondii is a parasite, a protozoan carried by cats. Man and other intermediate hosts may be infected. In the adult with the acquired infection systemic symptoms are usually mild. Similarly, the ocular symptoms of acquired toxoplasmosis may be mild. However, a severe form of acquired ocular toxoplasmosis has been recognised. In such cases there has been contact with wild cats in stables. In the case of infected pregnant mothers the child in utero may be infected by the more severe congenital form of the disease. The organism enters the brain as well as the eyes and may cause mental deficiency and epilepsy. A characteristic type of calcification is seen on skull x-ray or CT scan. In the eye a focal type of choroiditis often affects both eyes and this is usually at the posterior pole in the (macular region) (Fig. 18.4b), but may be anywhere in the fundi, and may be asymmetric. Histologically the Toxoplasma organism is found in the eye lesions. The diagnosis may be confirmed by sending some blood for serological tests. Four such tests are currently in use clinically: the toxoplasma dye test, indirect fluorescent antibody test, haemaglutination test and enzyme-linked immunosorbent assay (ELISA). These tests must be interpreted carefully because a high proportion of the population becomes infected at some point and the positive results increase with age, even in those with no clinical evidence of infection. For this reason the diagnosis may be less easy in acquired toxoplasmosis where evidence of systemic involvement may be slight or absent. It has been shown that there is a higher incidence of positive dye tests in patients with posterior uveitis than in the normal population, but in an individual case it is often necessary to demonstrate a changing titre in order to confirm the diagnosis. The most specific of these tests is the ELISA.

All the currently available anti-toxoplasma treatments have potential serious side effects. Therefore not all active toxoplasma retinochoroiditis lesions require treatment. Such treatment is required only if an active lesion involves or threatens the fovea and/or optic nerve. Treatment is also required when there is severe vitritis.

A combination of pyrimethamine and sulphadiazine has been recommended, but such treatment may cause a serious fall in the white cell count, which should therefore be monitored. An alternative anti-microbial treatment is clindamycin. This (clindamycin) needs to be given with a sulphonamide in order to reduce the risk of colitis. It is generally accepted that systemic steroids have some beneficial effect and may help to clear the vitreous more rapidly, but this treatment should be given only with antimicrobial cover. Steroids on their own will produce exacerbation or progression of the chorioretinitis. In fact the majority of cases resolve spontaneously, leaving more or less chorioretinal scarring at the macular region. Recurrences are fairly common, with or without treatment, and the fresh choroidal inflammation tends to arise at the edge of a previous scar.

Toxocariasis

Toxocariasis is caused by toxocara catis (from cats) or canis (from dogs). This nematode has been found in the enucleated eyes of young patients with a severe type of chorioretinitis. It is a unilateral disease found in children who are in close contact with puppies or eat dirt (through faecal contamination). The vitreous tends to be filled with a white mass of inflammatory cells so that the presence of a tumour may be suspected (e.g. retinoblastoma). Endophthalmitis tends to develop in these cases and the sight of one eye may be completely lost. During the acute stage the peripheral blood may show an eosinophilia. Treatment is unsatisfactory and includes a com-

bination of anti-helminthic agent taken by mouth (thiobendazole, mebendazole or diethylcarbamazine) and steroids.

Tuberculosis

In former years this was considered to be a common cause of posterior uveitis, clinicians having been impressed by the number of patients with a previous history of tuberculosis (TB). The relationship seems less likely now that TB has been almost eliminated from most populations. However, this diagnosis must not be forgotten especially in the immunosuppressed patient and patients with recalcitrant or atypical uveitis since there is currently a slight re-emergence of the disease. Choroidal tubercles are a well-described entity: these raised yellowish granulomatous foci were used as a diagnostic feature of miliary TB and occasionally chronic pulmonary TB. They are usually seen in extremely ill patients and the yellowish tubercles become pigmented as they heal.

Treatment is as for systemic TB, and requires liaison with an infectious diseases specialist physician.

Presumed Ocular Histoplasmosis

Histoplasmosis is a fungal infection (causative agent—Histoplasma capsulatum). Infection with this organism occurs throughout the world but is more common in the Mississippi Valley and is thought not to occur in the UK. A severe pneumonitis may occur but most cases are asymptomatic.

Presumed ocular histoplasmosis (POHS) is not seen in patients with active histoplasmosis. The evidence for infection in the originally described cases was necessarily circumstantial—hence the expression 'presumed ocular histoplasmosis'. The syndrome consists of a certain type of haemorrhagic macular lesion (choroidal neovascularisation) combined with discrete foci of peripheral choroiditis and peripapillary chorioretinal scars.

Treatment includes systemic steroids, and appropriate therapy for choroidal neovascularization, when present.

Syphilis

Syphilis is a chronic infection caused by Treponema pallidum. Iridocyclitis occurs in patients with secondary acquired syphilis. It is a bilateral disease, but may be asymmetric, in which the iris vessels are particularly engorged. This acute anterior uveitis may become chronic if inadequately treated. Chorioretinitis may be either multifocal or diffuse (sometimes referred to as posterior placoid) and involves the mid-periphery and peripapillary area. Retinal vasculitis (affecting mainly venules, but arteries also) is common, and optic disc swelling may also occur (Fig. 18.5a, b) OCT images may be helpful in quantifying the retinitis (Fig. 18.5c, d). The inflammation in syphilis can take several forms, and may have a different appearance in immuno-compromised patients. Systemic associations should be looked for. The fundi may return to normal appearances if adequately treated on time (before permanent changes occur). In the healed phase, perivascular bone spicule pigmentation may be seen similar to that observed in retinitis pigmentosa, but localized to particular parts of the posterior segment.

In congenital syphilis other possible features occur such as deafness and corneal scarring from previous interstitial keratitis. The scattered pigmentation in the fundus may suggest an inherited retinal degeneration but a careful family history together with electrodiagnostic testing of the eyes usually enables one to distinguish the two conditions. It is also important to carry out serological testing. The Treponema pallidum immobilisation test (TPI) and the fluorescent treponemal antibody test (FTABS) are the most sensitive and specific.

As it is a venereal or sexually transmitted disease, the Genito-Urinary Team should be involved, and contact tracing is important. Treatment is specific with intramuscular injections of benzyl penicillin. An alternative treatment is high dose tetracyclines given orally. Systemic steroids may be added on control of the infection.

Sarcoidosis

The eye is very frequently involved in sarcoidosis. Involvement usually takes the form of an anterior, posterior uveitis or panuveitis. The choroiditis is more often peripheral and accompanied by inflammatory changes in the retinal veins. Sheathing of the veins may be seen and the vision may be impaired by macular oedema. Similarly, the optic discs may be inflamed. The inflammatory changes may be similar to those seen in pars planitis. Skin lesions, including granulomas, indurated, violaceous rashes on exposed body parts including the face (called lupus pernio) may occur. Occasionally, central nervous system including meningitis, polyneuropathy may be seen. When the diagnosis is suspected, the conjunctiva and skin should be searched for possible nodules, which may be biopsied, and an x-ray of the chest may reveal enlargement of the hilar lymph nodes (usually), or interstitial lung disease. CT scan of the chest gives a better yield for detecting hilar lymphadenopathy and other forms of pulmonary involvement. Serum angiotensin converting enzyme (ACE) and calcium levels are elevated, and serve as good screening tools, although these changes are non-specific. The x-ray of the chest also helps exclude TB before commencing therapy.

The management of the ophthalmological problem may involve treatment with local and systemic steroids but the opinion of a physician specialising in sarcoidosis is essential and should be sought before embarking on treatment.

Behcet's Disease

Behcet's disease is a multi-system disease associated with HLA-B5. It was originally thought to occur only in the Mediterranean and Japan where the disease is most common, but is now known to occur in most populations to varying extents. The disease is characterised by an obliterative vasculitis affecting both arteries and veins. The clinical syndrome consists of oral and genital ulceration

Fig. 18.5 (**a1**) Fundus photo of right eye showing acute syphilitic chorioretinitis. There is a large oval placoid lesion extending across the fovea, and a cotton wool spot along the inferior temporal arteriole. (**a2**). Fundus photo of the left eye with acute syphilitic chorioretinitis. The macular placoid lesion is smaller. The disc is swollen. (**b1**) Syphilitic optic disc swelling in the right eye and placoid lesion. (**b2**). Syphilitic optic disc swelling in the

left eye of the same patient. Note the asymmetry between the 2 eyes. There is a flame shaped haemorrhage at the inferior temporal disc margin. (**c**) OCT of the right eye shown in (a). There is disruption of the outer retina-RPE complexc. (**d**) OCT of the same eye post-treatment. The outer retina-RPE morphology looks more normal. Mottling of the RPE is noticeable in the left image

Fig. 18.5   (continued)

in combination with recurrent uveitis and skin lesions. The uveitis consists of recurrent bilateral non-granulomatous anterior and/or posterior uveitis. Hypopyon is common in acute anterior uveitis in Behcet's disease. Central nervous system involvement occurs as a very serious form of the disease.

The management involves good collaboration between the ophthalmologist and immunologist. Prolonged treatment with steroids and non-steroidal immunosuppressive agents (e.g. tacrolimus) is required.

Birdshot chorioretinopathy

Birdshot chorioretinopathy is an uncommon, often missed form of chronic bilateral non-infectious uveitis which affects persons aged 40-70 years old, and is significantly associated with HLA-A29. The condition usually presents with floaters, photopsia and impaired night vision, and the course may last for 10 years. The patient usually has moderate vitreous inflammation with snow balls and banking, retinal vasculitis, yellowish oblong choroidal lesions at the posterior pole and mid-periphery. The older lesions become more distinct, and more easily

detectable, with occasional pigmentation (Fig. 18.6). Macular oedema, epiretinal membranes, progressive retinal atrophy, and occasionally retinal or choroidal neovascularisation are known complications.

Treatment is commenced with high dose systemic steroids, associated with introduction with steroid sparing agents, including azathioprine, mycophenolate mofetil, or tacrolimus.

Sympathetic Ophthalmia

This is a rare but dramatic response of the uvea in both eyes to trauma. The significance of the condition rests in the fact that although the trauma has only affected one eye, the inflammatory reaction occurs in both. It may follow perforating injuries, especially when uveal tissue has become adherent to the wound edges. It may occur following intraocular surgery. The injured eye, which is referred to as the 'exciting eye', remains severely inflamed and, after an interval of between 2 weeks and several years, the uninjured eye ('sympathising eye') becomes affected. The inflammation in the sympathising eye, which is granulomatous, usually starts in the region of the ciliary body and spreads anteriorly and posteri-

Fig 18.6 (a) Right fundus photograph of a patient with Birdshot chorioretinopathy. The image is blurred because of vitritis. The scattered yellowish oval spots typical of the choroiditis are noticeable. (b) Left fundus image of same patient with Birdshot chorioretinopathy. The yellowish spots (inflammatory lesions of varying ages) are more noticeable

orly. The granulomatous inflammation (Dalen-Fuch's nodules) affecting the fundal periphery may be missed unless the pupil is fully dilated

Careful wound toilet and repair of the injured eye may probably prevent many cases, as can the removal of blind, painful and inflamed eyes within the critical 2 week period following injury. Treatment with high dose steroids is required in order to control the inflammation and save the eye and vision. The treatment may be prolonged, and require non-steroidal immunosuppressants in order to reduce the systemic side effects of therapy.

Other Causes

A wide variety of infective agents have been shown to cause posterior uveitis on rare occasions. The leprosy bacillus and the coxsackie group of viruses are two examples chosen from many. Others include the Ebola virus (see Chap. 21).

An especially rare but intriguing form of non-infectious uveitis is known as the Vogt-Koyanagi-Harada syndrome, a multi-system disease, in which is seen the combination of vitiligo, poliosis, meningoencephalitis, bilateral uveitis

associated with multifocal exudative retinal detachments. Retinal vasculitis, and varying degrees of vitritis may occur, and involvement of the optic disc is not uncommon. Recurrent anterior uveitis may occur.

Endophthalmitis and Panophthalmitis

Endophthalmitis is an inflammation of the interior cavities and all layers of the globe except the sclera. Further extension of the inflammation into the sclera (i.e. inflammation of the entire globe, with or without possible extension into the orbit) leads to panophthalmitis.

Endophthalmitis may be infectious or non-infectious, although common usage implies infection, infectious endophthalmitis is more dangerous. Endophthalmitis may be endogenous (where there is haematogenous spread of infection from a distant [non-ophthalmic]) source), or exogenous (where infection is introduced into the eye through an opening: intraocular surgery, penetrating eye injury, corneal ulcer, periocular infection with breach of globe). Endogenous endophthalmitis accounts for approximately 10% of endophthalmitis.

Fig 18.7 (**a**) Hypopyon in endophthalmitis is represented by the yellowish debris within the inferior limbus, extending from 5.30 to 6.30 clock positions. Note the ciliary injection. (**b**) Fundus image in endogenous endopthalmi-tis, showing widespread haemorrhages, yellowish retinal patches, attenuated retinal vessels. Most of the time, the fundus image is obscured by the associated vitritis

Endophthalmitis may be bacterial fungal or viral, although the exogenous type is usually bacterial. Varying degrees of pain, inflammation and visual loss may be associated with endoge-nous endophthalmitis, whilst exogenous endo-phthalmitis is usually painful. Anterior uveitis with or without hypopyon may be seen (Fig. 18.7a, b).

Endophthalmitis is one of the feared results of infection after injury or surgery but it may prove reversible with prompt diagnosis and intensive antibiotic treatment. High degree of suspicion is required to make prompt diagnosis and treat-ment, which is an emergency. Vitreous biopsy is required for identification of the causative organ-ism (in addition to other investigations including blood cultures, exclusion of diabetes, MRIs) fol-lowed immediately by intravitreal injection of appropriate anti-infective agent, as well as sys-temic anti-infective agents. Systemic steroids are only introduced when appropriate anti-infective agent has been started. When endophthalmitis and panophthalmitis are not properly and aggres-sively treated, the sight is usually lost perma-nently and after months or years the whole eye begins to shrink.

Episcleritis and Scleritis

Both these conditions form part of the differential diagnosis of the red eye. The episclera is the con-nective tissue underlying the conjunctiva and it may become selectively inflamed, either diffusely or in localised nodules. In the case of episcleritis, close inspection of the eyes shows that the inflam-mation is deeper than the conjunctiva and there is a notable absence of any discharge. The eye is red and may be gritty but not painful. Episcleritis is seen from time to time in the casualty department and the patient may be otherwise perfectly fit and well. Such cases tend to recur and some develop signs of dermatological disease. The condition responds to local steroids, but systemic aspirin may also prove effective. Scleritis is less common and more closely linked with rheumatoid arthritis and other collagen diseases. It is a vasculitis. The eye is red (diffuse or localised) and painful (Fig. 18.8a). Scleral thinning may be noticed in areas with healed scleritis (Fig. 18.8b). In severe cases the sclera may become eroded with prolapse of uveal tissue (see Fig. 7.2). Occasionally, scleri-tis may be infectious, e.g. due to herpes simplex or zoster. Topical treatment is of no benefit in

Fig 18.8 (a) Active scleritis. Diffuse engorgement of the deep scleral blood vessels and episcleral/conjunctival oedema are seen superiorly. The associated anterior uveitis is depicted by the presence of posterior synechiae. (b) Resolved scleritis in the same eye shown in (a). The conjunctival and scleral congestion, is resolved. Areas of thinned sclera are obvious as the brownish-black patches across the superior sclera

scleritis. The condition responds to systemic anti-inflammatory agents, particularly oral flurbiprofen (Froben) which may be supplemented with systemic steroids and/or immunosuppressants. Infectious scleritis require specific treatment for the underlying pathogen.

Summary

- The reader should understand the different causes of ocular inflammation, and that,
- Inflammation of the eye can affect any of its layers as well as the ocular adnexae.
- Ocular inflammation may be due to immune abnormalities including allergy, autoimmune diseases, accompany non-infectious or infectious diseases elsewhere in the body.
- Inflammation of the uvea (uveitis) is divided into anterior, intermediate or posterior uveitis depending on which part of the uvea is predominantly involved: anterior uveitis (iritis or iridocyclitis) is inflammation predominantly affecting the anterior chamber and iris; intermediate uveitis (pars planitis) is inflammation predominantly affecting vitreous and ciliary body, and posterior uveitis (choroiditis) refers to predominant involvement of the choroid (and retina).
- Patients presenting with 'red eyes' require examination to exclude cause other than conjunctivitis.
- Eyes with presumed anterior uveitis should have fundus examination with pupil dilatation in order to exclude posterior segment inflammation.
- Good clinical acumen is required to characterize the inflammation.
- Investigations are directed by the clinical findings.
- Infectious causes, and systemic diseases which may present initially as uveitis need particular attention with high degree of suspicion for appropriate diagnosis and treatment.
- Treatment is guided by the diagnosis, based on clinical features, and confirmed as necessary with appropriate investigations.
- Infectious inflammation requires prompt treatment with particular agents directed at the causative organism.
- Collaboration between the ophthalmologist and other specialists including the chest and genitourinary physicians is important as necessary.
- Sympathetic ophthalmitis which occurs following trauma, or surgery, and is rare but devastating, if missed.

The Ageing Eye

19

Abstract

The eye and its supporting structures undergo well known changes with age. As the population continues to age, it is important to distinguish 'normal' involutional changes from aging pathology of these structures. This chapter describes the standard age changes, as well as diseases that occur in the eye and its adnexae with age. These include cataracts, age-related macular degeneration, glaucoma, giant cell (or temporal) arteritis, and eyelid changes.

Although the eye and its supporting structures undergo a number of well-defined changes with age, the distinction between these involutional changes and disease is not always clear cut. For the elderly patient it is often reassuring to know that the problem is part of a 'normal' process rather than the result of a specific illness and perhaps sometimes an artificial demarcation is drawn for the benefit of the patient.

The worldwide increase in number of elderly people presents problems in ophthalmology. A high proportion of elderly people instill drops into their eyes, either prescribed for them or as self-medication. It is important that adequate advice is available. Advising the elderly is often time consuming and may entail speaking to a younger relative or neighbour, but an adequate explanation of the disease or problems will avoid anxiety and probably the need for further subsequent unnecessary consultation.

The three commonest diseases of the elderly eye are cataract, glaucoma and age-related macular degeneration (AMD). The first can be cured, the second arrested or prevented, while the third generally tends to run a progressive course and treatment is unsatisfactory at present, especially for dry AMD, although significant progress has been made in the management of neovascular AMD recently. Attempts to measure the incidence of these problems have produced a wide range of figures. Out of a population of elderly persons complaining of impaired vision about 30% turn out to have a cataract and a similar number to have AMD, whereas 5% or less have chronic primary open angle glaucoma (POAG). It is estimated that vision loss occurs in 1:9 persons aged over 60 years, 1:5 aged over 75 years, and 1:2 in those aged 90 years and older. Visual impairment due to glaucoma is more prevalent and occurs at an earlier age in blacks than in whites. Although there is an unexpectedly high incidence of cataract in patients with POAG, the association of AMD with cataract or glaucoma is more random.

Changes in the Eyes with Age

The External Eye

The eyelids tend to lose their elasticity and become less firmly opposed to the globe. The upper and lower lid margins become progressively lower so that whereas in the infant the upper lid may ride level with or slightly above the upper corneal margin, in an elderly subject the upper lid may cross a significant part of the upper cornea. An area of white may be seen between the lower margin of the cornea and the lower lid. Some limitation of the ocular movements is accepted as normal in the elderly, especially limitation of upward gaze. The conjunctiva tends to become more lax and a thin fold of conjunctiva may be trapped between the lids when blinking if this becomes excessive. In some elderly patients there is loss of connective tissue around the lacrimal puncta so that the opening is seen elevated slightly from the rest of the lid, and the punctum slightly everted. Degenerative plaques are seen on the bulbar conjunctiva in the exposed region and the conjunctiva is especially prone to chronic inflammation.

The Globe

Arcus senilis is the name given to the circular white infiltrate seen around the margin of the cornea. The lens gradually loses its plasticity throughout life, resulting in a progressive reduction in the focusing power of the eye. This loss of focusing ability is also contributed to by the progressive loss of ciliary muscle tone. A child may be able to observe details of an object held 5 cm from the eye, but as a result of hardening of the lens and weakening of the ciliary muscle the nearest point (called the 'near point') at which an object can be kept in focus gradually recedes. This progressive degeneration tends to pass unnoticed until the eye is no longer able to focus to within the normal reading distance. This usually occurs approximately at the age of 45 years

if the eyes are otherwise normal, and the phenomenon is called presbyopia. Some degree of opacity of the lens fibres is very common in old age and only when this becomes more extensive is the term 'cataract' used. The pupil becomes smaller with age and does not show the wide range of adjustment to illumination seen in younger people. The vitreous shows an increase in small opacities visible to the subject as 'vitreous floaters'. A more dramatic degenerative change, which occurs in a high proportion of normal individuals in the 60–70 years' age group, is detachment of the vitreous. Vitreous degeneration and onset of floaters occurs earlier in eyes that are more myopic. The formed part of the vitreous separates from the retina, usually above at first, leaving a fluid-filled gap between the retina and posterior vitreous face. Movement of the vitreous face may cause troublesome symptoms, for example flashing lights and floaters, but often a vitreous detachment goes unnoticed and is an incidental finding on examination of the eye. In most eyes, posterior vitreous detachment is incomplete, and the vitreous remains attached at areas of firm vitreo-retinal adhesions, including the optic disc margin and the macular area. Such firm adhesions in the macula may result in vitreomacular traction (VMT) and macular hole formation. VMT is most easily appreciated on optical coherence tomography (OCT) (Fig. 19.1). The important association between sudden vitreous detachment and subsequent retinal detachment has already been discussed in Chap. 13. The appearance of the fundus also shows gradual changes; the retinal arterioles become straighter and narrower, as also do the venules. Colloid bodies or drusen are more commonly seen due to degenerative changes in Bruch's membrane and the pigment epithelium, and peripheral chorioretinal degeneration is more evident. The young retina is more shiny than the old retina and in the elderly the normal light reflex is less marked. The optic disc tends to become somewhat paler and a degree of optic atrophy is accepted by many clinicians as a senile change unrelated to disease.

Fig. 19.1 Vitreomacular traction: (**a**) colour photo (**b**) OCT showing foveal attachment of posterior hyaloid, significant traction and macular hole

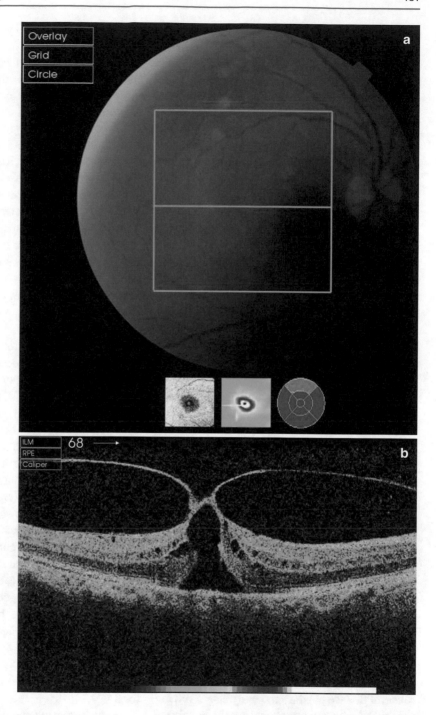

Eye Disease in the Elderly

The prevalence of blindness increases with age. The prevalence and causes of blindness also vary from one community to another depending on the age structure of the population and environmental conditions. In England and Wales (1980), the prevalence of blindness was found to be 9/100,000 under 5 years of age and 2324/100,000 above 75 years. In 2017, two million people were reported as sight impaired (visually impaired or severely visually impaired) in the UK, including 25,000 aged 16 years or younger. This included 1.7 million in England, 107,000 in Wales, 171,000 in Scotland, and 51,000 in Northern Ireland. These included persons awaiting treatment for cataracts, refractive errors needing glasses. Of these, 350,000 are registered as permanently visually impaired or severely visually impaired.

A recent survey in the United States has shown that the incidence of cataract in the 45–64 year old population is 5.6% for males and 2.1% for females. The incidence is slightly higher in the Black population, and rises to 21.6% for males and 26.8% for females in the 65–75 year old population. In the same age group (65–75) the incidence of AMD is 9.6% for males and 6.9% for females. Both of these conditions are therefore very common, and they demand time and medical expertise, both at the primary care level and in hospital.

With increasing longevity throughout the world especially in the developing countries, there will be a continuing increase in the number of blind people, especially those suffering from diseases related to age such as cataracts, glaucoma, and macular degeneration. It is estimated that by 2050, 4.1 million people will be affected by sight loss in the UK (compared to the two million in 2017).

Age Related Macular Degeneration

Age-related macular degeneration (AMD) is the most common cause of irreversible central visual loss in the elderly populations of the industrialised world. In the UK it accounts for approximately 48% of adult visual impairment. It is a bilateral disease in which the early stages are not associated with any symptoms, but the late forms of AMD are symptomatic and result in visual loss.

Visual loss in the first eye (from AMD) usually occurs at about 65 years of age (but may do so earlier, as early as 50 years). For the advanced forms of the disease, the second eye becomes involved at a rate of approximately 7–10% per annum from time of involvement of the first eye, and has accounted for approximately half of all registered visual impairments in the UK. Because of demographic changes (upward shift) in the elderly population, the prevalence of AMD is expected to increase in the future, placing even greater demands on health providers.

There are 2 main types of AMD: 'dry' or atrophic, and 'wet' or neovascular (nAMD). Severe visual impairment is usually associated with the nAMD, and among the eyes with severe visual loss, approximately 80–90% of cases are due to nAMD, whilst 10–20% of cases have the dry form. The atrophic form of AMD results in significant vision loss only when the atrophy affects the fovea.

AMD is a multi-factorial disease contributed to by interaction between genetic and environmental factors. This may account for the wide variation in different AMD phenotypes. In 2005, a major breakthrough in our understanding of the risks and pathogenesis occurred when a number of US laboratories including that of Hageman found a genetic link in AMD. They found that patients with a particular mutation in their *complement factor H* gene (on chromosome 1) had a dramatically increased risk of AMD. This discovery that the complement system in some way played a role in AMD confirmed the suspicions of many that an immune related mechanism was pivotal in the pathogenesis of the disease. Since then, a number of other gene mutations have been found, such as those in the *ARMS2/HTRA1* (on chromosome 10), *complement components 2* and *6*, as well as *complement factor B* which predispose to AMD. However, there are also complement-related genes that may be protective for AMD.

While increasing age is an undoubted risk factor, unfortunately this is not modifiable. Dry AMD (including the end stage of geographic atrophy) occurs in all populations. However, nAMD occurs more commonly in Caucasians and Asians, and about one-third give a family history of similar problems. Smoking has been shown to increase the risk of AMD by three to fourfold. Smoking cessation regimens therefore offer the prospect of dramatically reducing the incidence of severe visual loss secondary to AMD. Systemic hypertension, cardiovascular disease and low antioxidant intake including Vitamins A, C, E levels, as well as zeaxanthin, carotenoids are associated with increased risk of AMD.

Older people with macular degeneration complain of blurring of their vision and inability to read. Younger or more observant patients notice that straight edges may look kinked. Usually one eye is considerably more affected than the other by the time patients present to the hospital, although both eyes may be affected simultaneously. Because the advanced degenerative process is limited to the macula, the peripheral field remains unaffected and the patient can walk around quite normally. Difficulty in recognising faces or in seeing bus numbers is also a common complaint.

In the early stages of dry AMD, inspection of the fundus shows spots of pigment in the macular region. Drusen are also often seen (Fig. 19.2a, b). These are small round yellowish spots often scattered over the posterior pole. Unfortunately the word 'drusen' has been used rather loosely in ophthalmology to refer to two or three types of swelling seen in the fundus. It is used to describe the very rare mulberry-like tumours seen around the optic nerve head in tuberose sclerosis and it is also used when referring to the multiple shiny excrescences seen on the optic disc as a congenital abnormality (optic disc drusen - described in Chap. 22). Drusen, seen at the posterior pole of the eye, as in AMD are 'macular drusen', also known as `colloid bodies`, and perhaps this term is preferable to some clinicians. Under the microscope, colloid bodies are seen as focal degenerative changes (mainly thickening) in Bruch's membrane. Drusen are of varying sizes, and may have varying degrees of hyperpigmentation associated. Small drusen are considered

Fig. 19.2 Drusen: (**a**) small drusen; (**b**) larger more wide spread drusen

part of normal aging, whilst larger drusen (more than 63 microns in diameter), with softer edges (therefore, described as 'soft drusen') are more likely to progress to vision loss. Most eyes with macular drusen maintain good vision, but a significant number (especially larger drusen, as described above) will develop slow progressive atrophy of the retinal pigment epithelium (RPE) and choriocapillaris. In turn this leads to secondary atrophy of the overlying photoreceptors. The geographic atrophy (GA) lesions manifests as sharply demarcated localized areas. The initial symptoms reported by patients may be gaps in images or words. Over time, this focal atrophy spreads to involve large parts of the macula, leading to the so called 'geographic atrophy' (advanced dry AMD where there are well delineated areas of atrophy) which is associated with central or paracentral scotoma (Fig. 19.3), and a moderate loss of vision. The vision loss is more severe if the geographic atrophy involves the foveal centre. The atrophic change in the RPE, choroid and photoreceptors is referred to as "dry" AMD because there is no leakage of fluid or bleeding into the retina or subretinal space.

In the 'wet type' of macular degeneration or nAMD, a fan of new vessels arises from the choroid - choroidal neovascularisation (CNV) stimulated by growth factors such as vascular endothelial growth factor (VEGF). The growth of these new vessels seems to be important because they invade breaks in Bruch's mem-

brane, and grow through it into the subretinal space. Serous or haemorrhagic exudate tends to occur and this may be either under the pigment epithelium, subretinal space or into the retina (Fig. 19.4). A sudden loss of central vision may be experienced as the result of such an episode. Subsequently, 'healing' of the leaking vascular complex results in scar tissue formation which further destroys the central vision permanently similar to a scar resulting from a skin wound.

The terms 'classic' and 'occult' CNV describe the different patterns of CNV leakage on fundus fluorescein angiography (FFA). The classic CNV (also called Type 2 CNV) has an obvious lacy pattern in the early phases of the angiography,

Fig. 19.3 Dry age-related macular degenerationgeographic atrophy. (**a**) Colour fundus photograph showing early geographic atrophy with fovea sparing, soft drusen still obvious; (**b**) fundus photograph showing advanced geographic atrophy involving the fovea; (**c**) fundus fluo-rescein angiogram (FFA) showing window defects corresponding to the atrophic patches, which are more obvious than in colour alone in (**b, d**) OCT image showing atrophic patches in the outer retina and RPE (same eye as in **b**)

30/10/2014, OD
IR&OCT 30° [HS] ART(9) Q: 23

Fig. 19.3 (continued)

whilst in occult CNV (called Type 1 CNV) the vascular network pattern is not obvious despite the leak (hence the term occult). Other investigations undertaken in AMD include optical coherence tomography (OCT) in which the difference between types 1 & 2 are more obvious, OCT-A (Fig. 19.4f), and indocyanine angiography (ICG-A).

Management

Prevention Avoidance of smoking is the most important preventive measure against all forms of AMD. It may take up to 10–15 years for the risk of aggravating AMD for ex-smokers to return to that of non-smokers.

Dry AMD No effective treatment is available for established dry AMD at present. A large multicentre randomised placebo controlled trial (AREDS trial) suggested that progression to advanced AMD could be reduced by as much as 25% in high risk patients by daily supplements of vitamins C (500 mg) and E (400 IU), zinc (80 mg) and beta carotene (15 mg). On the basis of these results of the AREDS it is recommended that persons older than should have dilated eye examinations to determine their risk of develop-

ing advanced AMD then, those with high risk characteristics should consider taking supplements and antioxidants plus zinc. Importantly, this formulation is not recommended for smokers because beta carotene has been shown to increase the risk of lung cancer. The beta carotene has been replaced in recent formulations. There is also evidence to suggest that those individuals with a high intake of macular pigments lutein and zeaxanthin were at reduced risk of AMD. The recently completed large international trial of lutein/zeaxanthin and omega-3 fatty acid supplementation in AMD (AREDS 2) has confirmed the results from AREDS). The additive effect was not shown. However, it is still recommended that these nutritional supplements in combination offer the best chance of reducing the progression of dry AMD. They are thought to reduce the damaging effects of light on the retina through their reducing and free-radical scavenging actions.

Potential treatments for dry AMD directed at blocking the complement pathway are currently under investigation. Unfortunately, intravitreal injections of lampalizumab has failed to show efficacy, although other drugs including Pegcetacoplan are currently ongoing.

Neovascular or Wet AMD Some stages of nAMD are treatable. End stage disease in nAMD (so called 'disciform' CNV) characterized by fibrous scar arising from the earlier CNV is untreatable. However, there are a few clinically proven treatments for active nAMD (before the end stage) whilst several more are in the pipeline. The mainstay of contemporary nAMD treatments is pharmacologic, and dependent on early prompt diagnosis.

Fig. 19.4 Neovascular (wet) age-related macular degeneration. (**a**) Colour photograph of left macula showing haemorrhage, and yellowish elevation; (**b, c**) early and late phase fundus fluorescein angiogram of the same eye in a patient with early wet AMD; (**d**) OCT image of the same eye; (**e**) colour fundus photograph of eye with advanced wet AMD. (**f**) (1). Colour photo and OCT image showing choroidal neovascularisation (CNV). The B-scan (upper right) shows the irregular elevation of the RPE complex from the CNV, associated with subretinal hyperreflective material and fluid spaces. (**f**) (2). An OCT-A image of the same eye showing the CNV complex in the outer retina/choriocapillaris complex

Fig. 19.4 (continued)

Fig. 19.4 (continued)

Prior to 1999, the only treatment proven by a randomised controlled trial to provide long term visual benefit in nAMD was argon laser photocoagulation. Controlled trials of the effect of laser photocoagulation of the CNV showed that this treatment is useful in extrafoveal CNV i.e. when the leakage is not directly under or threatening the fovea. Laser photocoagulation ablates the CNV. It is important that those cases that are

likely to benefit from treatment are first identified quickly. This entails photography of the fundus and FFA, as well as ICGA. Very often patients present at the stage when new vessels have already advanced across the macular region to near or under the fovea, or where the fovea has already been permanently damaged by haemorrhage, exudate, or scar tissue making effective laser treatment impossible. Another limitation of laser treatment is the high rate of recurrence of the CNV within a short time following treatment. Only about 5–7% of CNV are eligible for laser photocoagulation by modern standards. However, laser photocoagulation is now superseded by pharmacologic treatments.

The second proven treatment is photodynamic therapy (PDT) with Verteporfin (Visudyne) became available in 1999. PDT specifically targets the CNV complex for damage by low energy laser, but avoids damage to the unaffected tissue including the photoreceptors. This treatment aimed to preserve vision, and was useful in eyes with predominantly classic CNV on FFA (approximately 20% of CNV), and in addition, repeated treatment is required at 3-monthly intervals, resulting in additive collateral damage to the RPE and photoreceptors and further visual loss with time. PDT is now mainly reserved for cases of idiopathic polypoidal choroidopathy (IPCV) which a variant of nAMD, where it has been found to be effective in closing the polyps especially when given with intravitreal anti-VEGF drugs (see below).

The discovery that VEGF was important in the development and progression of nAMD led to the recent developments of intravitreal injections of anti-VEGF drugs, similar to blocking blood vessel growth in cancer therapy. The first licensed drug was pegaptanib (Macugen, Eyetech/Pfizer). This is an aptamer that binds only one subtype of VEGF (VEGF 165 isoform). It is given every 6 weeks in the form of an intravitreal injection. Visual stabilisation in approximately 70% of patients after receiving the drug for 2 years whilst only 5% were noted to have improved vision. However, all nAMD lesion types were treatable. Subsequently, ranibizumab (Lucentis, Genentech/ Novartis) was licensed. This drug is a fragment of a monoclonal antibody that binds and inhibits the action of all subtypes of VEGF and is given every 4 weeks by intravitreal injection into the affected eye. Injection intervals may be extended after stabilization. Significant visual improvement occurs in approximately a third of adequately treated eyes, whilst vision is maintained in up to 95%. Similarly, aflibercept (Eylea, Regeneron/Bayer) is a fusion protein which binds all forms of

VEGF-A and B, and placental growth factor (PlGF), and licensed for the treatment on nAMD and gives similar visual benefits to that of ranibizumab. These benefits persist for several years as long as treatment is continued as necessary. Figure 19.5 shows OCT and OCTA images of CNV before and after the injection of ranibizumab.

Before ranibizumab received its FDA and EU licenses, many ophthalmologists began the intravitreal injection of bevacizumab (Avastin, Genetech/Roche). This is an anti-VEGF monoclonal antibody, formulated for the intravenous treatment of bowel cancer. On a dose for dose basis, it is much cheaper than ranibizumab, when split into smaller quantities required for intravitreal injections for AMD, and seems to be as effective. However, it is not licensed for intraocular use.

Brolucizumab (Beovu, Novartis) is another new anti-VEGF drug. It is a humanized single-chain antibody fragment which binds to VEGF, and shown to be superior to aflibercept in drying up the macular in nAMD. It also has a longer duration of action (compared to previously existing anti-VEGFs, particularly aflibercept in clinical trials) so that approximately 50% of eyes require 3-monthly injections after the initial three initiation doses. Brolucizumab, however, has a slight increase in the side effect of intraocular inflammation, which requires early detection and treatment.

Faricimab (Roche/Genentech) is a bispecific antibody designed to block 2 distinct pathways of angiopoietin-2 (Ang-2) and VEGF-A that drive a number of retinal conditions, including nAMD. Ang-1 stabilises blood vessels and reduces vascular permeability when bound to Tie1. Ang-2 has been shown to play a considerable role in angiogenesis, vascular instability and inflammation, similar to VEGF. As such, blocking Ang-2 in addition to VEGF will provide a more efficient and longer lasting treatment for nAMD (and possibly other retinal vascular diseases). Faricimab (Roche/Genetech) is thought to have a better drying effect, and longer duration of action (compared to aflibercept), lasting up to 4-monthly (or 12 weekly) repeat injections in

Fig. 19.5 (a) OCT image of the left eye shows a CNV complex with REP elevation and significant disruption of the outer and middle retina. The thickness map below the B scan provides supporting evidence. (b) OCT-A image of the same eye as in (a) shows a classic CNV network between the outer retina/choriocapillaris complex pre-treatment. (c) OCT image of the same as in (a) after 3 intravitreal injections of ranibizumab. The subretinal mass is more organised, and the black spaces depicting fluid have resolved. (d) OCT-A of the same eye after 3 intravitreal injections shows significant reduction in size of the CNV network. The pink colour in the left bottom image represents flow within the choroid, whilst the red depicts retinal blood flow

Fig. 19.5 (continued)

some patients. An antibody fragment based on the faricimab full antibody is in development.

KSI-301 (Kodiak Sciences, Palo Alto) is a new investigational intravitreal full length anti-VEGF antibody biopolymer conjugate, where a humanised IgG conjugated with an inert biopolymer to prolong vitreous availability and therefore duration of action, possibly up to 24 weeks. Phase III studies are ongoing.

OPT-302 (Opthea) is an anti-VEGF R3 receptor fusion protein that blocks VEGF-C and D (differing from other currently available anti-VEGFs). This drug is currently in Phase III studies in nAMD in combination with ranibizumab.

A refillable reservoir port delivery system (PDS) for ranibizumab 100 mg/mL is being developed by Genentech, and is designed to be refilled at 24-week or more intervals after the initial surgical insertion. It looks promising in delivering sustained drug concentrations over long periods without significant adverse events.

Other agents that block intra-cellular signalling pathways of growth factors thought important in angiogenesis, such as platelet derived growth factor (PDGF) are currently under investigation, as adjunct to treatment with anti-VEGF agents. Fovista (Ophthotech/Novartis) was not found to add or improve efficacy when given with ranibizumab in phase 3 trials. As such it has not been licensed for treatment of nAMD. Future, potential treatment modalities may also include the ocular use of gene therapy to enhance continuous production of anti-VEGF molecules in the eye (as a biofactory), or developing longer acting anti-VEGF molecules. Other strategies include targeted radiotherapy as a potent anti-angiogenic agent, macular translocation surgery and drugs designed to alter or overcome the genetic abnormalities in the complement system. On the far horizon, treatments such as retinal prosthesis, replacement of damaged photoreceptors by stem cells and the sub-macular replacement of retinal pigment epithelial cells hold promise.

In addition, biosimilars (biologic medical product very similar to another already approved drug) to approved anti-VEGFs (including ranibizumab and aflibercept) are currently in development. Theoretically, appropriate biosimilars should have similar efficacy and adverse event profile, but reduced costs compared to the original (generic) drug,

For patients with advanced dry AMD or nAMD unresponsive to treatment, visual rehabilitation techniques offer the potential of use the patient remaining vision to its maximal potential. Most hospital optometry departments and some community optometrists offer a low vision aid service. This encompasses the use of, or advice on large print books, lighting and the use and provision of hand and spectacle supported magnifying devises and CCTV devises. Practical measures can be taken in the management of these patients to alleviate their handicap. Telescopic lenses may be needed for reading or watching television and full consideration should be given to the question of blind registration. It is important to explain the nature of the condition and prognosis to the patient. This can alleviate considerable anxiety and fear of total blindness and help the patient come to terms with the problem. In most cases one eye is involved first, the other following suit within 1–3 years. There are also a small number of training courses for patients to learn to use eccentric fixation. This involves training in the use of areas of retina near the macular, outside the area affected by disease, for tasks such as reading. The visual acuity, progressively deteriorates to less than 6/60 Snellen (LogMAR 1.0), but the peripheral field remains unaffected so the patient is able to find his or her way about, albeit with some difficulty.

Referral Pathways for AMD

The advent of new anti-VEGF therapies for nAMD have been shown to be very successful in stabilising vision in the vast majority of patients and also offer the chance of restoring some of the vision lost by the disease processes. It has become extremely important therefore, that patients reporting new symptoms such as distortion in their central vision are rapidly referred to a local ophthalmology department with the facilities and expertise to evaluate and treat these patients.

Choroidal Neovascularistion from Non-AMD Causes

It is important to appreciate that other diseases or conditions may lead to CNV formation, usually in younger persons than in nAMD. These include myopic degeneration (myopic CNV), angioid streaks, different types of choroiditis (including punctate inner choroiditis, multifocal choroiditis, and birdshot), and choroidal rupture (which may occur from blunt trauma). Figure 19.6 shows images of an eye with CNV secondary to choroidal rupture from blunt trauma. Treatments for non-AMD CNV are extended from nAMD (especially anti-VEGF therapies), but may require less prolonged course of treatment.

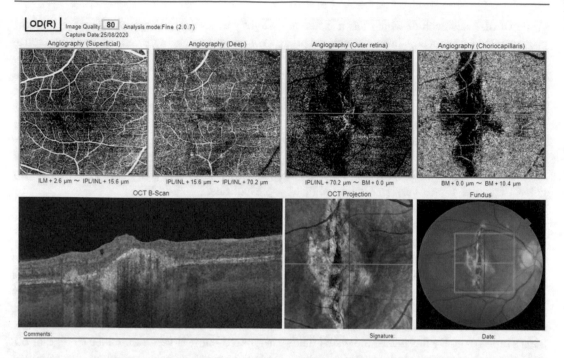

Fig. 19.6 Colour photo and OCT-A scans of CNV secondary to choroidal tear from blunt trauma. The CNV complex is seen as the lacy branching pattern in the outer retina/choriocapiilaris images (top right 2 images)

Cataract

This common condition in the elderly eye has already been considered, but it is important that every physician can identify and assess the density of a cataract in relation to the patient's vision. The physician must realise the potential of cataract surgery in the restoration of vision. Cataract surgery is required only if vision is sufficiently reduced so far as to interfere with the patient's normal lifestyle. The contraindications for cataract surgery are few and even in extreme old age the patient may benefit. Surgery may be delayed if the patient has only one eye or if there is some other pathology in the eye, which is likely to affect the prognosis. The need for someone to assist the patient in the instillation of eye-drops and the domestic chores during the post-operative period may require some attention but is not a contraindication. About one third of the population aged 70 years or more suffer from cataract, but the quoted figures may vary according to the diagnostic criteria, and the particular population.

If an elderly person has an opaque lens, which obscures any view of the fundus with the ophthalmoscope, and the pupil reacts quickly, then he or she is likely to do well after surgery. It is useful to remember that the reading vision is usually fairly well preserved even when the cataract is quite dense, and if the patient is unable to read, there may be coincidental AMD or other macular pathology, except if the cataract is of the posterior subcapsular type. It is also important to appreciate that clear media is important to allow monitoring and treatment of other disease affecting the ocular fundus e.g. AMD. Such clear media also allow optimization of the residual vision in the eye with macular disease. Cataract surgery, therefore, should not be withheld because of a co-existing or suspected macular pathology.

Glaucoma

The various types of glaucoma have also been considered already, and the reader would realise that glaucoma is simply the manifestation of a group of diseases each of which has a different prognosis and treatment. Chronic simple or primary open angle glaucoma (POAG) is the important kind in the elderly because it occurs more commonly and often remains undiagnosed. The physician and optometrist can play a vital part in the screening of this disease by becoming familiar with the nature of glaucomatous cupping of the optic disc. About 1% of the Caucasian population over the age of 55 is thought to suffer from POAG and the figure may rise to as high as 20–30% in those over 75. POAG prevalence is much higher in the African and Caribbean populations, and its occurrence is at a much earlier age. In most instances the treatment is very simple but requires the cooperation and understanding of the disease by the patient. The treatment is preventative of further visual loss rather than curative. POAG is best managed in an eye unit on a long term basis. By this means the visual fields and intraocular pressure can be accurately monitored and the treatment adjusted as required. More recently, the care of glaucoma patients is being shared between hospital units and selected (trained) optometrists in the community in UK and other countries. Continuity and consistency of care is paramount, in order for the patient to benefit from such shared care.

Deformities of the Eyelids

Both entropion and ectropion are common in the elderly and a complaint of soreness and irritation in the eyes as well as watering should always prompt a careful inspection of the configuration of the eyelids. Entropion is revealed by pressing the finger down on the lower lid so that the inverted lid becomes everted again to reveal the lash line. Sometimes entropion may be intermittent and not present at the time of examination, but usually under these circumstances, there is a telltale slight inversion of the lid, which is made apparent by comparing the two sides. Ectropion is nearly always an obvious deformity due to the easy visibility of the reddened and everted conjunctiva, but slight degrees of ectropion are less obvious. The lower punctum alone may be slightly everted, causing a watering eye, and the symptoms may be relieved by applying retropunctal cautery to the conjunctiva. Both ectropion and entropion respond very well to lid surgery and there is no reason why geriatric patients should put up with the continued discomfort and irritation when a complete cure is readily available. These lid deformities may recur sometimes and require further lid surgery, but careful surgery in the first instance should largely prevent this.

Temporal Arteritis

This condition, also known as giant cell arteritis (GCA), seen only in the elderly, may rapidly cause total blindness unless it is treated in time. The disease is more common than was originally supposed but it is very rare under the age of 60. Medium-sized vessels, including the temporal arteries, become inflamed and the thickening of the vessel wall leads to occlusion of the vascular lumen. Histologically the inflammatory changes are characterised by the presence of foreign body giant cells and the thickening of the vessel wall is at the expense of the inner layers so that the total breadth of the vessel may not be altered. Specifically, destruction of elastic fibres, splitting and fragmentation of the internal elastic lamina, severe intimal thickening and reduction in the vessel lumen, in addition to diffuse inflammation of the vessel wall are seen. In early disease, the inflammatory changes tend to be segmental so that a single biopsy of a small segment of the temporal artery does not always reveal the diagnosis.

Patients with GCA usually present in the eye department with blurring of vision or unilateral loss of vision. Typically these symptoms are accompanied by headache and tenderness of the scalp so that brushing the hair may be painful. Often there is low-grade fever and there may be aches and pains in the muscles and joints as well as other evidence of ischaemia in the brain and heart. Scalp ulceration and jaw claudication may occur in severe cases. The blurring of vision is due to ischaemia of the optic nerve head or occa-

Fig. 19.7 Giant cell arteritis: anterior ischaemic optic neuropathy'

sionally central retinal artery occlusion. The diagnosis rests largely on finding a raised erythrocyte sedimentation rate (ESR), elevated C-reactive protein (CRP) levels and a positive temporal artery biopsy in an elderly patient with these symptoms. Palpation of the temporal arteries reveals tenderness and sometimes thickening and the absence of pulsation is a useful sign. Polymyalgia rheumatica is a syndrome consisting of muscle pain and stiffness affecting mainly the proximal muscles without cranial symptoms. It belongs to the same disease spectrum as GCA.

Inspection of the fundus in a patient with visual symptoms shows pallor and often swelling of the optic nerve head and narrowing of the retinal arterioles (Fig. 19.7). Once the disease is suspected, a biopsy is essential and this should be done without delay. Delay may result in vision loss in the other eye, which will occur within 2 weeks in over 75% of cases. Treatment can be commenced immediately sometimes even before biopsy. However, it is advisable that the lag between starting treatment and biopsy is as short as possible (preferably less than 2 weeks). The symptoms disappear rapidly after administering systemic steroids, initially in a high dose of 1.5 mg/kg body weight, (for example Prednisolone 120 mg per day), and the dosage is then reduced rapidly according to the level of the ESR. Once the ESR is down to normal levels, a maintenance dose of systemic steroids is contin-

ued, if necessary for several months (on the average 24 months). Calcium and Vitamin D supplements will be prescribed as prophylaxis against side effects of long term steroid therapy. For patients with relapsing disease requiring a protracted course of steroids, the addition of tocilizumab (TCZ) (an IL-6 receptor antagonist) with steroid taper is recommended rather than continuing monotherapy with high dose steroids.

Temporal arteritis is recognised as a self-limiting condition. About a quarter of all these patients are liable to become blind unless adequate treatment is administered and in some instances extraocular muscle palsies causing diplopia and ptosis may confuse the diagnosis. For simplicity one might summarise the disease by saying it causes headache in patients aged over 70 with an ESR over 70, who require treatment with over 70 mg of Prednisolone.

Stroke

Patients who complain of visual symptoms after a stroke quite often have an associated homonymous hemianopia and the association between hemiplegia and homonymous hemianopia should always be borne in mind. A simple confrontation field test may be all that is required to confirm this in a patient with poor vision and normal fundi following a hemiplegic episode. The vertical line of demarcation between blind and seeing areas is very well defined and may cut through the point of fixation. Fortunately the central 2° or 3° of the visual field are often spared. When there is the so called macular sparing, the visual acuity as measured by the distance visual acuity (e.g. Snellen) chart may be normal. Patients tend to complain of difficulty in reading if the right homonymous field is affected rather than the left, and although they may be able to read individual words, they have great difficulty in following the line of print. Thus a patient with a right hemiplegia and a right homonymous hemianopia may have normal fundi and visual acuity of 6/6 (Snellen) and yet be unable to read the newspaper. The picture may be further complicated by true dyslexia and the patient may admit to being able to see the paper and yet be unable to make any sense of it. Dyslexia may be suspected if other higher functions such as speech have been affected by the stroke. One of the features of a homonymous hemianopic defect in the visual field is the patient's complete lack of insight into the problem, so that even a doctor may fail to notice it in himself. It is unusual for a homonymous hemianopia to show any signs of recovery, but once the patients understand the nature of the handicap they may learn to adapt to it to a surprising degree.

Summary

In summary, a significant number of eye diseases occur more commonly in the older population, including AMD, cataracts, and glaucoma. Changes also occur in the ocular adnexae including eyelids, which may not seem, at a cursory glance, to affect the eye sight directly.

It is important to remember that

- AMD is the most common cause of severe visual loss in the over 65 year old age group.
- Patients with severe visual loss in one eye from AMD have a 50% chance of the disease affecting the fellow eye in the subsequent 5 years.
- There is currently no effective treatment for established dry AMD, although progress is ongoing.
- Cessation of smoking offers the chance of significantly reducing the number of patients with severe visual loss secondary to AMD.
- The use of anti-VEGF agents such as ranibizumab, aflibercept, or brolucizumab offers the chance of stabilising the vision in the vast majority of patients with nAMD.
- Non-AMD causes of CNV occur in younger persons, and need care in diagnosis and treatment (similar to that of nAMD).

- Several newer intravitreal drugs for nAMD are now available or in development, including faricimab, and KSI-301.
- Gene therapy for production of anti-VEGF molecules in nAMD is under investigation.
- Effective treatment of nAMD relies on rapid referral and treatment.
- Vitamin supplementation offers the chance of reducing the risk of AMD progression by 25% in high risk patients.
- POAG results in slow progressive visual loss which is asymptomatic till late.
- The visual loss in POAG is irreversible.
- Early POAG diagnosis and treatment with anti-glaucoma medication is important in preventing visual loss.
- GCA is an inflammatory disease of medium and large blood vessels that may result in sudden irreversible visual loss in persons over 70 years old; the other eye becomes involved in over 70% of cases within 2 weeks if not treated adequately.
- It presents with headaches, scalp tenderness and ulceration, jaw claudication
- Urgent diagnosis and treatment with high dose systemic steroids is required.
- Recalcitrant cases of GCA are treatable with tocilizumab.
- Visual loss as part of the stroke syndrome should always be kept in mind especially in patients without obvious ocular changes.
- Cataracts are surgically treatable with excellent outcomes, and are still beneficial in eyes with associated other pathology.
- Cataract surgery is still useful in patients with macular disease, as such surgery enhances residual macular function and allows better monitoring of the macula disease activity and treatment.
- Correction of eyelid malposition in the elderly should not be withheld, and not purely cosmetic, but has functional implications.

The Child's Eye

20

Abstract

Special techniques for examining children's eyes and the differences between the infant and adult eye are discussed in this chapter together with various conditions which are found specifically in the eyes of children.

How the Normal Features Differ from Those in an Adult

At birth the eye is relatively large, reaching adult size at about the age of 2 years. One might expect that before the eye reaches its adult size, it would be long sighted (hypermetropic), being too small to allow parallel rays of light to be brought to a focus on the retina. In actual fact the immature lens is more globular and thus compensates for this by its greater converging power. None the less, more than three quarters of children aged under 4 years are slightly hypermetropic. The slight change of refractive error which occurs as they grow compares with the more dramatic change in axial length from 18 mm at birth to 24 mm in the adult. The slight degree of hypermetropia seen in childhood tends to disappear in adolescence. Myopia is uncommon in infancy but tends to appear between the ages of 6–9 years and gradually increases over subsequent years. The rate of increase of myopia is maximal during the growing years and this may often be a cause of parental concern. The incidence of myopia worldwide appears to be increasing dramatically in young people, and it is predicted to effect over 50% of people by 2050. While genetics may play a role, the cause of the recent increase remains unclear, however it is thought that low light exposure and prolonged close work can increase the risk.

The iris of the newborn infant has a slate gray colour due to the absence of stromal pigmentation. The normal adult colouration does not develop fully until after the first year. The pupil reacts to light at birth but the reaction may be sluggish and it may not dilate very effectively in response to mydriatic drops. The fundus tends to look gray and the optic disc somewhat pale, deceiving the uninitiated into thinking that it is atrophic. The foveal light reflex, that is the spot of reflected light from the fovea, is absent or ill-defined until the infant is 4–6 months old. By 6 months the movement of the eyes should be well coordinated, and referral to an ophthalmologist is needed if a squint is suspected. Soon after birth, a baby's visual acuity can be measured using the preferential looking test, initially using a grating chart (normal acuity approximately 6/120) or with pictures, using Cardiff cards up to the age of 2 (normal acuity approximately 6/18). From the age of 2 years Kays cards can be used to measure vision by a picture matching technique (normal acuity approximately 6/9 to 6/12). Once children learn to identify letters, at the age of 4 or 5 years, the crowded Logmar chart can be employed to measure visual acuity, which by this age is normally 6/6.

How to Examine a Child's Eye

The general examination of the eye has been considered already, but in the case of the child, certain aspects require special consideration. Before the age of 3 or 4 years, it may not be possible to obtain an accurate measure of the visual acuity, but certain other methods which attempt to measure fixation are available. The rolling ball test measures the ability of the child to follow the movement of a series of white balls graded into different sizes. Another test makes use of optokinetic nystagmus, which can be induced, by making the child face moving vertical stripes on a rotating drum. The size of the stripes is then reduced until no movement of the eyes is observed. In practice a careful examination of the child's ability to fix a light, and especially the speed of fixation, is helpful. The behaviour of the child may also be a helpful guide, such as, for example, the response to a smile or the recognition of a face. Sometimes grossly impaired vision in infancy is overlooked or interpreted as a psychiatric problem, but such an error can usually be avoided by careful ophthalmological examination. The reaction of the pupils is an essential part of any visual assessment. One of the difficulties in examining children is that they are rarely still for more than a few seconds at a time, and any attempts at restraint usually make matters worse. Before starting the examination it is useful to gain the child's confidence by talking about things that might interest him or her, not directly but in conversation with the parent. In fact it is sometimes better to ignore the very anxious child deliberately during the first few minutes of the interview. Once the young patient has summed you up, hopefully in a favourable light, then a gentle approach in a quiet room is essential for best cooperation. The cover test can only be performed well under such conditions and once this has been done the pupils and anterior

part of the eye can be examined, first with a direct ophthalmoscope but if possible with a portable or fixed slit lamp microscope. Fundus examination and measurement of any refractive error demand dilatation of the pupils and paralysis of accommodation. Cyclopentolate 1% or Tropicamide 1% are both used in drop form for this purpose. The indirect ophthalmoscope is a useful tool when examining the neonatal fundus, the wide field of view being an advantage in these circumstances. If the infant is asleep in the parent's arms, this may be beneficial because it is a simple matter to raise one eyelid and peer in without waking the patient. In the case of children between the ages of 3 and 6 years, fundus examination can be more easily achieved by sitting down and asking the standing patient to look at some spot or crack on the wall while the optic disc is located. On some occasions the child has become too excited or anxious to allow a proper examination and here one may have to decide whether it is reasonable to postpone the examination for a week or whether the matter seems urgent enough to warrant proceeding with an examination under anaesthesia. A casualty situation, which occurs from time to time, is when a child is brought in distress with a suspected corneal foreign body or perhaps a perforating injury. Here it is simplest to wrap the patient in a blanket so as to restrain both arms and legs and then examine the cornea by retracting the lids with retractors. Particular care must be taken when examining an eye with a suspected perforating injury in view of the risk of causing prolapse of the contents of the globe. Any ophthalmological examination demands placing one's head close to that of the patient and this can alarm a child unless it is done sufficiently slowly and with tact. It is sometimes helpful to make the child listen to a small noise made with the tongue or ophthalmoscope to ensure atleast temporary stillness.

Using modern ocular imaging techniques, it is often now possible for children to undergo retinal optical coherence tomography and autofluorescence scans thereby obtaining high resolution images of their maculae and optic nerves.

Screening of Children's Eyes

In an ideal world all children's eyes would be examined at birth by a specialist and again at 6 months to exclude congenital abnormalities and amblyopia. This is rarely achieved, although most children in Britain are examined by a paediatrician at birth and by a GP at 6 weeks. Thereafter the national guidelines suggest that the child is screened for poor vision between the ages of 4 and 5 by an orthoptist and referred for more detailed examination if required. This allows plenty of time for an intervention to take place before potentially irreversible amblyopia occurs around the age of 7 years. The commonest defect to be found is refractive error, that is simply a need for glasses without any other problem. Screening tends to include measurement of visual acuity alone but checking any available family history of eye problems would be very helpful. When there is a difference in the visual acuity of each eye, the screener shouldn't forget that there may be a possible treatable medical condition rather than just a refractive error.

Congenital Eye Defects

Lacrimal Obstruction

The watering of one or both eyes soon after birth is a common problem. The obstruction is normally at the lower end of the nasolacrimal duct where a congenital plug of tissue remains. Infection causing purulent discharge can be treated effectively by the use of antibiotic drops. Although the unpleasant discharge should be cleared by this, the eye continues to water as long as the tear duct is blocked. The parent can be shown how to massage the tear sac. This manoeuvre causes mucopurulent material to be expressed from the lower punctum when there is a blockage and can be used as a diagnostic test. If carried out regularly, this helps to relieve the obstruction. In most cases spontaneous relief of the obstruction occurs, but if this does not occur after about 12 months, probing and syringing of the lacrimal

passageway under general anaesthesia is an effective procedure, which can be done as a day case. It is important to remember that a watering eye may be due to excessive production of tears as well as inadequate drainage, and in a child, a corneal foreign body or even congenital glaucoma may be mistaken for lacrimal obstruction by the unwary.

Epicanthus

This relatively minor defect at the medial canthus is formed by a bridge of skin running vertically. This is seen normally in some oriental races. In Europeans it usually disappears as the bridge of the nose develops, but its importance lies in the fact that it may give the misleading impression that a squint is present. Severe epicanthus can be repaired by a plastic procedure on the eyelids.

Ptosis

Congenital drooping of the eyelid may be unilateral or bilateral and sometimes can be inherited. The ptosis may be associated with other lid deformities. Referral for surgery is indicated if there is significant head tilt and especially if the lid covers the visual axis as there is a risk of amblyopia if not corrected quickly. See Chap. 4 for more information about eyelid deformities.

Congenital Nystagmus

Children with congenital nystagmus are usually brought to the department because their parents have noticed that their eyes seem to be continuously wobbling about. Such abnormal and persistent eye movements may simply occur because the child cannot see (sensory nystagmus) or they may be due to an abnormality of the normal control of eye movements (motor nystagmus). It is important to distinguish congenital nystagmus from acquired nystagmus due to a space occupying intracranial lesion.

Sensory Congenital Nystagmus The roving eye movements are described as pendular, the eyes tending to swing from side to side. Examination of the eyes reveals one of the various underlying causes: congenital cataract, albinism, aniridia, optic atrophy, or other causes of visual impairment in both eyes. A special kind of retinal degeneration known as Leber's congenital amaurosis may present as congenital nystagmus. The condition resembles retinitis pigmentosa, being a progressive degeneration of the cones and rods, and occurs at a very young age. It tends to lead to near blindness at school age. It is important to diagnose it early as gene therapy is now possible for one sub type of the disease. Patients with congenital nystagmus usually need to be examined under general anaesthesia, and electroretinography (a technique that can detect retinal degenerations at an early stage) should be performed at the same time.

Motor Congenital Nystagmus The exact cause of this type of nystagmus is usually never ascertained but a proportion of such cases show recessive inheritance. Other abnormalities may be present, such as learning difficulties, but many children are otherwise entirely normal. The nystagmus tends to be jerky, with the fast phase in the direction of gaze to the right or left. The distance vision is usually impaired to the extent that the patient may never be able to read a car number plate at 23 m. The near vision, on the other hand, is usually good enabling many patients with this problem to graduate through university.

Spasmus Nutans This term refers to a type of pendular nystagmus, which is present shortly after birth and resolves spontaneously after 1 or 2 years. Like other forms of congenital nystagmus, it may be associated with head nodding.

Albinism Pigmentation of the eyes and skin is under genetic control. When the lack of pigmentation is limited to the eye, the patient has ocular albinism and when generalized, the patient has oculocutaneous albinism. The typical oculocutaneous albino has pale pink skin and white hair, eyebrows and eyelashes. There is often congenital nystagmus and reduced visual acuity. The optic fundus appears pale and the choroidal vasculature is easily seen (usually obscured by retinal pigment). In addition clinical and OCT examination often shows underdevelopment of the foveal pit (foveal hypoplasia) and electrophysiological tests demonstrate mis-routing of the optic nerves to the occipital cortex. The iris has a gray-blue colour but the red reflex can be seen through it giving the iris a red glow. Ocular albinism is inherited as an X linked recessive disorder while oculocutaneous albinism is inherited in an autosomal recessive manner and may be partial or complete. Albinos often need strong glasses to correct their refractive error, which is usually myopic astigmatism. Dark glasses are also usually required because of photophobia. Tinted contact lenses may also sometimes be helpful.

Structural Abnormalities of the Globe

There are many different developmental abnormalities of the globe but most of these are fortunately rare. Coloboma refers to a failure of fusion of the foetal cleft of the optic cup in the embryo. Coloboma of the iris is seen as a keyhole shaped pupil and the defect may extend into the choroid, so that the vision may be impaired. Inspection of the fundus reveals an oval white area extending inferiorly from the optic disc. Children may be born without an eye (anophthalmos) or with an abnormally small eye (microphthalmos). It is always important to find out the full extent of this type of abnormality and if the parents have noticed something amiss in the child's eye, then referral to a paediatric ophthalmologist is required without delay. Often a careful discussion of the prognosis with both parents is needed.

Aniridia Aniridia (congenital absence of the iris) may be inherited as a dominant trait and can be associated with congenital glaucoma, underdevelopment of the fovea and limbal stem cell failure which can lead to corneal opacification. The lens may be subluxated or dislocated from birth. This may be suspected if the iris is seen to be tremulous. This strange wobbling movement of the iris used to be seen in the old days after cataract surgery without an implant, but it is now still seen after injuries to the eye and signifies serious damage. Congenital subluxation of the lens is seen as part of Marfan's syndrome. (Congenital heart disease, tall stature, long fingers, high arched palate). Congenital glaucoma has already been discussed in the chapter on glaucoma; it may be inherited in a dominant manner and is the result of persistent embryonic tissue in the angle of the anterior chamber. When the intraocular pressure is raised in early infancy, the eye becomes enlarged producing buphthalmos ('bull's eye). This enlargement with raised pressure does not occur in adults.

Congenital Cataract The lens may be partially or completely opaque at birth. Congenital cataract is often inherited and may be seen appearing in a dominant manner together with a number of other congenital abnormalities elsewhere in the body. The condition may also be acquired in utero, the best known example of this being the cataract due to rubella infection during the first trimester of pregnancy: remember the triad of congenital heart disease, cataract and deafness in this respect. Minor degrees of congenital cataract are sometimes seen as an incidental finding in an otherwise normal and symptomless eye. The nature of the cataract usually helps with the diagnosis. The lens fibres are laid down from the outside of the lens throughout life. If the opaque lens fibres are laid down in utero then this opaque region can remain in the centre of the lens. Only when the cataract is very thick does it present as a white appearance in the pupil and often it is difficult to detect it. It is important to examine the red reflex and see whether the darker opaque lens fibres show up. The surgeon has to decide whether the vision of the child has been significantly affected and unless the cataracts are very dense it may be better to wait until the school years approach in order to obtain a more accurate measure of the vision. Sometimes the vision may turn out to be surprisingly good with apparently dense cataracts. The surgical technique is similar to that for cataract surgery in the adult use a contact lenses until a intraocular lens is inserted when they are older and the eye has however some-

times the child is left without an intraocular lens (aphakia) and the parents undergone most of its growth. When the cataract is unilateral, this presents a special case because the affected eye tends to end up having a degree of amblyopia even if an intraocular lens and regular changes of contact lenses are used to refine the vision.

Other Eye Conditions in Childhood

Abnormalities of Refraction

Nowadays children whose vision is impaired because they need a pair of glasses are usually discovered by routine school testing of their visual acuity. They may also present to the doctor because the parents have noticed them screwing up their eyes or blinking excessively when doing their homework. Some children can tolerate quite high degrees of hypermetropia without losing visual acuity simply by exercising their accommodation, and unless there appears to be a risk of amblyopia or squint, glasses may not be needed. By contrast, even slight degrees of myopia, if both eyes are affected, can interfere with school work. Myopia does not usually appear until between the ages of 5 and 14 years, and most commonly at about the age of 11. With the recent rapid increase in the incidence of myopia, interest has focused on ways to prevent or limit myopic progression in children. Two techniques that has shown some success are orthokeratology—the wearing of special contact lenses while asleep to temporarily reshape the corneal curvature and weak atropine drops.

Squint

This exceedingly common inherited problem of childhood has already been considered, but it is worth summarising some of the main features. All cases of squint require full ophthalmological examination because the condition may be associated with treatable eye disease, most commonly amblyopia of disuse. There is no reason why any patient, child or adult, should suffer the indignity of looking 'squint eyed' because the eyes can be straightened by surgery. In spite of this, it is not always possible to restore the full simultaneous use of the two eyes together (binocular vision). In general, the earlier in life that treatment is started, the better the prognosis.

Amblyopia of Disuse

This relatively common condition has been defined as a unilateral impairment of visual acuity in the absence of any other demonstrable pathology in the eye or visual pathway. This rather negative definition fails to explain that there is a defect in nerve conduction due to inadequate usage of the eye in early childhood. The word "amblyopia" means blindness and tends to be used rather loosely by ophthalmologists. It is most commonly used to refer to amblyopia of disuse ('lazy eye') but it is also used to refer to loss of sight due to drugs and toxins. Amblyopia of disuse is very common and some patients even seem unaware that they have any problem until they suffer damage to their sound eye. This weakness of one eye results when the image on the retina is out of focus or out of position for more than a few days or months in early childhood or, more specifically, below the age of 8 years. Amblyopia of disuse therefore arises as the result of a squint or a one sided anomaly of refraction, or it may occur as the result of opacities in the optical media of the eye. A corneal ulcer in the centre of the cornea of a young child may rapidly lead to amblyopia. Once a clear image has been produced on the retina, either by the wearing of spectacles or other treatment, the vision in the weak eye may be greatly improved by occluding or blurring the vision in the sound eye with atropine drops. The younger the patient, the better are the chances of improving the vision by occlusion, even so, normal stereoscopic vision may not be achieved. Beyond the age of 8 years it is unlikely that any significant improvement can be achieved by this treatment and, by the same token, it is unlikely that amblyopia will appear after the age of 8. An adult could suffer total occlusion of one eye for several months without experiencing any visual loss in the occluded eye.

Leucocoria

This term means 'white pupil' and it is an important sign in childhood. There are a number of conditions that may produce this effect in early childhood. The important thing to realise is that if a parent notices 'something white' in the pupil, the matter must never be overlooked and requires immediate investigation. The differential diagnosis includes congenital cataract, opaque nerve fibres in the retina, retinopathy of prematurity, endophthalmitis, some rare congenital abnormalities of the retina and vitreous and, not common but most important, retinoblastoma.

Retinopathy of Prematurity

During the course of oxygen therapy in premature infants, the development of retinal vessels is arrested. When oxygen treatment is reduced, the areas of arrested development become ischaemic and the pre-existing vessels become engorged and new vessels grow from the peripheral arcades of the fundus. This growth of abnormal vessels leads to vitreous haemorrhage, retinal detachment and retinal fibrosis. The infant can rapidly become blind. The management of the condition involves screening those babies at risk (premature and/or of low birth weight) and of monitoring of blood oxygen levels. When the condition occurs, treatment with cryotherapy used to be performed, however this has been largely replaced by retinal laser photocoagulation. Nowadays, the use of intravitreal injection of anti-VEGF agents is showing great promise and research is being conducted to find the most appropriate dose and time point for effective treatment. The treatment also has the advantage of being non-destructive on the retina.

Ophthalmia Neonatorum

It is important to realise that in the early part of this century, a large proportion of the inmates of blind institutions had suffered from ophthalmia neonatorum. The disease affects primarily the conjunctiva and cornea and is the result of infection by organisms resident in the maternal birth passage. The gonococcus was the most serious cause of blindness but a number of other bacteria have been incriminated including staphylococci, streptococci and pneumococci. It has also been shown that chlamydial infection of the genital tract may lead to the same problem as may also infection by the herpes simplex virus. The blindness, which resulted from this condition, was so serious that any excessive discharge from the eyes has been a notifiable disease in this country since 1914. Ophthalmia neonatorum is caused by unhygienic conditions at birth and its relative rarity nowadays is due to the fact that midwives are trained to screen for the condition. Bacterial conjunctivitis usually occurs between the second and fifth day after birth whereas chlamydial infection tends to occur a little later, between the sixth and tenth day. Purulent or mucopurulent discharge is evident and the eyelids may become tense and swollen so that it is difficult to open them and carry out the all important examination of the cornea. When the disease is suspected, the infant should be admitted to hospital, swabs taken and treatment started with systemic and topical antibiotics. The history of infection in the parents needs to be explored and managed by a genito-urinary specialist.

Uveitis

Uveitis is rare in childhood; it may take the form of choroiditis, sometimes shown to be due to toxoplasmosis or toxocara, or the form of anterior uveitis sometimes associated with Still's disease. The management of these cases is similar to that of the adult, but recurrences may result in severe visual loss in spite of treatment.

Optic Atrophy

One must be rather wary about the diagnosis of optic atrophy in very young children because the optic discs tend to look rather pale in normal individuals. Occasionally unilateral visual loss with or without a squint is found to be associated with pallor of the disc on one side. Confirmed optic atrophy, either unilateral or bilateral, requires a full neurological investigation. The causes of optic atrophy in childhood are numerous but the important ones may be listed as follows:

Optic Atrophy without Systemic Disease
- Hereditary optic atrophy.
- Drug toxicity

Optic Atrophy with Systemic Disease
- Glioma of the optic nerve secondary to neurofibromatosis
- Craniopharyngioma
- Post-meningitis
- Post-traumatic after head injury
- Hydrocephalus
- Hypoxic brain injury
- Disorders of lipid metabolism.

Juvenile Retinal and Macular Degenerations

Conditions such as retinitis pigmentosa (peripheral retina) and Stargart's disease (macula) are rare causes of progressive peripheral and central visual loss respectively. The diagnosis can easily be missed as fundus examination can be remarkably normal early on, however, with modern retinal imaging early cases may be detected. The inheritance of retinal and macular dystrophies can be dominant, recessive or sex linked so a thorough examination of other family members is essential .

The Phakomatoses

The three conditions: neurofibromatosis (Von Recklinghausen's,disease), tuberose sclerosis (Bournville's disease) and Von Hippel-Lindau disease are classed together under this name. They all involve the eye but may not become evident until later life. Often examination of the eye reveals the diagnosis. In neurofibromatosis, multiple neurofibromata are seen on the skin, and the eyelids may be enlarged and distorted. Gliomata may develop in the optic nerves and scattered pigment 'cafe au lait' patches are seen in the skin. Brown (Lisch) nodules are often seen on the iris. In tuberose sclerosis, learning difficulties and epilepsy are associated with a raised nodular rash on the cheeks and mulberry like tumours (astrocytomas) in the optic fundus. Von Hippel-Lindau disease presents to the ophthalmologist as angiomatosis retinae. Vascular tumours appear in the peripheral retina, which may leak and expand and lead to detachment of the retina. Similar tumours may be present in the posterior fossa (cerebellar haemangioblastomas) and the spine. Other important findings may include pancreatic cysts, renal and adrenal tumours. Patients often require life-long eye examinations and brain and abdominal scans.

Summary

The differences between the child and adult eye are described and the special methods needed to screen and examine children's eyes are outlined. An account is given of the commoner conditions that confront the paediatric ophthalmologist and finally some rare but important conditions to complete the picture.

Systemic Disease and the Eye

21

Abstract

Systemic diseases may affect the different parts of the eye. This is because the pathophysiologic processes that underlie disease manifestation elsewhere in the body are similar to those in the eye.

This chapter describes systemic diseases that commonly affect the eye, including diabetes mellitus, hypertension, thyroid disease, and acquired immunodeficiency syndrome, and other selected infectious diseases. Other diseases including those that manifest as uveitis, and neurological diseases are described in other appropriate previous chapters.

Introduction

Systemic diseases may affect different parts of the eye. These are generally diseases where the underlying pathophysiologic changes affect different tissues including the eye e.g. diabetes mellitus and hypertension. The specific ocular tissue predisposition varies from disease to disease. Similar to ophthalmic involvement, other specific organs including the kidneys and brain may be affected.

The several systemic diseases that may affect the eye are summarized in Table 21.1. Some of

Table 21.1 Systemic diseases with ocular manifestations

Class	Examples
Spondyloarthropathies	Ankylosing spondylitis, psoriasis
Connective tissue diseases	Rheumatoid arthritis, juvenile idiopathic arthritis, polyarteritis nodosa, pseudoxanthoma elasticum, systemic lupus erythematosus, Wegener, Marfan, stickler, Ehlers-Danlos
Inflammatory bowel disease	Ulcerative colitis, Crohn disease
Non-infectious multisystem inflammatory disease	Sarcoidosis, Behcet disease, VKH
Multisystem infections and infestations	HIV, toxoplasmosis, cat-scratch fever, lyme disease, syphilis, onchocerciasis, chlamydia, Ebola, Covid-19
Muco-cutaneous disease	Steven Johnson syndrome, acne rosacea
Cardiovascular disease	Systemic hypertension
Metabolic disease	Diabetes, Dysthyroid disease, acromegaly
Myopathies	Myasthenia gravis, myotonic dystrophy
Leukemias, and other blood dyscrasias	Chronic lymphocytic leukemia, myeloid dysplasia
Neurological disease	Multiple sclerosis, Phakomatosis, von Hippel-Lindau

N. R. Galloway et al., *Common Eye Diseases and their Management*,
https://doi.org/10.1007/978-3-031-08450-8_21

these diseases and their ocular manifestations are described in other chapters of this book, whilst the reader is referred to larger texts for those not described in detail here.

Diabetes Mellitus

Diabetes mellitus affects 6% of the UK population. This equates to 4.7 million of the UK population in 2019, including 90% type 2, 8% type 1, and 2% other (rare) types of diabetes. The disease is more prevalent in other countries, and the worldwide prevalence is approximately 463 million (9.3%) in 2019, and estimated to rise to 578 million (10.2%) by 2030. Approximately 50% of people with diabetes are unaware they have it. Diabetic retinopathy (DR) is the commonest cause of legal blindness in patients between the age of 20 and 65 years such that about 1000 people are registered blind from diabetes per year in the United Kingdom. That means 14% of severe visual impairment in working age group is due to diabetes. The management of diabetic eye disease has improved greatly over the past 20 years so that much of the blindness can now be prevented. In spite of this, most general practitioners are aware of tragic cases of rapidly progressive blindness in young diabetics. Approximately 7% newly registered sight loss occurs in diabetics. The more serious manifestations of diabetes in the eye tend to affect patients in the prime of life. The tragedy is even greater when one considers that this blindness is largely avoidable.

Diabetes is therefore the most important systemic (non-infective) disease which gives rise to blindness. Many diabetics remain free of eye problems, but a diabetic is 25 times more likely to become blind than other (non-diabetic) members of the population.

When taking an eye history from diabetic patients, it is especially important to note the duration of the diabetes and the age of onset as the incidence of DR is most related to the duration of diabetes. Other risk factors are listed in Table 21.2.

Table 21.2 Risk factors for diabetic retinopathy

- Age
- Duration of diabetes
- Smoking
- Hypertension
- Poor diabetic control
- Hyperlipidaemia
- Renal impairment
- Pregnancy

DR is extremely rare under the age of 10 years; it does not usually appear until the disease has been present for some years. Juvenile onset diabetics usually take longer to show eye changes than those with a late onset, probably because we are often unsure of the exact onset of the disease type 2 diabetes.

Although DR is the most serious ocular complication, the eye may be affected in a number of other ways and it is convenient to consider the various ocular manifestations of diabetes in an anatomical manner beginning anteriorly.

The systemic complications of diabetes include nephropathy, large blood vessel (including stroke) and coronary artery disease, neurological (sensory polyneuropathy) and increased infections.

Eyelids

It is usual to check the urine of patients presenting with recurrent styes but in practice it is unusual for diabetes to be diagnosed in this way. Xanthelasma of the eyelids is said to be slightly more common in diabetics.

Ocular Movements

Elderly diabetic patients are more prone to develop transient third and sixth cranial nerve palsies than non-diabetics of the same age group. Sometimes isolated third nerve palsy may be painful and the pupil is spared. A fasting blood sugar may be required in patients presenting with isolated third nerve palsies. Hypertension and arteriosclerosis need exclusion.

Cornea and Conjunctiva

Some diabetics have microcirculatory changes e.g. conjunctival vascular irregularity and dilatation. Tear film abnormalities are common in diabetics of all ages, although more obvious in the older age group. Corneal sensitivity is reduced in diabetes, and this reduction parallels the duration and poor control of diabetes. Corneal abrasions heal more slowly, and may be more recurrent compared to non-diabetics. Corneal ulcers in diabetics may prove particularly troublesome. Minor trauma to the cornea may lead to the formation of indolent chronically non-healing or infected ulcers, which respond very slowly to intensive treatment with local antibiotics. Inadequate treatment may lead to endophthalmitis and loss of the eye. This problem occurs especially in diabetics with severe vascular disease and typically in a patient who has had to have a gangrenous leg removed.

Anterior Chamber

A particular kind of iritis is occasionally seen in diabetics after cataract surgery when there is a severe plastic reaction. It is important that such cases are treated adequately to prevent the development of posterior synechiae, which will make subsequent fundal examination difficult. Some eye surgeons consider it advisable therefore to use mydriatic drops (Cyclopentolate) after cataract surgery in diabetics. In addition, higher frequency of post-operative steroid eye drops may be necessary to reduce inflammation.

Iris

The iris itself often shows degenerative changes in longstanding diabetics. The pupil may react sluggishly and fail to dilate very widely after the instillation of mydriatic drops. The ophthalmic surgeon can appreciate that pigment is easily lost from the iris when it is handled, and it is interesting that a characteristic vacuolation of the pigment epithelium lining the posterior

surface of the iris is seen in histological sections. When diabetes seriously interferes with the circulation of the eye, the iris may become covered on its anterior surface by a fibrovascular membrane. To the naked eye, the iris takes on a pinkish colour, but examination with the slit lamp biomicroscope or a magnifying lens soon reveals the minute irregular blood vessels on its surface. The appearance is known as 'rubeosis iridis' or neovasclarisation of the iris (Fig. 21.1). Special care is required in looking for fine iris neovascularization in persons with pigmented iridis, including African-Caribbean persons, as it is not as obvious. Iris neovascularization occurs in eyes with severe retinal ischaemia, which leads to production of high levels of vascular endothelial growth factor (VEGF) in the posterior segment, diffusing forwards to the iris and anterior chamber. Neovascular glaucoma occurs once the rubeosis involves the anterior chamber angle. If left untreated very few eyes with rubeosis iridis retain useful sight. The iris should be examined carefully before pupillary dilation, in order not to miss these fine new vessels as they become less obvious after pupil dilatation.

Lens

It was mentioned in an earlier chapter that diabetics tend to develop senile cataracts at an earlier stage than normal. Cataracts once developed also progress more quickly in diabetics compared

Fig. 21.1 Rubeosis iridis (iris noevascularisation)

to non-diabetics. In addition, a rapidly advancing type of cataract is seen in young poorly controlled patients. This is a true diabetic cataract. This cataract is bilateral and consists of snowflake posterior or anterior opacities, matures rapidly and is similar to the rare cataract seen in starvation from whatever cause. The routine testing of urine of patients with cataracts produces a good return of positive results, making this an essential screening test.

It was also mentioned in a previous chapter that the refractive power of the lens might change in response to a rise in the blood sugar level. This results from increased hydration of the lens in patients with high uncontrolled blood sugar levels. Similarly, known diabetics with fluctuating blood sugar (uncontrolled diabetics) will have intermittent blurring due to the hydration of the lens. Undiscovered diabetics quite often become short sighted due to this so-called index myopia. They may then obtain some distance glasses and subsequently consult their doctor, who treats their diabetes. By this time the glasses are made and, of course, turn out to be unsatisfactory, because the index myopia may improve with treatment. In some instances index myopia proves irreversible, being the first sign of cataract formation. Macular oedema may complicate cataract surgery more commonly in diabetics compared to non-diabetics, requiring treatment.

Retina and Vitreous

DR is the most serious complication of diabetes in the eye and often reflects severe vascular disease elsewhere in the body. There are two kinds of DR: background and proliferative. Background retinopathy (BGDR) is very common when diabetes has been present for some years and is less of a threat to the sight than the proliferative variety. Diabetic maculopathy is a special form of retinopathy that may occur with either background or proliferative disease. It is important that the doctor is able to recognise retinopathy, and it is especially important that he

or she should be familiar with the warning signs that indicate proliferative changes and significant maculopathy.

DR is essentially a small vessel disease affecting the retinal precapillary arterioles, capillaries and venules. The larger vessels may be involved. The vascular disease may take the form of vascular leakage, or closure with resultant ischaemia, or combination of both.

Background Retinopathy

There are usually no ophthalmic symptoms initially, but inspection of the fundi of most diabetics who have had the disease for 10 years or more reveals, at first, a few microaneurysms. They are often on the temporal side of the macula but often scattered over the posterior pole of the fundus (Fig. 21.2). These may come and go over months and the overall picture may be unchanged for several years. The vision is not affected unless the microaneurysms are clustered round the macular region and leak fluid resulting in macular oedema. Exudates are also seen and these tend to form rings around areas of diseased vessels, although only one part of the ring may be present at any given point. These are yellowish white deposits with well-defined edges, which are the result of precipitation of leaked lipoproteins from diseased blood vessels. Capillary dilatation is a more subtle sign of DR. Hemorrhages, which may be small ('dot') or large ('blot'), result from the venous end of capillaries and are in the deep retina. Flame-shaped haemorrhages may also occur in the retinal nerve fibre layer. 'Cotton wool' spots represent axoplasmic accumulation adjacent to microinfarction of the retinal nerve fibre layer. They are greyish white with poorly defined fluffy edges (similar to cotton wool—hence the name). Histological examination of diseased retina has shown areas of capillary closure and capillary microaneurysms. The vessel walls have thickened basement membranes and loss of mural cells (pericytes), with relative preservation of endothelial cells (Fig. 21.3).

Fig. 21.2 Background diabetic retinopathy. (**a**) Early: microaneurysms, haemorrhages (different sizes), scattered exudates. (**b**) Severe: extensive haemorrhages, cotton wool spots, and venous dilatation

Fig. 21.3 Trypsin digest of retina from a diabetic showing microaneurysms and loss of some mural cells (percytes)

The Pre-Proliferative Stage

Pre-proliferative retinopathy is typically seen in poorly controlled diabetics (usually type 1 diabetes). The situation may become very bad very quickly and it is important to be able to recognise the warning signs, which occur before proliferation. There are three of them: a large number of dark blot haemorrhages in all retinal quadrants, irregular calibre and dilatation of the retinal veins ('beading') and finally, the presence of intraretinal microvascular abnormalities (IRMA). These warning signs may herald the appearance of the retinal or optic discs new vessels (signs of proliferative retinopathy), which should not be confused with normal disc capillaries or with widened collateral vessels, which are enlargement of pre-existing veins following retinal vascular occlusions, in an attempt to improve circulation. Approximately 50% of eyes with pre-proliferative changes will progress to proliferative disease within 1 year.

Proliferative Retinopathy

Proliferative diabetic retinopathy (PDR) occurs in 5% of all diabetics. Younger onset diabetics have an increased risk of PDR after 30 years. Until recently 50–70% of PDR cases became blind within 5 years. This still pertains if these eyes not adequately treated.

PDR is characterised by the development of new blood vessels (neovascularisation) on the optic nerve head and/or the retina (Fig. 21.4). These occur as a response to retinal ischaemia, which leads to excessive levels of VEGF and other cytokines being released from the retina. These new vessels may appear as small tufts, which ramify irregularly. They may be fine, flat initially but enlarge and move forwards into the vitreous cavity as they grow. Once the new vessels form and grow, and because these new vessels are fragile, there is increased risk of an acute pre-retinal or vitre-

Fig. 21.4 Proliferative diabetic retinopathy: significant neovascularisation from the optic disc

ous haemorrhage. This is a significant threat to vision because the vitreous haemorrhages may become recurrent or dense preventing any meaningful examination and treatment. Retinal fibrosis associated with the neovascularisation, and traction retinal detachment, and neovascular glaucoma may occur at later stages of PDR (end stage PDR).

It is important to appreciate that PDR may be quite severe before the patient notices anything, as DR is asymptomatic, and the situation may have to be explained very carefully to him or her.

Diabetic Maculopathy

Diabetic maculopathy is the commonest cause of visual impairment in diabetics. It occurs more commonly in type 2 diabetics, although it can occur in all types. Three types of maculopathy are known and are due to retinal vascular leakage, closure, or combinations of the two. Leakage may be focal or diffuse, and may occur in isolation or in combination with other macular changes. The three types of maculopathy are:

Focal diabetic macular oedema (DMO), due to focal leakage from a microaneurysm or dilated capillaries and surrounding exudates are seen (Fig. 21.5a). OCT shows localized thickening of the retina, with or without intraretinal fluid or cysts, and subretinal fluid accumulation (Fig. 21.5b).

Diffuse DMO, caused by diffuse leakage from dilated capillaries at the posterior pole of the eye. The retinal oedema is diffuse and may be associated with microaneurysms and few haemorrhages but exudates are absent (Fig. 21.6a, b). OCT images show a more diffuse spread of retinal thickening, intraretinal as well as subretinal fluid compared to that seen clinically on biomicroscopy and colour photographs, and allows more objective assessment of the oedema following treatment (Fig. 21.6c).

Ischaemic maculopathy is due to closure of the perifoveal and surrounding vascular network. In addition to diffuse oedema several dark haemorrhages may be present (Fig. 21.7a). Fluorescein angiography may be required to confirm the ischaemia and determine its severity (Fig. 21.7b). OCT will not show the ischaemia, but in severe cases may show retinal thinning. This thinning may, however, be confounded by associated retinal oedema. OCT-A which depicts retinal capillary network may show the foveal ischaemia, although excessive oedema may confound such findings that assess flow rather true vascular morphology, or leakage.

Treatment

Control of diabetes. This aspect of treatment may seem self evident but in the past the value of careful control has not always been fully recognised. Some patients have the impression that eye problems develop anyway 'if the diabetes has been present long enough'. Nothing could be fur-

Fig. 21.5 (**a, b**) Focal maculopathy showing circinate exudates

Fig. 21.6 Diabetic macular oedema (DMO): (**a**) colour photo; (**b**) late phase fluorescein angiogram of same eye showing dye leakage characteristic of diffuse and cystoid dye leakage macular oedema; (**c**) OCT showing cystic spaces in the retina indicating oedema before treatment, and resolution of the oedema after intravitreal injection of ranibizumab

Fig. 21.7 Ischaemic diabetic maculopathy: (**a**) colour photograph; (**b**) fluorescein angiogram

ther from the truth. Control of the diabetic state needs to be sustained all the time. It is not the short-term, but rather the long-term control of the blood sugar that is important in determining the severity and progression of DR. Control or elimination of the known risk factors (Table 21.2) is also important in reducing DR severity.

Treatments for DMO

The current treatments for DMO target reducing vascular leak in the macula once it has occurred, and do not necessarily prevent it.

Laser photocoagulation. The use of a focused light beam to 'cauterise' the retina has been practiced for several years. The advent of more focused light in the form of lasers has enhanced such use, and the value of this treatment has been confirmed by extensive clinical trials for both PDR and some types of maculopathy. Laser photocoagulation has been the mainstay of treatment until recently when pharmacological treatments were introduced. The laser treatment of focal and diffuse maculopathy involves application of small number of burns (of 100-200 μ spot size)

to the leaking area, whilst avoiding the foveal avascular zone. (A laser burn to the fovea results in immediate central vision loss). Such treatment helps prevent further visual deterioration, but may need to be repeated. Despite this treatment, a significant number of patients still lost vision over several months to years afterwards. Ischaemic maculopathy generally is not amenable to laser treatment.

Pharmacological treatments for DMO target reducing vascular leak in the macula once it has occurred, they do not attempt to treat the underlying pathology. These pharmacological treatments are aimed at antagonizing VEGF (pegaptanib, ranibizumab, aflibercept and bevacizumab) or non-VEGF inflammatory pathways with steroids (fluocinolone, dexamethasone or triamcinolone), and are given by intravitreal injections. Each drug has its specific duration of activity, and therefore frequency of administration. These treatments are summarised in Table 21.3. These pharmacologic treatments are particularly useful in eyes where the oedema has affected the fovea and immediate surrounding area, so that laser photocoagulation is not recommended or will be damaging to the vision.

Table 21.3 Pharmacological treatments for DMO

Drug	Class of pharmacological agent	Frequency of intravitreal administration
Pegaptanib (Macugen, Pfizer)	Anti-VEGF: Blocks VEGF 165. Unlicensed for treatment of DMO.	6 weekly
Ranibizumab (Lucentis, Novartis)	Anti-VEGF: Blocks all VEGF isoforms	4–8 weekly
Aflibercept (Eylea, Bayer)	Anti-VEGF: Blocks all VEGF isoforms and PlGF	4–8 weekly
Bevacizumab (Avastin, Roche)	Anti-VEGF: Blocks all VEGF isoforms. Unlicensed for intravitreal administration	4 weekly
Dexamethasone implant (Ozurdex, Allergan)	Glucocorticoid (steroid)	3–6 monthly
Fluocinolone implant (Iluvien, Alimera)	Glucocorticoid (steroid)	2–3 yearly
Triamcinolone (Kenalog, Squibb; Trivaris, Allergan; Triescence, Allergan)	Glucocorticoid (steroid) Kenalog (Squibb) is unlicensed for intraocular administration; Trivaris not available in EU	2 months
Brolucizumab (Beovu, Novartis)	Anti-VEGF: Blocks all VEGF isoforms	Initially 4-weekly, then extending to 2–3 monthly
Faricimab (Roche/Genetech)	Bispecific antibody: Blocks all VEGF isoforms, and Ang-2	Initially monthly, extending to 2–4 monthly
KSI-601	Anti-VEGF biopolymer conjugate: Blocks all VEGF isoforms	2–6 monthly intervals
Others		

Treatments for Proliferative Diabetic Eye Disease

Laser Photocoagulation The value of panretinal laser photocoagulation (PRP) as treatment for PDR has been confirmed by extensive clinical trials. Laser burns to the retina destroy the ischaemic drive in the retina, and reduce VEGF production. The treatment must be applied promptly in the early proliferative stage or sometimes before. About 2500–3000 burns (of 500 μ spot size) or equivalent are needed in an eye with PDR. Larger number of burns are required if smaller spot sizes (than 500 μ) of laser are used. This may require several treatment sessions (Figure 21.8a, b).

Glaucoma Surgery Rubeosis iridis requires treatment, preferably before the intraocular pressure becomes elevated. Drainage surgery may be needed if neovascular glaucoma is not controlled by medical means. Rubeosis iridis initially requires panretinal laser photocoagulation. However, such eyes may have cloudy corneas, because of the high IOP. An initial intravitreal injection of off-license bevacizumab, or other anti-VEGF, in order to induce regression of the iris neovascularization and clear the cornea may be necessary before laser application. This also helps the glaucoma surgeon when he undertakes the drainage surgery. Primary open angle glaucoma may also be more common in diabetics. Drainage surgery in these cases is less successful than in non-diabetics. Special measures need to be taken to avoid failure. It is also vital to control rubeosis iridis before any attempts at cataract surgery in order to avoid catastrophic intraocular bleeding.

Vitreo-Retinal Surgery There have been dramatic advances in the technical side of vitreous surgery in recent years so that it is now possible to remove a persistent vitreous haemorrhage and to divide or remove fibrous tissue, even from the surface of the retina and relieve traction retinal detachment. Vitrectomy for vitreous haemorrhage tends to be performed sooner these days (within 1 month) because of the relative safety of

Fig. 21.8 (**a**) Panretinal laser photocoagulation in proliferative diabetic retinopathy. (**b**) Modern laser photocoagulation: less intense laser burns; treatment incomplete

the technique, and the higher risk of visual loss from delayed surgery. Preoperative ultrasonography may be helpful in planning the surgery. Vitrectomy may be combined with intraoperative PRP.

Prognosis

A better understanding of DR has resulted from advances in molecular biology, and the use of more accurate methods of investigation, especially fluorescein angiography, OCT, and OCT-A, and also the routine use of indirect ophthalmoscopy and slit-lamp biomicroscopy. Serial fundus photography and the use of ultrasound have also been important. The molecular changes driving onset and progression of DR are better understood. In particular, VEGF and non-VEGF pathways are known to play important parts in the development and progress of DR and DMO. This better understanding and modern technology have led to more effective treatments so that the more severe ocular complications are now largely avoidable or treatable. Blindness tends to be limited to those cases where social or other circumstances make management difficult. Patient education is vital in order to maintain continuing improvement in visual prognosis for diabetics. Approximately 75% of diabetics will

develop some form of retinopathy after 20 years of disease. About 70% of patients with PDR will progress to blindness if untreated in 5 years.

Thyroid Eye Disease

Dysthyroid eye disease is an autoimmune disease in which the manifestations may be notable in the hyperthyroid, euthyroid or hypothyroid phase. Although the ophthalmic features of thyroid disease are often diagnosed in the hyperthyroid phase, a significant number of patients may be euthyroid (i.e. have no other evidence of thyroid disease) or less often hypothyroid at the time of detection of the eye changes. Thus the ophthalmic disease may precede, be coincidental or follow the systemic manifestations and is usually progressive for 1–5 years after which it stabilises. The orbital involvement is an immunological disease that affects orbital muscles and fat.

Grave's disease is a term used to describe the most common form of hyperthyroidism that has an autoimmune basis. Hyperthyroidism may arise from other conditions e.g. thyroid tumour or pituitary dysfunction. It usually affects women more commonly, between 20 and 45 years (female: male ratio = 4:1). Usually it is characterised by goitre, infiltrative ophthalmopathy, thyroid acropathy (clubbing) and pretibial myxoedema.

When these ophthalmic changes occur in isolation the condition is described as Ophthalmic Grave's disease (OGD). Smoking has a major detrimental effect on thyroid eye disease.

The systemic features of hyperthyroidism include weight loss, high pulse rate, poor tolerance of warm weather and fine tremor. The eye signs of thyroid disease are eyelid retraction and lid lag, puffiness of the eyelids, chemosis, proptosis, exposure keratitis, double vision from muscle involvement and optic neuropathy (see Table 21.4).

Lid Retraction The eyelids are drawn up slightly, more on one side than the other. Reveals white sclera above corneoscleral junction (Fig. 21.9). Similarly, lower eyelid retraction may also occur. Eyelid retraction occurs in approximately 50% of patients with thyroid eye disease, and has been attributed to fibrotic contraction of the eyelid retractors: levator palpebrae superioris, and inferior rectus, secondary overaction of the levator palpebrae superioris, or the sympathetic Muller muscle.

Fig. 21.9 Dysthyroid eye disease: eyelid retraction

Lid Lag When instructed to follow a pencil as it moves downwards, the upper lid appears to lag behind the rotation of the eye, revealing more of the white above. The upper lid shows jerky movements as the eye rotates smoothly down. There is also reduction in the rate of blinking. The eyes tend to dry up more quickly compared to that in normal persons.

Table 21.4 The 13 possible signs of thyroid eye disease

- Proptosis
- Raised intraocular pressure when looking up
- Lid lag
- Lid retraction
- Lid swelling
- Chemosis
- Conjunctival congestion
- Double vision
- Exposure keratitis
- Corneal ulceration
- Optic disc swelling
- Impaired visual acuity
- Constriction of visual field

Fig. 21.10 Dysthyroid eye disease: bilateral eyelid oedema, worse on the right than left

Lid Swelling Puffiness of the eyelids may be present (Fig. 21.10).

Chemosis This means conjunctival oedema. To the naked eye it appears as though the eyes are brimming with tears, and the expression 'the tear that never drops' is sometimes used. When severe, the conjunctiva overhangs the lower lid margin.

Proptosis Eyelid retraction may give the false impression of proptosis but measurement of the position of the globe in relation to the bony orbit can be achieved by means of an exophthalmometer. Any relative protrusion can thus be measured for future reference. Dysthyroid disease is the commonest cause of unilateral or bilateral proptosis. Forward protrusion of the globe may lead to severe exposure keratitis demanding urgent attention.

Exposure Keratitis Punctate staining with fluorescein across the lower part of the cornea is characteristic and due to inadequate closure of the retracted upper lid.

Limitation of Extraocular Muscle Action The muscles become infiltrated (with inflammatory cells, including lymphocytes, plasma cells and macrophages, as well as increased glycosaminoglycans with fluid retention) and thickened producing a characteristic appearance on CT or MRI scan, which helps to distinguish this form from other causes of diplopia. The muscle thickening is confined to the bellies so that the tendons are not affected. The main restriction of movement is due to infiltration then subsequently tethering of the inferior recti with limitation of upward gaze. The resulting pressure on the globe may cause the intraocular pressure to rise on looking up and this has been used as a diagnostic test. The other extraocular muscles are involved less frequently.

Optic Nerve Compression This condition occurs only in 5% of cases of thyroid eye disease. However it is important because of the seriousness of the condition. It is due to the increased pressure within the orbit, where enlargement of the extraocular muscle causes crowding of the orbital apex with subsequent compression of the optic nerve. The first sign may be swelling of the optic disc, followed by optic atrophy. It is therefore vitally important to monitor the visual acuity and central visual field in these cases.

Management

Laboratory tests required to confirm dysthyroid state are listed in Table 21.5.

Patients should be advised to stop smoking. Reassurance is all that may be required in the mild forms of the disease. In some cases treatment is usually limited to that of the exposure keratitis or dryness due to the reduced blink reflex. Ocular lubrication with artificial tear drops, and an antibiotic ointment instilled at night is often sufficient. Sometimes a small lateral tarsorrhaphy on each side can greatly improve the appearance of a young girl with lid retraction. Lid retraction may also be improved by the use of guanethidine eye drops, which are thought to provide sympathetic antagonism. More severe cases may need surgery, or injection of botulinum toxin to weaken action of the eyelid retractors.

If there is visual deterioration (from optic nerve compression or significant proptosis) large doses of systemic steroids are probably the best line of treatment (e.g. prednisolone 120 mg/day). Initial recovery is usually dramatic and rapid but then the side effects of systemic steroids ensue. The dose should be reduced as soon as feasible but it may be necessary to continue with a maintenance dose for many months. Some ophthalmolgists may use other immuno-suppressive agents e.g. azathioprine or orbital radiotherapy in severe cases of proptosis and or optic nerve compression. If there is no response between 24 and 48 h, surgical decompression of the orbits is required. If double vision persists beyond the

Table 21.5 Routine tests for thyrotoxicosis

- Serum thyroxine (T4)
- Thyroid autoantibodies
- T3 assay

acute stage, extraocular muscle surgery may be helpful, in addition to operations designed to deal with lid retraction (see previous paragraph).

Hypertension

Although the effects of raised blood pressure on the appearance of the fundus of the eye were recognised in the nineteenth century, the nature of the detailed changes have been disputed for a long time. Certain characteristic features, such as the 'nipping' of the veins at arteriovenous crossings, narrowing of the arterioles, haemorrhages, papilloedema and exudates, are beyond doubt. Some confusion can be avoided if it is realised that the effects of raised blood pressure are modified by other changes in the eye due to natural ageing. It is now accepted that the exact cause of the raised blood pressure does not by itself influence the fundus appearance. However, the appearance of the retinal vessels and associated changes serve as a good guide to the severity of the disease and urgency of treatment. The changes observed in the fundus represent retinal, choroidal, and optic nerve damage following prolonged elevation of systemic blood pressure, as well as the speed with which they occur.

The Effect of Age on the Retinal Blood Vessels

In older patients the retinal arteries are seen to be narrower and straighter and the veins are also narrower than in younger patients. The term 'retinal arteriosclerosis' is used to describe these changes.

The Effects of Raised Blood Pressure on the Retinal Vessels

In younger patients, irregular narrowing of the retinal arterioles is seen, and is thought by many to be due to spasm of the blood vessel walls. This is seen as focal constriction and dilatations of the retinal arterioles, which may also become slightly more tortuous. This hypertonicity leads in time to more permanent changes in the vessel walls so that the vessels resemble those of an older patient. The arterioles may also have increased wall reflex, with reduction in the visibility of blood column within the arterioles (referred to by some as 'copper wiring'). Nipping of the veins at arteriovenous crossings is seen, and on the distal side of the crossing the vein may be distended. Occasional flame haemorrhages, cotton wool spots and exudates, may indicate more severe vascular damage, but do not necessarily lead to 'malignant' hypertension (Fig. 21.11a).

In older persons, the already narrowed retinal arterioles tend to show less dramatic changes. Hypertonicity of the vessel walls is not seen, unless there is severe elevation of the blood pressure, but arteriovenous nipping remains an important sign, and haemorrhages may be present in more severe cases. The cotton wool spots of hypertension reflect ischaemic damage to the nerve fibre layer due to obstruction of the retinal pre-capillary arterioles. Exudates are due to abnormal increased vascular permeability.

Other changes that may occur secondary to chronic systemic hypertension include retinal vascular occlusions, retinal macroaneurysms, and non-arteritic anterior ischaemic optic neuropathy.

'Malignant' Hypertension

Occasionally patients with a severe hypertensive problem present directly to the ophthalmologist because their main symptom is blurring of the vision, the other more usual symptoms being less evident. Similarly, patients who present to the physician with malignant hypertension, with or without ocular symptoms should have their eyes examined. On examination, the visual acuity may be only slightly reduced unless there is significant macular oedema, vascular occlusion, or optic nerve involvement, and there may be some enlargement of the blind spot and constriction of the visual fields. Inspection of the fundus reveals marked swelling of the optic disc; the oedema often

Fig. 21.11 Hypertensive retinopathy: (**a**) retinal haemorrhages, exudates, cotton wool spots, and irregular and generalised arteriolar narrowing; (**b**) fundus in malignant hypertension showing optic disc swelling with peripapillary haemorrages and cotton wool spots (as well as in all quadrants), constricted arterioles, macular oedema and exudates; (**c**) chorioretinal changes in treated chronic malignant hypertension showing Elschnig spots, pale optic disc, attenuated white (silver-wired) retinal arterioles, narrowed veins, and an atrophic fovea

extending well away from the disc with scattered flame shaped haemorrhages, and cotton wool spots (Fig. 21.11b). Hypertensive changes in the choroid initially may manifest as choroidal ischaemia and leakage. Focal occlusions of the choriocapillaris lead to greyish-whitish lesions in the acute stage, which may be associated with focal RPE detachments, and subsequent focal hyperpigmentation; these are called Elschnig spots. (Fig. 21.11c). Siegrist's spots are linear pigmentations along choroidal arteries and develop similarly to Elschnig's spots.

If the diastolic blood pressure is above 110–120 mmHg, there is little doubt about the diagnosis, but below this level it is essential to bear in mind the possibility of raised intracranial pressure from other causes. When hypertension is as severe as this the patient should be treated as an acute medical emergency and referred without delay to the appropriate physician.

The optic neuropathy in hypertension is seen clinically as optic disc oedema, and results from constriction/obstruction of the posterior ciliary arteries, which supply the optic nerve.

Retinal Vascular Occlusions

Retinal vein occlusions (RVO) are the second
commonest type of retinal vascular disease (after
diabetic retinopathy), and is due to obstruction of
the retinal veins. It usually occurs in persons over
50 years old, but can occur earlier. This is more
common in hypertensive patients compared to
normotensives. It is also associated with diabetes,
hyperlipidaemia, and other cardiovascular risks,
as well as increased intraocular pressure. Factors
that predispose to increase blood viscosity e.g.
leukemia may also predispose to RVO. However,
it should be noted that retinal vein occlusions
may occur in the absence of any known systemic
disease associations. Obstruction of a branch of
the central retinal vein, called branch retinal vein
occlusions (BRVO) is more common than central retinal vein occlusion (CRVO). RVO may be
further divided into ischaemic and non-ischaemic
types. RVOs that are initially ischaemic may
convert to ischaemic types with further drop in
vision.

The fundus appearance in CRVO is dramatic
with numerous scattered haemorrhages, cotton
wool spots and dilated tortuous retinal veins in
all four quadrants, and swelling of the optic disc,
and the patient experiences sudden blurring of
vision in one eye (Fig. 21.12). The level of vision
reduction is dependent on the level of retinal
ischaemia. In addition, ischaemic CRVO may
progress to iris neovascularization.

In BRVO, the venous dilatation, retinal
haemorrhages, and cotton wool spots are confined only to the distribution of the occluded
vein. The obstruction in BRVO usually occurs
at an arterio-venous crossing. BRVO that are
secondary to other disease (other than arteriosclerosis or hypertension) do not occur at
arterio-venous crossings, as in inflammatory
diseases e.g. sarcoidosis, Behcet's disease, and
toxoplasmosis. Ischaemic BRVO of sufficient
size will predispose to retinal or optic disc
neovascularization.

Fig. 21.12 (**a**) Central retinal vein occlusion, and (**b**)
macular branch retinal vein occlusion

Visual loss in RVO is due to ischaemia, macula oedema or both.

Management

Any underlying disease (as above) should be
treated adequately to prevent a recurrence of vascular occlusions in the same or other eye, as well
as improve general health and well being.

Macular oedema in CRVO does not respond
to laser photocoagulation. Recent clinical trials
have shown that the macular oedema in CRVO
responds to multiple intravitreal injections of

anti-VEGFs or steroids similar to the situation in diabetic macular oedema (Fig. 21.13). Iris neovascularization and neovascular glaucoma should be treated along similar lines as described for that in advanced diabetic eye disease, and involves anti-VEGF therapies and PRP.

Macular oedema in BRVO responds to modified grid laser photocoagulation. However, more recent advances have shown that intravitreal injections of anti-VEGF drugs and/or steroids e.g. Ozurdex may lead to significant resolution of the oedema, and visual improvements compared to or better than achieved with laser photocoagulation (Fig. 21.14). However, these injections need to be repeated at different intervals for a long time (similar to that in DMO).

Retinal Artery Occlusions

Retinal artery occlusions result from a sudden reduction of central retinal artery perfusion (CRAO) or a branch of the central retinal artery (BRAO) causing ischaemia of the inner retina in the distribution of the affected blood vessel. Retinal arterial occlusions are less common and the prognosis is uniformly worse than vein occlusions, due to the significant infarction of the inner retina.

Arterial occlusions manifest as a sudden, painless loss of vision. Sometimes, there is blurring of vision which recovers within 24 hours, a phenomenon described as amaurosis fugax. On fundoscopy, there is whitening of the affected retina (due to oedema/swelling of the inner retina. This appears as a cherry red spot in CRAO,

Fig. 21.13 Central retinal vein occlusion; (**a**) colour photo, (**b**) OCT before (showing intraretinal and subretinal cysts/oedema) and after treatment (showing resolution of oedema, and restoration of normal architecture) with intravitreal injection of ranibizumab

Fig. 21.13 (continued)

whilst in BRAO the whitening is restricted to the retinal area supplied by the occluded vessel (Fig. 21.15). The retinal whitening disappears at approximately 4 weeks after the occlusion. An embolus may be seen in arterial branch or the CRA at the optic disc. The occluded arteriole will be narrowed, and blood flow disrupted and seen as cattle-tracking of the blood column in the occluded vessel. In BRAO, a visual field defect

corresponding to the distribution of the occluded vessel is observed.

Retinal artery occlusions may be caused by arterial wall thickening, thrombus or emboli. The potential sources of emboli are similar for CRAO and BRAO and include calcified emboli from cardiac valves and atheromatous plaques in the carotid arteries; platelet or fibrin emboli may also be observed. These emboli are however, seen more frequently in BRAO than CRAO. In giant cell arteritis, the vascular lumen is obstructed by the thickened CRA wall due to progressive inflammation. Similarly, vasculitis from varicella zoster, and orbital infections in diabetes (e.g. mucormycosis) may lead to CRAO. Increased blood coagulability may also result in CRAO or BRAO.

There is no satisfactory treatment for BRAO or CRAO. The visual loss is therefore permanent, except for cholesterol emboli that move on.

Ischaemic Optic Neuropathy

Some elderly patients complaining of visual loss in one eye are found to have a pale swollen optic disc and sometimes evidence of branch retinal artery occlusion, giving an altitudinal defect of the visual field. This appearance should suggest the possibility of giant cell (temporal) arteritis and an ESR & CRP, and a temporal artery biopsy should be considered as urgent investigations (Fig. 21.16).

However there is a group known as 'non-arteritic' or idiopathic anterior ischaemic optic neuropathy (AION) which occurs in patients between 50 and 75 years old, individuals who may have diabetes or hypertension, but may be healthy. An acute loss of vision occurs. There may be sectorial optic disc swelling, and a few peripapillary haemorrhages. An altitudinal visual field defect may be seen. In these patients retinal arterial occlusion is absent. About one third of these patients develop bilateral disease. There is no known treatment for non-arteritic AION but giant cell arteritis needs exclusion, as its management is different, and urgent.

Anaemia

When the haemoglobin concentration in the blood is abnormally low, this becomes apparent in the conjunctiva and ocular fundus. The conjunctiva, similar to oral mucosa is pale. The retinal vessels become pale and the difference

Fig. 21.14 Hemispherical retinal vein occlusion; (a) colour photo, (b) OCT before (showing intraretinal cysts/oedema) and after treatment (showing resolution of oedema, and restoration of normal architecture) with intravitreal injection of Ozurdex

Fig. 21.14 (continued)

between arteries and veins becomes less apparent. The fundus background also appears pale but this sign is dependent upon the natural pigmentation of the fundus and may be misleading. In severe cases small haemorrhages are usually seen, mainly around the optic disc. The haemorrhages tend to be flame-shaped but a special feature of anaemic retinopathy is the presence of white areas in the centre of some of the haemorrhages. The haemorrhages may be due to associated low platelet counts. In pernicious anaemia, retinal haemorrhages and bilateral optic neuropathy which manifests as centrocaecal scotomas are seen. In severe cases the optic nerves are atrophic. Anaemia secondary to blood loss may give rise to ocular hypoperfusion, which leads to anterior ischaemic optic neuropathy. Examination of the conjunctiva is perhaps of more value or at least is certainly an easier way of assessing the haemoglobin level and this part of the examination of the eye should, of course, precede oph-thalmoscopy. The cause of the anaemia should be sought and treated in collaboration with the general practitioner or haematologist.

The Leukaemias

All ocular tissue may be involved in leukaemia. The eye changes may occur at anytime during the course of leukaemia, or they may comprise the presenting features of the disease. These changes are more common in the acute leukaemias than in the chronic types.

Two groups of ophthalmic manifestations are recognised in leukaemias. The first group con-sists of leukaemic infiltration of ocular structures for example, retinal and pre-retinal infiltrates or anterior chamber and iris deposits. All of these are quite uncommon. The second group of manifestations is considered to be second-ary to the haematological changes for example, thrombocytopenia, increased blood viscosity and highly increased leucocyte count. These changes include subconjunctival haemorrhages, intra-retinal haemorrhages which may be white cen-tred, cotton wool spots, 'slow flow retinopathy', (Fig. 21.17), and retinal venous occlusions (espe-cially CRVO).

Less common manifestations include choroi-dal and optic disc infiltrations, retinal and optic disc neovascularisations. Apart from the eye

Fig. 21.15 Retinal arterial occlusions. (**a**) Central retinal artery occlusion showing 'cherry-red spot', and multiple retinal arterial emboli; (**b**) branch retinal arterial occlu-sion, whitish oedematous superior retina, and an embolus in the superior retinal artery branch at optic disc; (**c**) same fundus as in (**b**) showing resolution of the retinal oedema 6 weeks after the acute obstruction, note embolus is still present; (**d**) OCT image of the same eye with BRAO in acute phase and after resolution of the retinal swelling

Fig. 21.15 (continued)

Fig. 21.16 Anterior
ischaemic optic
neuropathy. The superior
part of the disc is pale

Fig. 21.17 The fundus in leukemia. Note dilated, tortuous veins and haemorrhages

changes, patient's vision may be impaired by leukaemic infiltrates elsewhere in the visual pathway (leading to field defects).

Ocular disease may also occur as complications of treatment of the leukaemia e.g. opportunistic infections e.g. Herpes zoster, graft-versus-host reactions, and subconjunctival and intraocular haemorrhages.

Sickle Cell Disease

This condition is mentioned separately because of the severe and devastating effect it may have on the individual's vision. The sickle cell haemoglobinopathies are inherited, and due to the affected person having one or more abnormal haemoglobins as recognised by the electrophoretic pattern which are labelled alphabetically. Haemoglobins S and C are the most important ophthalmologically. Thalassaemia (persistence of foetal haemoglobin) can also cause retinopathy. The abnormal haemoglobins occur either in combination with normal haemoglobins resulting in AS (sickle cell trait) or in association with each other as SS (sickle cell anaemia or disease)

or SC (sickle cell haemoglobin C disease), and S thal (Thalassemia). Individuals with sickle cell trait usually lead a normal life and do not have any systemic or ocular complications. The red blood cells in patients with sickle cell (SS, SC, SThal) disease adopt abnormal shapes under hypoxia and acidosis. These abnormal red cells are less deformable compared to normal and lead to occlusion of the small retinal blood vessels including capillaries especially in the retinal periphery.

Sickle cell retinopathy can be divided into two types: (1) non-proliferative and (2) proliferative. In non-proliferative sickle retinopathy there is increased venous tortuosity, peripheral chorioretinal atrophy, peripheral retinal haemorrhages, peripheral haemosiderin deposits which appear refractile, and peripheral arterial occlusion (Fig. 21.18a). These lesions are usually asymptomatic. When central retinal arterial or venous occlusion, macular arteriolar occlusion or choroidal ischaemia occur there is significant visual deficit.

When significant ischaemia is present retinal neovascularisation occurs (proliferative sickle cell retinopathy—PSR (Fig. 21.18b, c). This is generally in the retinal periphery. Such periph-

Fig. 21.18 Sickle cell (SC) retinopathy: (**a**) non-proliferative SC retinopathy showing occluded peripheral retinal arterioles; (**b**) sea-fan neovascularisation in proliferative SC retinopathy (PSR); (**c**) vitreous haemorrhage in eye with PSR in (**b, d**) SCR maculopathy. Inner retinal thinning of temporal macula without obvious clinical retinopathy. OCT B-scan shows inner retinal thinning; OCT-A shows focal loss of the deeper retinal capillary network with normal inner retinal capillary network

eral neovascularisation may respond to laser photocoagulation or cryotherapy of the retina. Occasionally, PSR may result in vitreous haemorrhage or traction retinal detachment, and in some cases, vitrectomy is required. Occlusion of choroidal vasculature in Sickle Cell Disease has also been described. OCT and OCT-A images shows the capillary closure and thinning of the retinal layers without any obvious changes on fundoscopy (Fig. 21.18d).

Onchocerciasis

Onchocerciasis, commonly known as river blindess, is caused by the filaria onchocerca volvulus. The name 'river blindness' is derived from the occurence of the disease in focal areas along rivers and streams where the blackfly (Similium) breeds in fast flowing water. The blackfly can travel several kilometers and does not respect international borders.

The disease is characterised by a few adult worms encased in nodules and the invasion of the body by microfilaria produced by the adult worms. It is endemic in Equatorial Africa—West and Central, Central and South America. It is estimated that there are about half a million blind people due to onchocerciasis. Significant inroads have been made by international Onchocerciasis Control Programmes.

The adult worm has a lifespan of 15–30 years. The microfilaria is sucked up by the blackfly when it takes its blood meal. Subsequently, division within the blackfly gives rise to latter stages of the larva, which are re-injected, into the skin of the next victim of the blackfly's bite. The microfilariae migrate under and through the skin and may mature in about 1 year. Newly produced microfilariae migrate to the eye through the skin or blood.

Clinical manifestations of onchocerciasis may be divided into extraocular and ocular manifestations.

Extraocular Features

Skin: pruritis—a maculopapular rash, which may be associated with hypo- or hyper-pigmentation, dermal, and epidermal atrophy or 'onchodermatitis'.

Subcutaneous nodules—which are firm, round masses in the dermis and subcutaneous tissue, especially close to joints in the head and shoulder.

Ocular Features

Intraocular microfilariae may be seen in the anterior chamber. Dead microfilaria are usually seen in the cornea (especially peripherally).

Punctate keratitis and sclerosing keratitis.

Anterior uveitis, usually of the nongranulomatous type with loss of the pigment frill, and posterior synechiae are common. Secondary cataract and glaucoma may develop.

Chorio-retinitis of the chronic non-granulomatous type with secondary degenerative changes in the RPE neuroretina and the choriocapillaries. There may be granular atrophy of the RPE, subretinal fibrosis, retinal arteriolar attenuation and vasculitis. Optic atrophy and neuropathy are not uncommon.

Diagnosis is confirmed by (1) Skin snip and (2) The Mazzoti Test which depends on a Herxheimer reaction to a single dose of diethyl-carbamazine (DECM). Care is required with this test since the reaction could be very severe.

Management

1. Vector control: An international (WHO) programme, the Onchocerciasis Control Programme (OCP) has been successful in reducing the endemicity of the disease in the Volta River Basin.
2. Chemotherapy of infected patients now uses Ivermectin, which in a single dose rids the

patient of microfilaria for one to 2 years. This medication needs to be repeated over several years in mass administration projects.

Diethylcarbamazine is the older treatment for the microfilaria but is more toxic and requires to be taken over a 2–3 week period. Adult worms can only be killed by Suramin, or removed surgically.

Acquired Immune Deficiency Syndrome (AIDS)

AIDS refers to the final stages of infection by the Human Immunodeficiency Virus (HIV). The earlier stages of the disease are often asymptomatic. (Table 21.6).

In the Western countries, AIDS commonly affects homosexuals, haemophiliacs, and intravenous drug abusers, although there is now a significant heterosexual and paediatric pool of patients. In Africa and the rest of the world, it is generally a heterosexual disease, and a significant paediatric population is also known. Transmission is through sexual intercourse, parenteral or transplacental routes. Once infected, the HIV virus targets the CD4+ T lymphocytes of the host resulting in a steady decline in the numbers of these cells, and reduced immunity to pathogens.

According to the Centres for Disease Control and Prevention (CDC), Atlanta (USA), an adult individ-

ual who is infected with HIV and has a CD4+ T cell count of <200/µL or a CD4+ T cell count of <14% of the total lymphocyte count, or has one of the several known opportunistic infections, tumours, or other manifestations (wasting syndrome or encephalopathy) associated with the disease.

In children, HIV status may be classified according to infection, clinical, and immunologic status, allowing for better management. In infants, born to HIV mothers, the situation is even more complicated because of maternal transmission of anti-HIV Ig G antibodies to the infant, although true infection occurs only in up to 15% of them.

Ocular features occur in 75% of patients with AIDS. The major ocular complications of AIDS occur later in the disease and can be predicted by CD4+ T cell levels. At CD4 level >200 µ/L common ocular complications are toxoplasmosis and Herpes zoster ophthalmicus and retinitis whilst at CD4 levels <50/µL CMV retinitis is common.

AIDS microangiopathy (non-infectious) occurs in about 50% of patients (in both developing and Western countries). It consists of microaneurysms, telangiectasia cotton wool spots and a few retinal haemorrhages. Retinal peripheral perivascular sheathing may sometimes occur in the absence of intraocular infections.

Other ocular involvement of AIDS includes infections with opportunistic and non-opportunistic organisms (e.g. CMV, cryptococcus, molluscum contagiosum, syphilis, toxoplasmosis) (Figs. 21.19 and 21.20). Neoplasms of the conjunctiva, lids and orbit, and neuro-ophthalmic complications are other features.

In Western countries, the commonest ophthalmic complications of AIDS is CMV retinitis whilst in developing countries (as Africa), CMV is not a major problem; Herpes zoster ophthalmicus and conjunctival carcinoma are common in AIDS patients in Africa and AIDS patients die of other complications for example tuberculosis. Therefore, short term survival from AIDS itself is a problem in developing countries whilst in Western countries quality of life for the longer term is the main problem. The advent of anti-retroviral treatments has prolonged life expectancy in AIDS patients.

Table 21.6 Phases of human immunodeficiency virus (HIV) infection

Phases	Manifestations
I	Acute infection: Asymptomatic with seroconversion
II	Asymptomatic carrier
III	Generalised, persistent lymphadenopathies; usually good state of general health
IV	Symptomatic HIV infection (AIDS) Subgroups (a) Constitutional (cachexia, fever, etc.) (b) Neurological (c) Infections diagnostic of AIDS (d) Malignancies (e) Others: e.g. CD count<200/µL

Fig. 21.19 Cytomegalovirus retinitis in acquired immune defi ciency syndrome (AIDS)

Treatment with HAART regime (involving 2 nucleoside reverse transcriptase inhibitors) or 1 or 2 protease inhibitors leads to significant elevation of CD4+ T cell levels such that the ocular complications, especially opportunistic infections are less commonly encountered. The treatment regimens continue to evolve, and are better left to trained specialists.

Ophthalmological Signs of AIDS
1. Non Infectious Retinopathy:
   (a) Cotton-wool spots.
   (b) Retinal haemorrhages.
   (c) Microvascular changes.
2. Opportunistic Infections:
   (a) Involvement of posterior segment.
      • Cytomegalovirus retinitis
      • Acute retinal necrosis (Herpes simplex, zoster).
      • Progressive outer retinal necrosis
      • Toxoplasmic chorioretinitis.
      • Pneumocystis carinii choroiditis.
      • Tuberculous choroiditis.
      • Endophthalmitis caused by Candida albicans—usually intravenous drug users.

   • Cryptococcus chorioretinitis.
   • Syphilitic retinitis.
   (b) Involvement of anterior segment.
      • Chronic keratitis and keratouveitis caused by herpes zoster and simplex.
      • Keratoconjunctivitis caused by cytomegalovirus, microsporum and gonococcus.
      • Corneal ulcer caused by Candida albicans, and bacteria (Pseudomonas aeruginosa, Staphylococcus aureus, and Staphylococcus epidermidis).
      • Syphilitic and toxoplasmic iridocyclitis.
      • Conjunctivitis caused by CMV, herpes zoster and simplex.
      • Bacterial conjunctivitis.
3. Neoplasms:
   (a) Conjunctival, palpebral and orbital Kaposi sarcoma.
   (b) Intraocular lymphoma.
   (c) Other neoplasms.
      • Conjunctival squamous carcinoma.
      • Palpebral and orbital lymphoma.
4. Neuro-Ophthalmological Signs:
   (a) Involvement of cranial nerves.

Fig. 21.20 Human immunodefi ciency virus retinopathy

- Internuclear ophthalmoplegia.
- third, fourth and sixth cranial nerve palsies.
- Retrobulbar neuritis and papillitis.
(b) Homonymous hemianopia.
(c) AIDS-dementia complex with cortical blindness.
HIV Encephalopathy and progressive multifocal leucoencephalopathy
5. Other Signs:
  (a) Conjunctiva.
    - Non-specific conjunctivitis.
    - Keratoconjunctivitis sicca.
    - Non-specific conjunctiva microvascular changes in the inferior perilimbal bulbar region (haemorrhages, microaneurysms, column fragmentation, dilatation, and irregular vessel diameter).
    - Bacterial conjunctivitis.
  (b) Cornea
    - Non-specific punctate keratitis.
  (c) Sclera:
    - Necrotizing scleritis.
  (d) Retina.
    - Talc-induced retinopathy (only intravenous drug users).
  (e) Eyelids

- Herpes zoster ophthalmicus.
- Palpebral molluscum contagiosum.
- Palpebral cryptococcosis.
(f) Orbit
  - Orbital apex granuloma.
  - Orbital pseudotumour.
  - Orbital infiltration by Aspergillus, pneumocystis carinii.
  - Orbital cellulitis.
(g) Visual and refraction defects.
  - Night blindness due to vitamin A and E malabsorption.
  - Progression of myopia.
  - Decreased accommodation.
(h) Acute closed-angle (bilateral) glaucoma caused by choroidal effusion.

Ocular Manifestations of Coronavirus (Covid-19)

Corona virus disease 2019 (Covid-19) became a global pandemic in December 2019 after originating in Wuhan, China. It is due to a highly transmittable severe acute respiratory syndrome coronavirus 2 (SARS-CoV-2), which is an enveloped positive single stranded RNA virus and follows previous outbreaks in Singapore in 2003. Covid-19 has resulted in many deaths worldwide due to severe systemic illness. The reader is referred to the extensive text available elsewhere on the systemic effects of Covid-19.

Covid-19 virus particles have been detected in tear film and conjunctival swabs by reverse-transcriptase polymerase chain reaction (RT-PCR). Similarly, nasal and nasopharyngeal detection of Covid-19 virus is well documented. As such, possible disease transmission through aerosol spread, and direct examination by an ophthalmologist has to be carefully managed. Wearing of appropriate facial (nose and mouth) protection by the patient as well as the ophthalmologist is important, in addition to the Perspex/plastic guards or shields on the slit lamp biomicroscope. The slit lamp and protective shields should be wiped down with disinfectant (preferably 70% ethanol) after every patient examination. Single use tonometer heads, or sterilisation with 10% sodium hypochlorite between patients is advised, if available. It is also preferable to have patient seats that are wiped down after each use.

Ocular manifestations of conjunctivitis, anterior uveitis, retinitis and retinal vasculitis as well as optic neuritis have been described in animals infected with coronaviruses including Covid-19.

Clinically, follicular conjunctivitis, with unilateral or bilateral conjunctival hyperemia, watery discharge, and mild eyelid oedema have been described. The conjunctival hyperemia seems to be marked in critically ill patients. The frequency of conjunctivitis is unclear but varies from 1 to 32% in different studies. As such the conjunctiva may be an infection portal as well as an entry point for Covid-19 infections.

In the ocular fundus, retinal changes include hyper-reflective lesions in the inner layers (ganglion cell and inner plexiform layers) on OCT, cotton-wool spots, and microhaemorrhages have also been reported. Retinal haemorrhages occur because of the increased coughing episodes, especially in patients who have received anticoagulation (Fig. 21.21). Vasalva (pre-retinal) haemorrhages have been described, and rarely central retinal artery occlusion may be seen. Other findings include cotton wools spots, venous dilatation and increased tortuosity. Neuro-

Fig. 21.21 Retinal images in a Covid-19 patient

ophthalmology complications are uncommon but have been reported, and include diplopia, III cranial nerve palsy, and abnormal MRI findings of cranial nerve perineural inflammation.

In the earlier phase of Covid-19, patients who are receiving intensive care treatment, risks of forced ventilation and prone positioning may result in other ocular risks and manifestations, including ocular surface disorders, secondary infections, and less frequently acute ischaemic optic neuropathy, as well as exposure to multidrug resistant bacteria. There is a significant intraocular pressure elevation in the prone patient that may result in optic nerve damage, if prolonged. Subconjunctival haemorrhages may also occur in severely ill patients because of forced ventilation and or anticoagulation.

Potential toxicity of drugs used (current and potential) in the treatment of Covid-19 need to be at the back of clinician's mind at all times.

Ocular Manifestations of Ebola Virus Disease

Ebola virus disease (EVD) or Ebola is a haemorrhagic fever of humans and other primates caused by ebolaviruses (filiviridae, an enveloped single-strand, filamentous RNA virus). The virus spreads through direct contact with body fluids, such as blood from infected humans or other animals, or human fluid or items recently contaminated. Ebola virus has been detected in the aqueous humour at day 63, and conjunctival fluid at day 22. The virus has been detected in intraocular fluids at 6 months after initial disease onset. Virus RNA was not detected in the aqueous at 19–34 months after infection.

The systemic disease has an acute onset, usually 2–21 days after exposure, with fever, sore throat, muscular pain, and headaches at presentation. Vomiting, diarrhoea, and a skin rash occur, and are followed by internal and external bleeding. Fluid loss with hypovolaemic shock occurs in a few days, and fatality follows in 25–90% of infected persons.

Ebola disease survivors have a high risk of developing complications in different organs.

This may be because of persistence of the virus in immune privileged tissues including the anterior chamber of the eye and cerebrospinal fluid. These complications include fatigue, vision loss, hearing loss, headaches, memory loss, sleep disorders, mood disturbances, abdominal pain, amenorrhea, miscarriages, and arthralgia. Ocular complications have been reported in 13–34% of survivors, where cataract, uveitis and optic atrophy are the main findings. Ocular motility disorders, and colour vision deficiencies have also been described. Ocular changes were noted within 2 months after EVB onset in 75% of cases. Uveitis consisted of anterior, uveitis, intermediate, posterior uveitis (focal choroiditis with or without macular involvement), or panuveitis, and may be unilateral or bilateral. Macular oedema, intraretinal fluid, epiretinal membrane, and traction retinal detachments and phthisis bulbi have also been described. Approximately 40% of survivors with eye disease had vision impairment. Eyes with uveitis had worse vision than those without it. Uveitis has also been described in close contacts of Ebola patients.

Topical and oral steroids, and immunosuppressive therapy have been effective in resolving the intraocular inflammation. It is thought that combination with anti-viral therapies may lead to earlier resolution, but not confirmed.

Connective Tissue Disease

Several connective tissue diseases affect the different parts of the eye, and to varying degrees. These include inflammatory diseases (e.g. juvenile idiopathic arthritis, spondyloarthropathies, rheumatoid arthritis, Sjogren syndrome, systemic lupus erythematosus, polychondritis, Wegener's granulomatosis, inflammatory bowel diseases), non-inflammatory (e.g. Marfan syndrome, Elhers-Danlos syndrome, and pseudoxanthoma elasticum [PXE]).

Marfan Syndrome Marfan syndrome is an autosomal inherited disease that affects the fibrillin gene on chromosome 15q. It has widespread effects including musculoskeletal, cardiovascular, dermatological and ophthalmic features. Marfan syndrome patients are tall and thin, with disproportionally long limbs compared to the trunk, and narrow high-arched palates. They have aortic dilatation with aortic and mitral incompetence. Ophthalmologically, patients have subluxation of the lens (ectopia lentis), anterior chamber angle abnormalities, hypoplasia of the dilator pupillae muscle, myopia, and high incidence of rhegmatogenous retinal detachments, and, infrequently, corneal changes.

Stickler Syndrome Stickler syndrome is a disease associate with changes in chromosome 12, and inherited as an autosomal dominant disease with variable penetrance. Genetic mutations occur in *COL2A1, Col11A1 or CO11A2*. Patients with Stickler syndrome have a 'marfanoid habitus', arachnodactyly, joint hyper-extensibility, and have a flat nasal bridge, with sensorineural deafness. In the eye, high myopia, and vitreopathy occur.

Pseudoxanthoma Eleasticum Pseudoxanthoma elasticum is inherited as an autosomal or recessive disease, where there is progressive fragmentation, and calcification of elastic tissue in different body organs, including the skin, cardiovascular system, gut and eye. Typically, the skin shows a 'chicken pluck' maculopapular appearance in the neck, axilla, antecubital fossa and groin. In addition, the skin may show hyperelasticity. Calcification of vascular intima leads to cardiac valvular and ischaemic heart disease, intermittent claudication, renal artery disease. Some manifest gastrointestinal bleeding due to calcified mucosal vasculature, which may go undiagnosed for some time. In the eye, typically, angioid streaks, which represent breaks in the calcified Bruch's membrane develop, and may be complicated with retinal atrophy over the streaks, or choroidal neovascular membranes.

Ehlers-Danlos Syndrome Ehlers-Danlos sundrome is a rare autosomal inherited disease. It is due to deficiency of the procollagen lysyl hydroxylase, and has several clinical subtypes. The skin is hyperelastic and bruises easily and is slow to heal, with increased scarring. The joints are hyperextensible with lax ligaments that predispose to frequent recurrent dislocations. The cardiovascular system is affected with mitral valve prolapse, dissecting aneurysm and rupture of large blood vessels. Abnormalities of scoliosis, diverticular disease and diaphragmatic hernia have been described. In the eye, angioid streaks are seen; keratoconus, microcornea, blue sclera, ectopia lentis, high myopia, retinal detachments occur.

Mucocutaneous Diseases

Mucocutaneous diseases that commonly involve the eye include acne rosacea, pemphigoid, Stevens-Johnson syndrome, and atopic eczema.

Acne Rosacea Acne rosacea is a common skin condition affecting sun exposed areas of the body. Clinically, erythematous papules appear on the forehead, nose, malar areas, and chin. The rash may be itchy and may develop telangiectasia, and pustules; rhinophyma is well known in this condition. In the eye, significant meibomitis may occur, and alongside the tear film instability result in corneal vascularization.

Steven-Johnson Syndrome Steven-Johnson's syndrome (S-JS) is a rare but severe adverse event affecting the eyes, skin and mucous membranes. Typically, it is a blistering disease affecting the mucocutaneous system. S-JS may blend to the more severe 'toxic epidermal necrolysis'. S-JS is a delayed hypersensitivity to different molecules which may be drugs or epithelial antigens modified by drugs and infections. Drugs associated with S-JS are sulphonamides and derivatives (including acetazolamide), azithromycin, lamotrigine, carbamazepine, allopurinol, diclofenac and nevirapine. It should be remembered that different infections can also trigger S-JS, particularly viral (Epstein-Barr, upper respiratory viruses) and bacterial infections (group A beta-haemolytic streptococci, diphtheria, brucellosis, typhoid, lymphogranuloma venereum, mycobacteria, Mycoplasma pneumoniae, and rickettsiae).

S-JS may present with a flu-like illness: fever, malaise, sore throat, and sometimes arthralgia. Blisters occur in the nasal and oral mucosa, and lips with haemorrhaging. Generalised erythematous skin rash with a haemorrhagic blistering, membranous conjunctivitis occur, and result in scarring of lacrimal gland openings. Inadequate treatment leads to conjunctival scarring, symblepharon, tear deficiency, cicatrical entropion, and corneal scar formation.

Treatment requires prompt diagnosis. In the acute phase, ocular lubrication, topical steroids and haptic contact lenses may be required, depending on severity. Systemic steroids have been advocated. In the healed phase, ocular lubrication and punctal occlusion may suffice in mild cases. Bandage, or gas-permeable contact lenses may be required. In severe cases, conjunctival or mucous membrane grafting, and limbal cell transplants, or lamellar corneal grafting are necessary, and require specialist expertise.

Summary

- After completing this chapter, the reader should appreciate that systemic diseases may affect different parts of the eye.
- Systemic diseases as expected affect a widespread of organs in the body, and include metabolic, non-infectious inflammatory, infectious, collagen, dermatologic, haematologic, and hereditary diseases.
- Particular diseases have predilection for particular tissues in the different organs, depending on the underlying pathophysiology. As example, the vasculature of the retina and choroid show the most marked changes in diabetes and hypertension, although other ocular tissues are affected. In acne rosacea, the eyelids, cornea and conjunctiva are more affected, whilst leukemia may affect any part of the eye. Mucocutaneous, connective tissue, and haematologic diseases have specific ocular predilections.
- The ocular changes may be the first manifestation or presentation of some of these diseases, such that the eye specialist has to remain vigilant.
- Systemic infections can have significant effects on the eye, including old as well as recently known diseases, such as Ebola virus and Covid-19. Survivors of EVD have virus particles detected in intraocular fluid for several months after the initial disease.
- Ocular tissues and fluid may be a source of transmission of infections including EVD, and requires care.
- The management of the ocular manifestations should be alongside that of the systemic disease, and therefore requires cooperation with other medical teams.
- The management may require local as well as systemic treatment as necessary.

Neuro-Ophthalmology

22

Abstract

Neuro-ophthalmology deals with disease of the visual and pupillary pathways from the optic disc and beyond, as well as control of eye movements. These result in abnormalities of eye movements, visual field defects, pupillary size and/or reactions, or abnormal optic disc appearances. This chapter describes the common neuro-ophthalmic abnormalities that the practitioner will come across in clinical practice.

Most ophthalmic departments find it necessary to retain a close liaison with neurological and neuro-surgical departments, and neuro-ophthalmology is now in itself a bona fide ophthalmology subspecialty. Retrobulbar (optic) neuritis, for example, is a condition, which presents quite commonly to eye casualty departments and usually requires further investigation by a neurologist. Less common but equally important are the pituitary tumours which can present in a subtle way to the ophthalmologist and which may require urgent medical attention, including neurosurgical services. There are many other, sometimes rare, conditions, which find common ground between the disciplines.

The Optic Disc

Normal Disc

One must be familiar with some of the variations found in otherwise normal individuals before being able to diagnose pathological changes. The optic disc marks the entrance of the optic nerve to the eye and this small circular part of the fundus is non-seeing, as there are no photoreceptors (light sensitive cells) in it; it corresponds with the blind spot in the visual field. The vertical optic disc diameter is approximately 1.5mm. When examining an optic disc, five important features are to be noted: the colour, the margins or contour, the central cup, the blood vessel entry, and the presence or absence of haemorrhages. The optic disc is larger in the myopic, and smaller in the hypermetropic eye.

Colour The optic disc is pink but often slightly paler on the temporal side. That of the neonate may be deceptively pale and some elderly discs appear atrophic without evidence of disease. Pallor of the disc is due to loss of nerve tissue and small blood vessels of the surface of the disc. In very severe optic atrophic cupping, there is exposure of the underlying lamina cribrosa. The myopic disc is relatively pale, whereas the hypermetropic disc is more pink and smaller than normal (Fig. 22.1).

Contour or Margins The margin of the optic disc is normally well defined. There are subtle differences depending on the size of the globe (and therefore refractive error). The disc margins are better defined in myopic than in hypermetropic subjects. In hypermetropes the edges of the disc may appear raised, sometimes resembling papilloedema. It is common to see a crescent of pigment on the temporal side of the disc called *pigmented crescent*, and if present makes it easier to determine the optic disc margin. Frequently an area of chorioretinal atrophy is present at the disc margin in myopes and may give rise to difficulty in deciding where the true disc margin is (Fig. 22.1a, b).

Central Cup The centre of the disc is deeper, i.e. further away from the observer, than the peripheral part. The peripheral part of the optic disc (called the neuroretinal rim) is not uniform and broadest superiorly. The central cup occupies about a third (or less) of the total disc diameter in normal subjects. The cup margin is best determined by observing where the blood vessels bend as they cross the surface of the optic disc. The ratio between the vertical diameter of the cup compared to the total disc diameter is known as the *cup-disc ratio*. Thus the normal cup-disc ratio is <0.3. Irreversible loss of nerve fibres (and supporting tissue) will result in increased (pathological) cupping of the optic disc.

Vessel Entry In general, a central retinal artery and vein divide into upper and lower branches (immediately on emerging from the disc) which in turn divide into nasal and temporal branches close to the disc margin. Many variations in the pattern are seen normally. The veins are darker and wider than the arteries and, unlike the arteries, can be seen to pulsate spontaneously in 80% of the population if examined carefully. In the other 20% of normals, venous pulsation at the disc can be induced by gentle pressure on the globe.

Haemorrhages Haemorrhages are never seen on or adjacent to normal discs. If present, they warrant further investigation.

Congenital Disc Anomalies

A number of minor congenital abnormalities are seen on the disc. In an astigmatic eye the disc is often oval. The central cup may be filled in by 'drusen'—small hyaline deposits, which may be found on the surface or buried in the substance of the disc. This appearance of optic disc drusen may mimic papilloedema until the drusen

Fig. 22.1 Normal optic disc in (**a**) myope and (**b**) hypermetrope

become exposed (Fig. 22.2). Alternatively, the central cup may be hollowed out further by a congenital pit in the disc. Optic disc pits are usually located temporally, but can be central, and the optic disc may be larger than normal. Eyes with optic disc pits often develop a serous retinal detachment. The central cup may be filled in by persistent remnants of the hyaloid artery which runs in the embryo from disc to lens, with or without associations of fibrous tissue (Bergmeister's papilla). Hypoplasia of the optic nerve, which may be unilateral or bilateral, may occur in isolation or be associated with other ocular or midline brain abnormalities. In coloboma of the optic disc, there is an

Fig. 22.2 Optic disc drusen. (**a**) Colour photo: the disc looks swollen, with indistinct margins, and the central disc looks full; some of the drusen are obvious but not uniformly. No disc haemorrhages are present. (**b**) red-free photo of the same disc showing autofluorescence of the drusen which are more obvious than in the colour photograph

obvious excavation of the inferior part of the optic disc, and remaining normal tissue displaced superiorly. The Morning Glory syndrome is a rare condition which manifests as a large excavation of the optic disc with surrounding abnormal glial tissue, and emergence of blood vessels at the margin, resulting in resemblance to the morning glory flower. This abnormality may be associated with brain abnormalities, including absence of the corpus callosum and pituitary deficiency, as well as frontonasal dysplasia. Some of these and other congenital abnormalities of the disc may be associated with visual field defects which are not progressive but which can cause diagnostic confusion. Myelinated retinal nerve fibres are recognised by their strikingly white appearance, which obscures any underlying vessels, and their fluffy margin (Fig. 22.3). Occasionally, a normal optic disc may be surrounded by an excavated sclera, and overlying atrophic choroid and retinal pigment epithelium. This is referred to as a peripapillary staphyloma.

Pale Disc

Optic Atrophy

Optic atrophy means loss of nerve tissue on the disc, and the resulting abnormal pallor of the disc (Fig. 22.4) must be accompanied by a defect in the visual field, but not necessarily by a reduction in the visual acuity. The optic disc margin is clearly defined, but the number of fine blood vessels on the surface are reduced. The number of countable small vessels, is sometimes used as an index of atrophy in difficult cases. The whole disc or part of it may be atrophic, depending on the cause. It must be remembered that the disc tends to be somewhat pale and the cup of disc tends to be larger in short-sighted eyes and care must be taken in diagnosing optic atrophy in such cases.

Classification of the causes of optic atrophy usually includes the term 'consecutive optic atrophy', referring to atrophy following retinal degeneration. The terms 'primary' (without any previous optic disc swelling) and 'secondary'

Fig. 22.3 Myelinated nerve fibres. There is an extensive fluffy edged whitish appearance extending from the superior optic disc margin, and obstructing underlying structures including blood vessels

(preceded by previous optic disc swelling) optic atrophy are also used but because these terms are confusing a simple aetiological classification will be used here. However, it is said that there is more gliosis in secondary than when it is 'primary' optic atrophy. Gliosis makes the appearance of the disc more grey or yellowish-grey than white and the cribriform markings often seen in optic atrophy may not be evident. It should be borne in mind that it is not usually possible to determine the cause of optic atrophy by the appearance of the optic disc. Even the cupped, pale disc of chronic glaucoma may be mimicked by optic atrophy due to chiasmal compression.

The following are the important causes of optic atrophy:

- *Glaucoma.*
- *Vascular.* Following obstruction of the central retinal artery or vein, giant cell arteritis and non-arteritic anterior ischaemic optic neuropathy.

- *Following disease in the optic nerve,* for example optic neuritis or compression of the nerve by an aneurysm or tumour (Fig. 22.4b).
- *Following papilloedema.* The disc may become atrophic as a direct result of the chronic swelling, irrespective of its cause.
- *Inherited.* Retinitis pigmentosa is an inherited retinal degeneration in which there is a progressive night blindness, constriction of the visual field and scattered pigmentation in the fundus. As the condition advances towards blindness, the discs become atrophic. Optic atrophy may also appear in certain families without any other apparent pathology, for example Leber's Hereditary Optic Neuropathy (LOHN), and autosomal dominant or recessive optic atrophies. LOHN results from a maternally inherited mitochondrial DNA mutation which presents with painless loss of vision, and subtle optic disc swelling and dilated capillaries, followed later by optic

Fig. 22.4 Optic atrophy. (**a**) diffuse atrophy (pallor) of the disc; (**b**) optic atrophy caused by pituitary compression of the left optic nerve

atrophy. Optic atrophy is also seen in the rare but distressing cerebro-retinal degenerations, which present with progressive blindness, epilepsy and dementia.

- *Toxic.* A number of poisons can specifically damage the optic nerve; methyl alcohol is a classical example. Tobacco amblyopia is a type of progressive atrophy due to excessive smoking of coarse tobacco, usually in a pipe and often in association with a high ethyl alcohol intake. This may, in fact, be an expression of vitamin B (especially B12) deficiency. Reversal may be achieved by abstention in the early phases of the disease, and administration of vitamin B12 and multivitamin supplementation. Other toxic agents include lead and drugs: ethambutol, isoniazid, digitalis.

- *Trauma.* The optic nerve may be damaged by indirect injury if bleeding occurs into the dural sheath. This may result from a fracture in the region of the optic foramen or rarely, from contusion of the eye itself. After the nerve has been damaged, a period of a few weeks elapses before the nerve head becomes atrophic, so that initially the eye may be blind but the fundus normal. The pupil reaction to direct light is impaired from the time of the injury. Such an injury may result in complete and permanent blindness in the affected eye but a degree of recovery is achieved in a small proportion of cases, if decompression of the nerve sheath is undertaken early.

Swelling of the Optic Disc

This is a serious sign because it may be due to raised intracranial pressure and an intracranial space-occupying lesion. There are, however, a number of other more common causes.

Apparent Swelling

The margins of the optic disc may be ill-defined and even appear swollen in hypermetropic eyes. Other congenital abnormalities of the disc such as optic drusen (Fig. 22.2) or myelination (Fig. 22.3) may also be mistaken for true swelling as described above.

Vascular

The disc may be swollen in congestive cardiac failure or in patients with severe chronic emphysema. Marked swelling of the disc with numerous haemorrhages is seen in occlusion of the central retinal vein and this compares with the pale and less haemorrhagic swelling that is seen in anterior ischaemic optic neuropathy. In the latter instance, swelling of the disc occurs in association with arterial disease and one must take pains to exclude temporal arteritis in the elderly.

Unilateral swelling of the optic disc may also occur due to compression of the nerve which results in interruption of axoplasmic transport.

Postoperative

Swelling of the disc is not uncommon in the immediate post-operative period after intraocular surgery. It is due to ocular hypotony, and may be associated with choroidal folds and effusions. The disc swelling may persist for longer periods if the intraocular pressure remains low. It is not usually regarded to be of serious significance, since the swelling regresses following normalisation of the intraocular pressure.

Papilloedema ('True Papilloedema')

Papilloedema is swelling of the optic discs due to increased intracranial pressure. By definition, the optic disc swelling must be bilateral, although it may be asymmetrical. Every doctor must be aware of the triad of headache, papilloedema and vomiting as an important feature of raised intracranial pressure. The optic disc may be markedly swollen and haemorrhages are present around it, but not usually in the peripheral fundus (Fig. 22.5a). In chronic papilloedema, the disc is paler and haemorrhages may be few or absent (as result of resorption) (Fig. 22.5b). Although these patients may complain of transient blurring of the vision, the visual acuity is usually normal and testing the visual fields shows only some enlargement of the blind spots. It is important to realise that the word 'papilloedema' refers to the non-inflammatory swelling of the disc, which results from raised intracranial pressure. Other signs of increased intracranial pressure should be looked for and include VIth cranial nerve palsies, and hearing loss. The most common causes of raised intracranial pressure are cerebral tumours, hydrocephalus, idiopathic ('benign') intracranial hypertension, subdural haematoma, malignant hypertension and cerebral abscess. Diagnosis of papilloedema entails careful examination of the optic disc, which must be backed up with visual field examination and colour fundus photography, and OCT. The fundus imaging is especially helpful when repeated, to show any change in the disc appearance. Fluorescein angiography may also be of great diagnostic help in difficult cases when abnormal

Fig. 22.5 Papilloedema. (**a**) acute papilloedema; (**b**) the optic disc is swollen with old peripapillary exudates, striae, and dilated retinal veins, but there are no haemorrhages

disc leakage occurs. This, however, is not usually required.

Optic Neuritis

Optic neuritis is inflammation of the optic nerve. This most commonly occurs in association with a plaque of demyelination in the optic nerve in patients with multiple sclerosis, but may be due to other aetiology (see under other causes), including non-infectious, infections (syphilis, cat-scratch fever, Lyme disease, Herpes zoster), post-virus infection syndromes (measles, mumps, chicken pox, whooping cough). The central vision is usually severely affected, in contrast with papilloedema, but optic neuritis occurs in many instances without any visible swelling of the disc (retrobulbar neuritis). When the inflammation affects the optic disc it is referred to as papillitis, which may complicate viral illnesses. Where there is inflammation of the retinal nerve fibre layer surrounding the disc, and or macular exudates in association with papillitis, the condition is called 'neuroretinitis'.

Other Causes

Chronic intraocular inflammation such as anterior, intermediate or posterior uveitis may be complicated by disc swelling. Severe diabetic eye disease may sometimes be marked by disc swelling (diabetic papillopathy). In severe cases of thyroid orbitopathy, the orbital congestion may cause disc swelling (dysthyroid optic neuropathy). In both instances the doctor should be warned that serious consequences might ensue unless prompt treatment is applied. Infiltration of the disc by leukaemia or lymphoma or chronic granulomata (as in sarcoidosis) and systemic vasculitis may also cause disc swelling.

Multiple Sclerosis

This common (in some parts of the world) and important neurological disease may often present initially as an eye problem and its proper management requires careful coordination at the primary care level. It is important to realise that multiple sclerosis (MS) should not be diagnosed after one single attack of optic or retrobulbar neuritis since this could cause unnecessary alarm about something that may never happen. Studies have shown that between 45 and 80% of patients with optic neuritis will develop MS after 15 years of follow up. Furthermore, optic neuritis has causes other than multiple sclerosis. The diagnosis of MS should be made by a neurologist and is based on finding additional evidence of the disease elsewhere in the body.

The cause of multiple sclerosis is not known, but the disease is characterised by the appearance of multiple inflammatory foci in relation to the myelin sheaths of nerves throughout the central nervous system. Myelin is engulfed by macrophages and microglial cells, initially. Subsequently, fibrous tissue plaques are gener-ated by astrocytes. The demyelination plaques are detectable on MRI scans of the brain. The optic nerve between globe and chiasm is commonly involved at an early stage and there may be a delay of several years before other features of the disease appear. Young or middle-aged people are mainly affected and the prognosis is worse when the disease is acquired at an early age. It should be noted that diseases other than MS may cause demyelination resulting in optic neuritis. These include isolated optic neuritis, neuromyelitis optica (Devic disease), and Schilder disease.

Ocular Findings

Optic or Retrobulbar Neuritis

This is an important cause of unilateral sudden loss of vision in a white eye in a young person. Optic neuritis occurs commonly (20–40% of cases), and usually in whites (85%), and women have a 3x higher frequency than men. The patient complains of pain behind the eye on attempting to move it and there is often a grey or coloured patch in the centre of the field of view. In severe cases the sight of the affected eye may be lost completely. On examination a relative afferent pupil defect on the affected side may be the only objective evidence of disease. It is essential to test the pupil before dilating it with eyedrops. The fundus is often normal initially (retrobulbar neuritis), although there may be slight swelling of the optic disc (optic neuritis). After two or three weeks the optic disc starts to become pale. The visual prognosis is generally good. Visual deterioration does not last longer than 1 week normally, and recovery is well under way in 4 weeks. Most patients make a complete or nearly complete recovery after six to twelve weeks. The attack is unilateral in 90% of cases although there is a risk, that the other eye may be affected at a later date and recurrent attacks in one or both eyes may cause permanent damage to the vision. Fortunately it is uncommon for a patient to be made blind by multiple sclerosis. Approximately 10% of patients develop a chronic progressive optic neuritis.

The diagnosis at the time of the acute attack relies on the history and noting the pupil reaction. It is often advisable to make the diagnosis in retrospect. The patient may give a history of visual loss in one eye, which has recovered and at a later date presents with other non-ocular signs and symptoms of demyelinating disease. If it can be confirmed that the patient has had a previous attack of optic neuritis, this may help in the confirmation of the diagnosis of disseminated sclerosis. Under these circumstances the pallor of the disc may be helpful, but careful assessment of the colour vision, visual acuity and measurement of the visually evoked potential may provide conclusive evidence. At the time of the acute attack, testing the visual field may reveal a central scotoma. The size of this defect diminishes as healing occurs, often leaving a small residual defect between blind spot and central area.

Magnetic resonance imaging (MRI) of the brain and orbits shows white matter lesions of demyelination plaques. Lumbar puncture (LP) may be undertaken by the neurologist as necessary. Other diseases that may cause optic nerve infiltration should be excluded, including sarcoidosis, systemic lupus erythematosus (SLE) and neoplasia, as well as anterior ischaemic optic neuropathy (AION), and neuroretinitis.

Treatment Usually, no treatment is required as visual recovery occurs in over 80% of patients. Corticosteroids, particularly high dose intravenous methylprednisolone may speed up recovery of vision. However, the final visual outcome is unchanged by such treatment. Oral prednisolone should be avoided as it may be associated with higher recurrence rates. Interferon beta1α given at the first episode of optic neuritis is thought to significantly reduce recurrence of demyelination.

Nystagmus
This usually appears at a later stage than optic neuritis and may only be evident in lateral gaze. It is often horizontal.

Internuclear Ophthalmoplegia
Whereas double vision is a common symptom in multiple sclerosis, it is unusual to see an obvious defect of the ocular movements. Sometimes it can be seen that one eye fails to turn inwards when the patient is asked to look to the opposite side, and yet when the patient is made to converge the eyes on a near object, the medial rectus moves normally. This failure of the muscle action with certain coordinated eye movements only i.e. limitation of adduction, whilst the opposite abducting eye shows nystagmus is termed 'internuclear ophthalmoplegia' (INO). It is very characteristic of multiple sclerosis when seen in young people (when the internuclear ophthalmoplegia is usually bilateral and is caused by a demyelinating lesion in the pons) but usually has a vascular cause in the elderly (when it is usually unilateral). The underlying lesion in INO is located in the median longitudinal fasciculus (MLF).

Other Features
Other types of ocular muscle dysfunction, for example, a lateral rectus palsy or ptosis, are rare. Careful inspection of the fundi in some cases reveals inflammatory changes around the retinal vessels especially in the periphery (peripheral retinal vasculitis), and intermediate uveitis. Demyelination of the optic chiasma, and optic tracts are uncommon, but may occur, as well as trigeminal and facial nerve involvement.

Defects in the Visual Fields

The pattern of a visual field defect gives useful localising information for lesions in the visual pathway. Localised abnormalities in the retina produce equivalent localised defects in the visual field on the affected side only. Defects due to ocular disease are relatively common as for example those seen in the elderly with glaucoma. Care must be taken to interpret field defects with this possibility in mind. The right half of each retina is linked by nerves to the right occipital cortex and the splitting of nerve fibres from each half occurs at the chiasm. Lesions in the optic nerve anterior to the chiasm (e.g. vascular lesions, sphenoid or olfactory groove meningioma) tend to cause unilateral defects whereas those posterior to the chiasm produce hemianopic or quadrantianopic defects (Fig. 22.6).

The Optic Chiasm The optic chiasm is located above the diaphragma sellae housing the pituitary gland. There are anatomic variations to the exact relationship, which may affect detailed clinical presentation of pathology. However, the basic principles remain unchanged. Chiasmal disease may be due to tumours (pituitary adenomas, craniopharyngiomas [Rathkes pouch lesions] meningiomas [tuberculum sellae or sphenoid ridge], nasopharyngeal tumours, or metastases), nonneoplastic growths (aneurysms, sphenoidal sinus pathology) or other causes (inflammation, trauma). A special type of field defect is seen with expanding pituitary tumours, the resulting pressure on the centre of the chiasm producing a bitemporal defect which progresses from above. Defects in the visual field due to craniopharyngioma will produce a bitemporal hemianopia with denser loss below as the chiasma is compressed from above.

Optic Tract Lesions behind the optic chiasma lead to field defects in both eyes involving the same side of the visual space (described as homonymous). However, the details vary depending on the particular lesion location. The visual field changes between the two eyes are usually incongruous, when the lesion is more anterior, e.g. in the optic tract.

Optic Radiation The optic tract extends from the lateral geniculate body to the occipital lobe. These fibres divide into 2 portions, some coursing the temporal lobe (temporal radiation) and represent the contralateral homonymous superior quadrantinopia, and parietal lobe (parietal radiation), representing for the contralateral homonymous inferior quandrantinopia.

Striate Cortex Cortical lesions tend to be more congruous, that is to say the blind areas on each side tend to be similar in shape and size. Anterior occipital lobe lesions produce a congruous contralateral homonymous defect, with preservation of central vision or sparing of the macula ('macular sparing'). Lesions of the occipital cortex tip lead to a congruous homonymous macular defects. Other features associated with cortical lesions include visual hallucinations, and denial of visual loss (Anton syndrome).

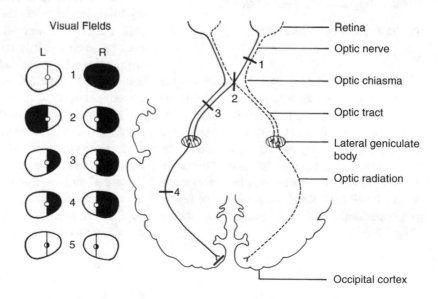

Fig. 22.6 The visual pathway and possible field defects

My car keeps knocking my gate post.
(Hemianopes should never drive)

Fig. 22.7 The effects of hemianopia

Notice from the diagram in Fig. 22.6 that the right half of the visual field is represented in the left half of each retina and thus the left half of the brain. This complies with the general rule that events occurring on the right side of the body are represented on the left side of the brain. It is surprising how patients may be unaware of a severe visual field defect, especially in hemianopia providing that the macula is spared (Fig. 22.7).

Abnormalities of the Pupil

The pupil constricts and dilates largely under the action of the sphincter pupillae muscle, which lines the pupil margin. It is supplied by parasympathetic fibres traveling within the IIIrd cranial nerve. The afferent stimulus is conveyed along the optic nerves and decussates at the optic chiasm and continues as the optic tract. The specific pupillomotor nerve fibres leave the optic tract without synapsing in the lateral geniculate nucleus and pass to the pretectal nucleus of the midbrain where they synapse with interneurones. The interneurones project to both Edinger-Westphal nuclei (which is part of the III cranial nerve nucleus). The pupillomotor (efferent) fibres then travel within the IIIrd cranial nerve to the pupil constrictor muscles of the ipsilateral eye via the ciliary ganglion (Fig. 22.8).

The dilator pupillae muscle is arranged radially within the iris and responds to the sympathetic nerves conveyed in the sympathetic plexus overlying the internal carotid artery. These fibres in turn arise from the superior cervical ganglion. The sympathetic supply to the dilator muscle therefore runs a long course from the hypothalamus to the midbrain and spinal cord and then up again from the root of the neck with the internal carotid artery.

Miosis refers to a small (constricted) pupil, mydriasis to a large (dilated) pupil (big word, big pupil). The pupil becomes smaller with age as does its reactivity. In young children the pupils are relatively large and sometimes anxious parents bring up their children because they are concerned about this. During sleep, the pupils become small. When examining the eye with the ophthalmoscope it is evident that the pupil constricts more vigorously when the macula is examined than when the more peripheral fundus is stimulated with the ophthalmoscope light. When an eye is totally blind, usually there is no light pupil reaction but as a general rule, the pupils remain of equal size. It should be apparent from

Optic nerve

Ciliary ganglion

Optic tract

III nerva

Red nucleus

Lateral geniculate nucleus

Edinger Westphal nucleus

Pretecto-oculomotor tract

Pretectal nucleus

Fig. 22.8 The pupillary pathway

Fig. 22.8 that the patient with cortical blindness (lesion within the occipital cortex) may have a normal pupil reaction. We must also remember that a pupil may not react to light because it is mechanically bound down to the lens by adhesions (posterior synechiae), or because of damage to the pupillary sphincter. When both maculae are damaged by age-related macular degeneration, the pupils may be slightly wider than normal and may show slightly sluggish reactions. A relative afferent pupil defect (also known as a Marcus Gunn pupil) implies optic nerve or severe retinal disease.

The Abnormally Dilated Pupil

The commonest reason for unilateral mydriasis is drugs in the form of locally administered eye drops, either prescribed by an ophthalmic department or obtained from a friend's medicine cabinet. The next commonest cause is probably the Adie pupil, a condition which is more common in young female patients. The affected pupil is usually dilated and contracts very slowly in response to direct and indirect stimulation. In bright light the pupil may constrict slowly on the affected side and take some time to dilate in the dark. The vision may also be blurred particularly at near because of the effect of the disease process on the ciliary muscle (necessary for accommodation). The pupillary constriction to near fixation is tonic and prolonged and worm-like. When this tonic pupil reaction is combined with absent tendon jerks in the limbs it is known as Holmes-Adie syndrome. When the vision is blurred and the pupil widely dilated, the symptoms may be partially relieved by the use of a weak miotic. After a delay of months or years the other eye may become affected. The overall disability is minimal and the condition has not so far been related to any other systemic disease. It is thought to have an underlying viral aetiology. Acute narrow angle glaucoma can occasionally present in this manner and confusion may arise if the eye is not very red; however closer examination of the eye should make the diagnosis obvious. Since the nerve fibres, which cause constriction of the pupil, are conveyed in the oculomotor nerve, oculomotor palsy if complete is associated with mydriasis. For this reason dilatation of the pupil may be a serious sign of raised intracranial pressure after head injury. One pupil may be wider than the other as a congenital abnormality (congenital anisocoria).

The Abnormally Constricted Pupil

Again, drugs are a common cause. Miotic drops are still encountered in the treatment of glaucoma and the constricted pupils of the morphine addict are well known if not so commonly seen. When a constricted pupil on one side is observed it is important to note the position of the eyelids. A slight degree of associated ptosis indicates the possibility of Horner syndrome. The total syndrome comprises miosis, narrowing of the palpebral fissure due to paralysis of the smooth muscle in the eyelids (Muller muscle), loss of sweating over the affected side of the forehead, a slight reduction of the intraocular pressure and enophthalmos (sunken globe). Horner syndrome may be caused by a wide diversity of lesions anywhere along the sympathetic pathway. While a Pancoast apical lung tumour is classically associated with Horner Syndrome, it is quite often noted in the elderly as an isolated finding and investigation fails to reveal a cause. The Argyll Robertson (AR) pupil is a very rare but famous example of the miosed pupil, which responds to accommodation but not to direct light. This type of pupil reaction was originally described as being closely associated with syphilis of the central nervous system. Visual acuity is normal in such patients.

Summary of Common Pupil Abnormalities

- *Third cranial nerve palsy*
  - Affected pupil is larger than normal
  - Efferent pupillary defect
  - Pupil inequality is more apparent in bright light
  - Complete ptosis
  - Eye looks down and out.

The course of third nerve is closely associated with the posterior communicating artery (PCA). Painful third nerve palsy with pupil involvement is due to compression of the nerve by an aneurysm of PCA. This condition needs to be investigated urgently with MRI or MRA for confirmation due to potential risk of aneurysmal rupture. This condition would require surgical intervention for treatment of aneurysm as prevention of intracranial haemorrhage and/or stroke.

- *Horner syndrome*
  - Lesion of sympathetic pathway
  - Affected pupil is smaller than normal
  - Pupil inequality is more pronounced in the dark
  - Patient may have neck scars, partial ptosis and the eye may appear to be sunken in (apparent enophthalmos).

- *Argyll Robertson pupils*
  - Congenital syphilis
  - Pupils often small and irregular
  - Sluggish light responses
  - Light near dissociation
  - May be blind from optic atrophy.

Double Vision

Double vision (diplopia) means that a person sees two images instead of one. Some patients say that they can see double when they mean that the vision is blurred. A clear distinction must therefore be made. Diplopia may be monocular or binocular. Monocular diplopia, that is, diplopia that is still present when one eye is closed, is quite common and is usually due to a cataract or corneal disease. Binocular double vision of recent onset should always be treated as a serious symptom. It is usually disabling, preventing the patient from working or even walking about. Some patients discover that the symptoms are relieved by placing a patch over one eye. Slight degrees of double vision may be compensated by a head tilt or turn and the nature of the adopted head posture can help to identify the cause of the double vision. In the same way, if the history is elucidated carefully, noting, for example, whether the diplopia is worse for near or distance vision or whether there is horizontal or vertical displacement of the second image, then a possible cause may be suspected even before examining the patient.

Assessment of Eye Movements in Diplopia

The complaint of double vision suggests that the separate eyes are not both fixed on the point of regard. The eye that is 'off line' sees the object of regard but it appears displaced. This failure of the eyes to work together is due to malfunction of one or a group of eye muscles or the neurological mechanisms that control them.

From the clinical point of view it is convenient to divide the eye muscles into horizontal and vertical groups. The horizontal muscles, the medial and lateral recti, are easy to understand because their actions are in one plane and they simply adduct (turn in) or abduct (turn out) the globe. The vertical recti are best considered as having primary and secondary actions. It is important to realise that the action of the vertical recti changes with the position of the globe. For example, when the eye is abducted the superior rectus elevates the globe but when the eye is adducted the superior rectus rotates the eye inwards round an anterior-posterior axis (intorts). In a similar manner the inferior oblique elevates the adducted eye and extorts the abducted eye (Fig. 22.9). In order to test the action of the superior oblique muscle, one must first ask the patient to adduct the eye and test for depression in adduction. That is to say a superior oblique palsy prevents the eye from looking down when it is turned in. The main line of action of the vertical recti is seen when the eye is abducted and that of the obliques is seen when the eye is adducted.

Examination of a patient with double vision entails, first of all, testing the gross eye movements in the cardinal positions of gaze and then noting the degree of separation of the images in these various positions. The Hess chart is one of several ingenious methods of recording the abnormal eye movements. The principle is to place a green filter before one eye and a red filter before the other and to ask the patient to look at a screen on which are placed a number of small illuminated white dots. The patient is then asked to localise the dots with a pointer. The amount of false localisation can then be measured in all positions of gaze. This technique is invaluable when assessing the recovery of an ocular muscle palsy.

Young children adapt to double vision very rapidly by suppressing the image from one eye, and under the age of eight years the suppression may lead to permanent amblyopia if the situation is not relieved. In adults the double vision may persist and be disabling for months or even years if not treated by incorporating prisms into the spectacles or by muscle surgery.

Causes of Diplopia

Ocular Muscle Imbalance It will be recalled from the chapter on squint that some patients have a latent squint, which is controlled much of the time but sometimes becomes overt. A typical example is the hypermetrope with esophoria who begins to complain of double vision when working for an examination. This problem may be solved simply by prescribing suitable spectacles. Sometimes anxious patients who have had a squint since childhood begin to notice their double vision again, having suppressed one image for many years. The symptoms are usually relieved with the cause of the anxiety.

Sixth (VIth) Cranial Nerve Palsy The affected eye is converged due to a weakness of the lateral rectus muscle. The eye is unable to abduct. It occurs most commonly as an isolated microvascular episode in hypertensive elderly patients and heals spontaneously in 3–6 months. Elderly diabetics are also more prone to VIth cranial nerve palsies. In young patients the possibility of multiple sclerosis or even raised intracranial pressure must be borne in mind.

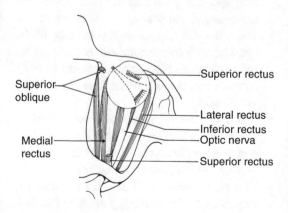

Fig. 22.9 The extraocular muscles

Fourth (IVth) Cranial Nerve Palsy The eye fails to look down when it is turned in and may be turned slightly up when the other eye is looking straight ahead. As such, the diplopia is worse when looking down and inwards. Trauma (a blow over the head) is an important cause in younger patients but a full investigation for an intracranial space-occupying lesion is usually needed. A head turn is more likely in bilateral cases.

IIIrd Cranial Nerve Palsy The eye is turned out and slightly down, the pupil is dilated and ptosis is usually severe enough to close the eye. Trauma is an important cause is young people but a posterior communicating aneurysm should also be considered, particularly if it is associated with pain. Other causes include demyelination, diabetes, microvascular occlusion and Herpes zoster infection. Recovery of nerve function particularly after compressive lesions may lead to a phenomenon known as aberrant regeneration. This may manifest as atypical pupil or lid responses on attempted eye movement.

Thyrotoxicosis Patients with this condition develop double vision because the extraocular muscles become infiltrated with inflammatory cells. The action of the inferior recti in particular becomes impaired and diplopia on upward gaze is a common sign. The other extraocular muscles may be subsequently affected. When the inflammation has settles, the infiltrating cells are replaced by fibrous tissue, further restricting muscle action.

The occurrence of other features of thyroid eye disease often helps in the diagnosis.

Myasthenia Gravis Myasthenia gravis is an autoimmune disease where the body produces antibodies to the acetylcholine receptor located at the motor end plate. This leads to excessive muscle fatigue, which can affect only ocular muscles, or may be systemic and involve other muscles.

This disease presents sometimes with diplopia with or preceded by ptosis, which becomes worse as the day goes by. Any one extraocular muscle or group of muscles may be affected, and the weakness worsens by the end of the day. The symptoms and signs show a transient improvement seconds after the intravenous injection of edrophonium chloride (Tensilon). Diagnosis may be confirmed by high serum titres of acetylcholine receptor antibodies. Approximately 10% of cases are associated with a thymoma which can become malignant. A chest CT scan is therefore mandatory in any patient suspected of having myasthenia gravis. Treatment is with an anticholinesterase such as pyridostigmine, supplemented with steroids as necessary.

Blow-Out Fracture of the Orbit A special cause of double vision following injury is the trapping of extraocular muscles, usually the inferior rectus in the line of fracture of the orbital floor especially, or other orbital wall. The patient experiences double vision on looking upwards and the limitation of movement is evident. There may be a relative enophthalmos. Surgical intervention to repair the orbital wall defect may be required if the patient suffers from prolonged diplopia or marked enophthalmos.

Summary

- The reader should understand and appreciate the common causes of neuro-ophthalmic problems that are seen by the ophthalmologist, and that good liaison between the ophthalmologist and neurologist is important.
- The optic disc represents the entrance of the optic nerve into the eye, and as there are no light sensitive cells (photoreceptors) in it, its location corresponds to the blind spot of the visual field.
- The optic nerve characteristics are defined by the colour, definition of contour or margin, cup, and supplemented by vessel entry and the presence or absence of haemorrhages.
- The characteristics of the optic nerve are important in determining presence of pathology in the eye or the anterior visual pathway.
- Congenital abnormalities can affect the optic disc.

- Optic atrophy is seen clinically as a pale disc, and indicates loss of optic nerve tissue and function, of variable degrees.
- Optic disc swelling may be due to papilloedema (bilateral disc swelling, by definition), optic neuritis, inflammation (uveitis), dysthyroid disease or diabetes, infiltration as in leukemia, lymphoma, or granulomatous inflammation eg sarcoid.
- Multiple sclerosis may present with optic neuritis, but more often, retrobulbar neuritis.
- Other features of demyelination may be present and need to be looked for, including nystagmus, internuclear ophthalmoplegia, extraocular muscle dysfunction, and systemic features.
- Pupillary abnormalities are important in determining local ocular disease, as well as important neurologic abnormalities. The particular type of pupillary defect may localize pathology.
- Visual field defects provide useful localizing information in visual pathway disease.
- Pathology affecting the anterior visual pathway (retina and optic disc) is unilateral, whilst pathology affecting the optic chiasma and beyond result in bilateral visual field defects.
- Diplopia may be uniocular or binocular. Monocular diplopia is never due to extraocular muscle problems, but rather ocular media problems (cataract or corneal disease). Binocular diplopia is due to malfunction of the extraocular muscles or their nerve supply.

Abstract

Many eye diseases are now known to be either inherited in a Mendelian fashion or genetic factors play an important part in their pathophysiology.

This chapter describes the up to date information available on the different patterns of disease inheritance, and relates this to ophthalmic diseases, including the different types of glaucoma, corneal dystrophies, age-related macular degeneration and retinal dystrophies. The application of gene therapy to ophthalmic diseases is also explored.

Many eye diseases are inherited or have familial clustering. It is therefore always advisable to enquire about the family history when taking a history from a patient with an ophthalmological complaint. Some types of inherited eye disease lead to blindness and relatives of patients with such conditions often seek advice concerning their risk of developing the disease. Patients may also consult with a view to prenatal testing, particularly if the disease leads to blindness at a young age.

Recent advances in molecular biology have led to a dramatic increase in our understanding of eye diseases. The discovery and the unraveling of the role of numerous ocular disease genes has also helped in our understanding of normal eye development and functioning. Because of the advances made in ophthalmic molecular genetics we are now able to refer to an inherited ocular condition not only by the mode of inheritance but also to denote the abnormal chromosome, the abnormal gene's position on the chromosome and its nucleotide sequence. To date over 270 different genes have been associated with retinal diseases alone (https://sph.uth.tmc.edu/retnet/) (accessed 5th September 2021). For many disorders we also now know the role the abnormal gene plays in the pathogenesis of the disease, either because it leads to the production of an abnormally functioning protein or because the gene defect leads to the abnormal regulation of nearby or distant genes. Once the abnormal gene product (protein) associated with a disease can be identified, then drugs can be designed specifically to either suppress its production or replace the lost function or gene therapy can overcome the abnormally functioning gene.

Examples of eye disease that have been mapped out to different chromosomes are shown in Table 23.1.

Several methods are used in molecular biology to link disease to particular gene loci. Traditionally, work usually starts by finding and classifying the disease in question in a large family or series of families. Next, the disease chromosome is sought (unless the inheritance pattern

Table 23.1 Chromosome mapping for common eye diseases

Chromosome	Eye disease
1	Leber's congenital Amaurosis, Stargardt's disease, open angle glaucoma (type 1A), congenital cataract, retinitis Pigmentosa,
2	Congenital cataract, iris coloboma Aniridia type 1, AR retinitis Pigmentosa, congenital glaucoma,
3	Usher' syndrome, AD retinitis Pigmentosa
5	Treacher Collins Mandibulo-facial dysostosis Dominant corneal dystrophies (Chr5q31)
7p	Goldenhar's syndrome
11	Aniridia type 2 (sporadic Aniridia / Wilm's tumour), Best's disease
12	Stickler's syndrome, congenital cataract
13q	Retinoblastoma
17	Neurofibromatosis type (NF1) (Von Recklinghausen's disease)
22q12	Neurofibromatosis type 2 (NF2)
X chromosome	Ocular albinism Juvenile retinoschisis Norrie's disease Choroideremia Retinitis Pigmentosa
(Xq 22–28)	Colour blindness—red cone, green cone

is X linked, then this step can be omitted) and then the position of the gene in question is gradually narrowed down (by the use of linkage analysis followed by chromosome walking). This usually produces a region of the chromosome on which a number of candidate genes are found. Sequencing of these genes and comparison with normal individuals or animal models usually allows the disease gene to be identified (this can be a very time consuming operation). Once the sequence of the gene is known, this can be compared on computer databases with similar known genes and the putative structure and function of the disease gene and its product can be determined. Nowadays, whole genome sequencing is often used in conjunction with very powerful computers to perform bioinformatics and in silico analysis to identify disease causing mutations very quickly. The potential of this approach has been brought about by the project to sequence the

entire human genome and more recently in the UK, the 100,000 genome project.

Eye screening in selected patients at risk of inherited disease may detect important life threatening conditions, for example Familial adenomatous polyposis (bowel cancer), retinoblastoma (eye cancers), Marfan's syndrome (heart abnormalities), neurofibromatosis (optic nerve tumours) and von Hippel Lindau disease (brain and renal tumours).

Basic Genetic Mechanisms

In order to be able to give advice about the appearance of inherited disease in future generations, it is essential to have a basic knowledge of the mechanism of genetic transmission.

The nucleus of each cell in the body contains 46 chromosomes arranged as 23 pairs. The 23rd pair comprises the sex chromosomes (the remainder being known as autosomes). These sex chromosomes are responsible for the transmission of sex characters but also carry a number of other genes unrelated to sex. In a woman the sex chromosomes are the same length but in a man one is shorter than the other. The shorter one is known as the 'Y' chromosome and the longer one, which is the same as the female sex chromosome, is the 'X' chromosome. When the sperm or ova are formed in the body, the pairs of chromosomes separate and the nuclei of the gametes (i.e. sperm or ova) contain only 23 chromosomes. When fertilisation occurs the 23 chromosomes from each gamete reunite as pairs. Genetic material is thus equally provided from each parent. Genes are arranged along the length of a chromosome and each one is known to bear special influence on the development of one or more individual characteristics. Genes are arranged in pairs on adjacent chromosomes. The two genes of the pair may be similar (homozygous) or different (heterozygous). If different, one may exert an overriding influence and is said to be dominant. The gene that is overridden is said to be recessive.

Genetic disorders can be divided into three broad groups:

1. Abnormalities of chromosomes - numerical or structural.
2. Abnormalities of individual genes, which are transmitted to offspring.
3. Abnormalities involving the interplay of multiple genes and the environment.

Pathological genes can carry abnormalities, which are transmitted to the offspring in the same way as (other) normal characteristics. In a given individual, the abnormal gene may be recessive and masked by the other one of the pair. The individual would thus not appear to have the disease but could transmit it. There are also some other terms that are important when describing genetic abnormalities: penetrance refers to the proportion of individuals who carry the gene and who express the disease, while expressivity refers to the clinical spectrum of severity of a particular genetic condition. The five important patterns of inheritance are:

1. Autosomal recessive
2. Autosomal dominant
3. Sex-linked recessive
4. Mitochondrial inheritance
5. Digenic (polygenic) inheritance

Autosomal Recessive Inheritance

If an abnormal recessive gene is paired with another abnormal one on the opposite chromosome, it will have an effect, but if the opposite gene is normal, the abnormality will not become manifest. Recessive disease in clinical practice usually results from the mating of heterozygous carriers. If the normal gene is 'A', and the abnormal gene is represented by 'a', then the disease will appear in the individual with genetic configuration 'aa' (homozygote), but not with the configuration 'aA' (heterozygote). When two heterozygotes mate the likely offspring can be considered as in the diagram (Fig. 23.1). If a patient has recessively inherited disease, their parents are likely to be normal but there may be brothers or sisters with the disease. It is important to enquire whether the parents are blood relatives because this greatly increases the likelihood of transmission. If an individual with recessive disease has a child with someone with the same recessive disease, then all the offspring will be affected. If one partner is a carrier and the other has the disease then there is a risk that 50% of the offspring would be carriers and 50% would be affected. When a carrier has a child with a normal individual, 50% of the offspring are carriers.

Fig. 23.1 Recessive inheritance

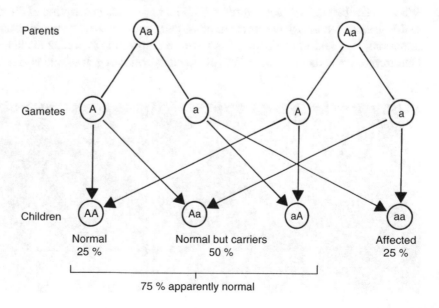

These expected findings could be calculated quite easily using the type of diagram shown in (Fig. 23.1). Common diseases inherited in this manner include sickle cell disease and cystic fibrosis and Stargardt disease.

Stargardt Disease

Stargardt disease is the most common macular dystrophy affecting approximately 1:8–10,000 people. It is inherited in an autosomal recessive manner and is usaually caused by mutations in a gene called ABCA4. Disease onset is usually in childhood with gradual blurring of the central reading vision which gradually worsens into adulthood although later onset (milder) forms of the disease are well recognized. The genetic mutation leads to a build up of a waste product called lipofuschin underneath the retina in the macular area which can be seen clinically as yellow "flecks". These can be seen more easily by shining a blue light on the macula, which causes them to autofluoresce (see Fig. 23.2a, b) By their third decade, many patients are registered severely sight impaired and currently there is no effective treatment.

Autosomal Dominant Inheritance

When a gene bearing a defect or disease gives rise to the disease even though the other one of the pair is normal, it is said to be dominant. An affected heterozygote may therefore have 50% of affected children when having a child with a normal partner Dominant inheritance can only be shown with certainty if three successive generations show the disease and if about 50% of individuals are affected. Also one sex should not be affected more than the other (Fig. 23.3). Examples of this type of inheritance are hereditary retinoblastoma and Marfan's disease.

Sex-Linked Recessive Inheritance

It has been mentioned already that males have the 'XY' configuration of sex chromosomes whereas females have 'XX'. Because of the unpaired nature of much of the male sex chromosomes, some recessive genes may have an effect in males when they do not do so in the female. Certain important eye conditions are carried in this way in pathological genes on the X chromosome and the pattern of inheritance is termed X-linked recessive. Examples of this type of inheritance are seen in ocular albinism and colour blindness. Retinitis pigmentosa may also show this pattern in some families. When inheritance is X-linked, only males are affected and there is no father-to-son transmission of the disease. Instead it is conveyed through a carrier female to the next generation (Fig. 23.4).

This description of the three important modes of inheritance should make it apparent that it is possible to predict the likely disease incidence in offspring. It should also be realised that such pre-

Fig. 23.2 (a, b) Colour fundus and autofluorescence images of a patient with Stargardt disease

Fig. 23.3 Dominant inheritance

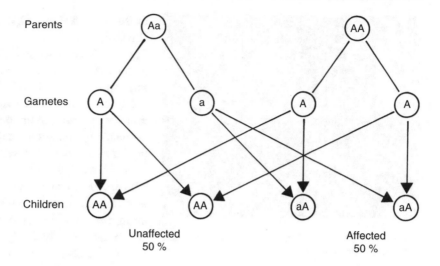

Fig. 23.4 X-linked recessive inheritance

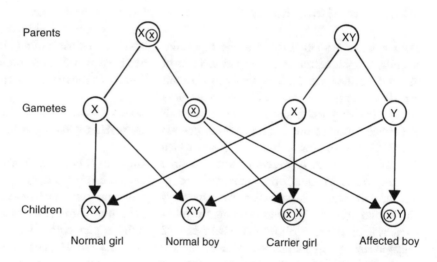

dictions can only be based on careful and extensive investigation of the family. Although some eye diseases are known to follow a fixed pattern of inheritance, others, notably retinitis pigmentosa, may be inherited in different ways in different families. In most large centres, genetic clinics are now in existence in which time is devoted specifically to the investigation of families and also to the detection of carriers.

Retinitis Pigmentosa

Retinitis pigmentosa is the name for a group of progressive conditions that initially have degeneration of the cells that patients see with in dim light (rods). Patients complain of worsening difficulty

seeing at night (nyctalopia). Later on, the disease causes degeneration of the cells used in bright light (cones). The disease affects approximately 1:4000 people. Patients often complain of progressive visual field constriction to the point that they have tunnel vision, where they only have functioning retina in their central macula. Clinically, patients have mid peripheral black bone spicules in their retina, pale, waxy optic discs and marked retinal vascular arteriolar attenuation (Fig. 23.5). Because mutations in over 100 different genes have been found to cause retinitis pigmentosa, it makes the development of treatments very problematic however, research on gene therapy for a small number of causes is being pursued.

Fig. 23.5 Wide angle colour fundus image of a patient with retinitis pigmentosa

Mitochondrial Inheritance

Mitochondria are small cytoplasmic organelles of cells. Mitochondria are the only organelles of the cell besides the nucleus that contain their own DNA. They also have their own machinery for synthesizing RNA and proteins. Instead of individual chromosomes, mitochondria contain circular DNA similar to bacteria, (from which they are thought to be derived). Mitochondrial DNA contains 37 genes, predominately encoding the enzymes necessary for the respiratory chain, and include 13 genes coding for mitochondrial proteins, 2 ribosomal RNAs and 22 transfer RNAs. All mitochondria in the zygote are derived from the ovum, therefore a mother carrying a mitochondrial DNA mutation will pass it on to all of her children (maternal inheritance) but only her daughters will pass it on to their children. Mitochondrial DNA mutations are usually manifest clinically in tissues with a high metabolic demand eg brain, nerve, retina, muscle and renal tubule. Examples of ophthalmic diseases caused by mitochondrial DNA mutations include Leber's Hereditary Optic Neuropathy, Chronic Progressive External Ophthalmoplegia (CPEO), Maternally Inherited Diabetes and Deafness (MIDD) and Kearns-Sayre syndrome.

Leber's Hereditary Optic Neuropathy (LHON)

Leber's Hereditary Optic Neuropathy is the most common inherited mitochondrial disorder, affecting approximately 1:50,000 people. For reasons unknown it tends to affect males much more than females by a ratio of up to 9:1 in some studies. It is caused by mutations in 4 of the 37 mitochondrial genes. Disease onset is usually in the late teens or early twenties and starts as a sudden painless loss of central vision in one eye followed a few months later by the fellow eye. In the acute stage, the optic disc is swollen and hyperaemic which later on, typically becomes pale in the temporal sector, next to the macula. In most cases, the visual loss is permanent, however a few cases have been reported in which partial recovery occurs. Until recently, no treatment was possible, but trials of an oral drug called idebenone have shown some limited benefit and a phase 2 trial of gene therapy is currently underway.

Digenic or Polygenic Inheritance

Digenic (or polygenic) inheritance occurs when a person has heterozygous defects in 2 (or more) different genes and the combination of defects are required to cause disease. Examples include retinitis pigmentosa where mutations in peripherin and ROM1 genes are required together for disease. Other ophthalmic diseases with complex inheritance include AMD, myopia and adult onset primary open angle glaucoma (POAG).

Adult POAG has complex inheritance where one gene may modify another in order to determine the severity of disease. It should be noted that juvenile POAG is inherited as an autosomal recessive disease with the gene located on Chr1q23, whilst congenital glaucoma is recognized as having both autosomal recessive (with genes on Chr1p36 and 2p21)and dominant patterns of inheritance. Similarly, several genes are (at least 32 at present) known to be associated with RP. The genetics of RP is therefore complex as the disease may be sporadic, autosomal dominant or recessive, sex-linked or digenic.

Chromosomal Abnormalities

Microscopic studies of the chromosomes themselves have revealed that abnormal numbers of chromosomes may be produced by a fault at the moment of fertilisation. These may be due to changes in numbers or structure of chromosomes. Numerical chromosomal changes include the absence of a chromosome (monosomy) e.g. as in Turner's Syndrome or an extra chromosome (trisomy) as in Down's Syndrome. In Down's Syndrome, cytogenetic studies have shown that these patients have an extra chromosome, which is indistinguishable from chromosome 21. Down's syndrome is more common in children born to older women and the eye changes include narrow palpebral fissures with a characteristic slant, cataract, high myopia and rather intriguing grey spots on the iris known as Brushfield's spots. Brushfield's spots are sometimes seen in otherwise normal individuals. Turner's syndrome (one missing X chromosome) and Klinefelter's syndrome (an extra X chromosome) are further examples of disease in which there are known to be abnormalities of the chromosome which are visible under the microscope. People with these last two diseases are of interest to the ophthalmologist on account of the abnormal but predictable manner in which they inherit colour blindness.

Structural abnormalities occur when recombination or reconstitution in an altered form follows chromosomal breaks. Such changes may be in the form of deletions, duplication inversions, translocations or isochromosomes.

Multifactorial Diseases

These are disorders that arise from an interplay of genetic and environmental influences. The genetic contribution is made up of at least two abnormal genes acting in concert to express a 'dosage related' type effect, which is significantly influenced by several environmental factors. This leads to variable phenotypic expression. Examples include diabetes mellitus, some malignancies and perhaps age-related macular degeneration.

In certain diseases including AMD, combinations of different genes and environmental conditions are required to result in disease. Specifically, complement factor H (CFH) and the ARMS2/HTRA1 are known genetic risk factors for AMD. When combined with the environmental risk of smoking, the risk is highly increased resulting in clinical disease.

Gene Therapy

Genetic diseases arise because a particular gene or groups of genes are abnormal leading to products that are detrimental to the particular cell and its function (dominant negative effect).or to a loss of the functional protein (haploinsuffiency).

Gene therapy currently involves delivery or replacement of a normal gene to tissues containing the abnormal disease gene in order to restore function. Theoretically, a simple replacement of a gene is all that is required. However, this is not easy to achieve in practice.

Current methods for such replacement involve the insertion of the normal or wild type gene into a viral vector (usually a modified adenovirus) and this is inserted into the target tissue (in the eye this is usually the photoreceptors or RPE cells). This is brought about by an operation to remove the vitreous from the eye and the modified virus is injected under the retina to be taken up by the target cells. The modified viruses are adapted such that they cannot divide or replicate and cause disease, but the new DNA is incorporated into the diseased target cell and the desired gene is expressed.

Currently, clinical trials are ongoing for a number of rare inherited eye diseases such as Leber's Congenital Amaurosis (LCA), X linked retinitis pigmentosa, choroideramia and LHON. Recently, a gene therapy for a rare type of LCA caused by mutations in a gene called RPE65 has been approved by NICE and is called Luxterna (voretigene neparvovec). It is now in routine use in the NHS to treat both children and adults.

In another approach to genetic diseases, particularly those of dominant inheritance where the mutation produces a protein that damages the host cell, the introduction of genes that may antagonize or inactivate the abnormal gene (called 'antisense' therapy) are introduced into the diseased cell. This then allows the normal or wild type gene on the other chromosome to be expressed and the cells to be undamaged and to function normally.

Summary

- There has been significant improvement in our understanding of the genetic basis of disease, including diseases of the eye recently. Many eye diseases are inherited.
- Several diseases arise through interplay of genetic inheritance and the environment.
- Different eye diseases have different inheritance patterns, e.g. congenital glaucoma has autosomal dominant and recessive patterns, whilst juvenile POAG has an autosomal recessive pattern, and adult onset POAG and AMD may be digenic or complex, and corneal dystrophies are predominantly dominant.
- Genetic manipulations may offer potential treatments for ophthalmic disease in the future.

Drugs and the Eye

24

Abstract

This chapter describes the effect of different drugs on the eye, whether administered topically or systemically. These include drugs that modulate pupil size, reduce intraocular pressure, or are used in the treatment of allergic eye diseases, dry eyes etc. Alternatively, these ocular effects may be unintended and therefore classified as adverse events.

Introduction

It is possible to achieve a high concentration of many drugs in the eye by applying them as eye drops. In this way, a high local concentration can be reached (particularly in the anterior segment of the eye) with minimal risk of systemic side effects. However the systemic side effects of drops cannot be discounted, particularly in susceptible individuals. For example, timolol drops can precipitate asthma and slow the heart rate in elderly patients, whilst pilocarpine drops can cause sweating and nausea. The action of local medications may be prolonged by incorporating them in an eye ointment but for most purposes drops are supplied in 10 ml or 5 ml containers. After the container has been opened it should not be kept for longer than a month because of the risk of infection. In order to avoid undue stinging, drops may be buffered to near the pH of tears and they contain a preservative or other excipient such as benzalkonium chloride, disodium edetate, or propylene glycol. It must be borne in mind that patients who develop an allergic reaction to drops may be reacting to the preservative, rather than the pharmacologic active component. There are some specially designed bottles that reduce contamination of eye drops and allow use up to 3 months without increased risks of infection. Single application containers are also used which do not contain a preservative but are expensive.

Eye lotions are usually prescribed in 200 ml quantities and are used to irrigate the conjunctival sac. Sodium chloride eye lotion is used in first aid to flush out foreign bodies or irritant chemicals. Fresh mains tap water is an adequate substitute for flushing the eye in an emergency, if the appropriate bags are not available.

One of the major drawbacks of using eye drops is that although high local concentrations of the drug are achieved in the anterior segment of the eye, little if any drug penetrates to the posterior segment. Eye drops are therefore of little use in treating diseases of the vitreous and retina. One way of delivering a drug to the posterior segment is to give it systemically. An example of this is the use of systemic prednisolone for posterior uveitis. This treatment method has the drawback of systemic side effects. Such side effects may be reduced by delivering the drug to the posterior segment by local injection either directly into the vitreous, along the orbital floor, within the sub-Tenon's space or in the sub-conjunctival space. For periocular injections, the drug has to penetrate the sclera in order to enter the intraocular compartments

Treatment of Infection

Chloramphenicol is rarely used as a systemic drug nowadays, but it has been useful for many years in the form of eyedrops. It remains a drug of choice in the UK and other countries for superficial eye infections. Other broad spectrum antibiotics in use include gentamycin, framycetin, tobramycin and neomycin as well as ciprofloxacin and ofloxacin. When an infection of the eye is suspected, a culture is taken from the conjunctival sac and treatment started with a wide spectrum antibiotic. Systemic and intravitreal administration may be needed if the infection is intraocular.

A number of antiviral drugs are now available but acyclovir in the form of acyclovir 3% (Zovirax) ointment is the most widely used treatment of herpes simplex keratitis. This preparation is different from that used on the skin. Recently ganciclovir (0.15%) eye gel has been introduced, as an alternative to acyclovir. The use of systemic acyclovir and famcyclovir for herpes zoster ophthalmicus has made a great impact on the severity of ocular complications. Valacyclovir is a more recent antiviral agent that may be administered orally and is active against herpes zoster as well as simplex.

Povidone iodine (5%) in aqueous solution is now preferred as the safest antimicrobial agent in the antisepsis of the conjunctiva especially as prophylaxis for intraocular surgery. The appropriate formulation in aqueous solution must be administered. It is important that the alcohol preparation used for skin preparation is avoided in the conjunctival sac on account of toxicity. The drops should be applied at least 3 mins prior to surgery.

Chlorhexidine (0.05 05 0.1%) is used as an alternative in ocular surface antisepsis in patients who are truly allergic to povidone iodine.

Table 24.1 Anti-infective agents commonly used in ophthalmology

Anti-infective agent and indication	Preparation
Chloramphenicol for conjunctivitis	Drops or ointment—broad spectrum for use in routine conjunctivitis of bacterial origin or for prophylaxis in viral cases and ocular trauma—cheap! May induce acute allergic reaction
Gentamicin, Soframycin, Norfloxacin, Neomycin, Ofloxacin, Ciprofloxacin, Moxifloxacin—for use as alternatives in conjunctivitis	Drops
Cefuroxime and Ciprofloxacin used for more severe infections of the cornea	Drops. Cefuroxime usually prepared fresh in pharmacy
Azithromycin—most useful in chlamydial infections	Ointment
Acyclovir (3%) (Zovirax) for herpes simplex keratitis	Ointment. Apply 5x daily. May cause redness of the eye and corneal epithelial toxicity.
Gancyclovir (0.15%) (Virgan)	Eye gel. Apply 5x daily. Use in acute herpes keratitis. May cause stinging and punctate keratitis

Chlorhexidine (0.02%) eye drops are also used in treatment of acanthamoeba keratitis (Table 24.1).

Drops Which Widen the Pupil

The pupils can be dilated either by local blockade of the parasympathetic pathway or by local stimulation of the sympathetic pathway. These drops which dilate the pupils are called mydiatrics, and usually cause paralysis of the ciliary muscles (cycloplegia), except phenylephrine.

Parasympathetic Antagonists

Routine mydriasis to allow examination of the fundus is best achieved by Tropicamide 0.5%

drops because the effect only lasts for about three hours. Cyclopentolate 1% (0.5% in babies) can last for 24 h, but because of its cycloplegic effect (blockade of accommodation) is preferable for the examination of children's eyes when refraction is also needed. Dilating the pupil runs the risk of inducing an attack of acute narrow angle glaucoma in a predisposed individual. Since the vision may remain blurred, driving should be avoided within the first 6–8 h after mydriasis. Atropine 1% in drop form is a long acting mydriatic, which is used when it is necessary to prevent or breakdown adhesions between iris and lens in acute iritis (posterior synechiae). It is also used in the treatment of amblyopia in children. Its effect lasts for about 7 days. Allergic reactions are quite common and occasionally systemic absorption may cause central nervous system symptoms of atropine toxicity.

Sympathetic Agonist

Phenylephrine (2.5 or 10% drops) is a sympathomimetic amine. It is used with a parasympathetic antagonist when extremely wide pupil dilation is required e.g. for intraocular surgery or for peripheral retinal examination. There are reports of severe acute hypertension after use of 10% drops (Table 24.2).

Indications, Effects and Adverse Events for Mydriatics

1. Diagnostic:
   (a) To enhance examination of lens, vitreous and fundus. Short acting agents preferred: tropicamide, cyclopentolate, and phenylephrine. (Note topical phenylephrine especially 10% may cause elevation of blood pressure. Use 2.5% which has less side effects).
   (b) Cycloplegia—enhances more accurate refraction especially in children: cyclopentolate, or rarely atropine.
2. Treatment of:
   (a) Iritis/Iridocyclitis: to break down or prevent posterior synechiae formation, and relieve ciliary spasm
   (b) Severe corneal epithelial defects: to relieve spasm of ciliary muscle and iris sphincter.

The clinician may use cyclopentolate, homatropine, or atropine depending on severity (stronger/longer acting agents for more severe disease). Atropine and homatropine may cause contact dermatitis of eyelid skin. They may also produce systemic effects in some patients.

Drops Which Constrict the Pupil

Drugs that constrict the pupil are called miotics. They may be associated with spasms of the ciliary muscles, and reduce intraocular pressure. Miotics have in the past been widely used for the treatment of chronic open angle glaucoma. Pilocarpine is available in 1%, 2%, 3% or 4% solutions. Although it is effective in reducing the intraocular pressure, the side effects of dimming of vision and accommodation spasm can be very disabling and mean that this treatment has largely been superceded. Pilocarpine is still used in the treatment of acute glaucoma attacks to constrict the pupil and open up the closed drainage angle. Sometimes it is necessary to constrict the pupil rapidly during the course of intraocular surgery and this is achieved by instilling acetyl choline

Table 24.2 Comparison of duration of action of several commonly used parasympatholytic drugs

Drug	Time Max-Effect	Duration of Max Effect	Patient able to read	Accommodation normal
Atropine	1–2 h	8–48 h	3–4 days	10–14 days
Homatropine	40 min	50 min	6 h	36h
Cyclopentolate (Mydrilate)	25 min	50 min	3 h	18 h
Tropicamide (Mydrilacyl)	20 min	15 min	45 min	4 h

Table 24.3 Miotics

Miotic	Effect	Use
Pilocarpine	causes direct stimulation of iris sphincter and ciliary body	In treatment of glaucoma or to constrict pupil (after dilation)
Acetylcholine	Choline ester: very short acting miotic	Mainly to constrict pupil in intraocular surgery e.g. cataract (when required)
Carbachol (carbamylcholine)	Choline ester: longer acting miotic (compared to acetylcholine) cholinergic agonist	Treatment of glaucoma May be used in pupil constriction after cataract surgery
Anticholinesterases, including Physostigmine (Eserine) and Phospholine iodide (Ecothiopate)	Eserine: miotic (reversible anticholinesterase). Phospholine iodide: long acting miotic (irreversible anticholinesterase)	Treating open angle glaucoma or accommodative esotropia. Less often used in modern clinical practice.

directly into the anterior chamber. Strong miotics run the risk of causing retinal detachment in susceptible individuals. Miotics have been used to reverse the effect of mydriatic drops used for fundus examination but this practice is no longer recommended as a routine because it is unnecessary and the symptoms of meiosis may make matters worse (Table 24.3).

Drugs in the Treatment of Open Angle Glaucoma

There has been a small revolution involving the type of eye drops used for the treatment of glaucoma in recent times. For years the mainstay of treatment was pilocarpine and the topical beta blockers e.g. timolol, but the potential systemic side effects of these drugs has led to the introduction of other novel types of ocular hypotensive agents. In general these new agents can be divided into α_2 adrenergic agonists, carbonic anhydrase inhibitors and prostaglandin analogues.

The production of aqueous humour can be reduced by either blockade of the β receptors on the ciliary body epithelial cells (i.e. with a β blocker) or by agonism of the α_2 receptors. Brimonidine and apraclonidine are both α_2 receptor agonists and show good efficacy compared with timolol. A significant number of patients however do develop an allergy to these agents and this has limited their widespread use.

Acetazolamide was introduced as a diuretic many years ago but although not a very good diuretic it has proved to be a potent ocular hypotensive when given orally. It is a sulphonamide derivative that is a carbonic anhydrase inhibitor. Acetazolamide is very effective in reducing intraocular pressure but systemic toxicity is common—parasthesiae of fingers and toes, malaise, confusion, renal stones, abdominal pain. Because of these side effects its use has been restricted to short term treatment. In 1995, dorzolamide was introduced and more recently brinzolamide has become available. These are also carbonic anhydrase inhibitors but they are available in drop form and are able to penetrate the cornea. Their ocular hypotensive effects are generally not as great as topical β blockers but they are useful as adjuvant agents.

It has recently been discovered that a second aqueous outflow route exists in the eye—the uveoscleral route. It is known that certain prostaglandins increase the flow of aqueous via this route and a number of topical prostaglandin $F_2\alpha$ analogues are now available. latanoprost, travoprost, bimatoprost and tafluprost have all been shown to as effective as topical β blockers with minimal side effects.

All these medications have the problem of compliance. Elderly patients may forget to instil drops on a regular basis. There are different combination therapies i.e. eye drops that contain a prostaglandin and a beta-blocker or beta-blocker plus a carbonic anhydrase inhibitor. In some cases even installation of 3 different glaucoma drops fails to control the intraocular pressure. In these instances the only sure way of lowering the

Table 24.4 Drugs used in treatment of glaucoma

Type of drug	Examples	Notes
Adrenergic beta blockers	Timolol 0.25%, 0.5% – Betaxolol 0.5%, – Levobunolol 0.5% – Carteolol 1%.	Introduced late 1970s; good IOP reduction Cardio-selective safer in chest disease
Miotics	Pilocarpine 1–4% Physostigmine Phospholine Iodide	See Table 24.3
Alpha2 adrenergic agonists	Brimonodine Aprachlonidine	Descrease aqueous humor production and increase uveoscleral flow
Prostaglandins	Latanoprost	Increase uveoscleral flow
Prostaglandin analogues	Travaprost Bimatoprost Tafluprost	Increase uveoscleral outflow
Carbonic anhydrase inhibitors (CAIs)	Acetazolamide— systemic Dorzolamdide— topical Brinzolamide— topical	Reduce aqueous humor production
Combination therapies	Combinations of beta blockers and topical CAIs, or prostaglandins and beta blockers or CAIs	Combined mechanisms to enhance IOP reduction

pressure is by glaucoma drainage surgery. Drugs used in treatment of glaucoma are summarised in Table 24.4.

Drugs in the Treatment of Acute Angle Closure Glaucoma

Angle closure glaucoma is a surgical problem. Once the acute attack has been aborted by the use of intensive pilocarpine drops and acetazolamide (Diamox) intravenously and/or orally, then a small hole is made in the iris with the YAG laser to allow redirection of the flow of aqueous. In many patients this provides a permanent cure. Beta blockers may also be used during the acute

stage and more recently the α2agonist apraclonidine has been shown to be a useful adjunct.

Drugs in the Treatment of Allergic Eye Disease

With the increasing incidence of atopy, the treatment of allergic eye disease has gained in importance in recent years. Treatments are designed to interfere with either the type 1 (IgE mediated response) or type 4 (delayed) hypersensitivity response, both of which are thought to be important in disease pathogenesis. For mild disease, initial treatment should involve antigen avoidance (if known) and frequent use of artificial tears (hypromellose) to wash away antigens from the ocular and conjunctival surface. Treatment of more severe disease involves the use of systemic or topical antihistamines (Levocabastine, Emedastine and Azelastine) which are helpful for relief of symptoms and topical mast cell stabilisers (sodium cromoglycate, nedocromil sodium and lodoxamide) which are useful in disease prevention if used regularly. There are several new anti-allergic eye drops that have become available recently, including Azelastine, Epinastine, Levocabistine, and Olopatidine. The treatment of very severe (sight threatening) disease involves the use of courses of topical and occasionally oral steroids. Anti-inflammatory drugs e.g. diclofenac, ketorolac, and nepafenac are reserved for more specific indications including prevention of intraoperative miosis, and prevention or treatment for post-cataract surgery macular oedema, as well as pain in corneal epithelial defects.

Local Anaesthesia in Ophthalmology

Proxymetacaine (Ophthaine) is a useful short acting anaesthetic drop that is comfortable to instill and so is particularly useful when examining children. Tetracaine (Amethocaine) and oxybuprocaine (Benoxinate) are also widely used but are longer acting and sting quite markedly. Local anaesthetic drops should not be used as pain relievers on a long- term basis because the anaesthetised cornea becomes ulcerated and severe infection of the eye may occur. Lignocaine (1 or 2%) with or without adrenaline is injected into the eyelids for lid surgery. Local anaesthesia for intraocular surgery is obtained by either topical route (drops), sub-Tenon's injection, periorbital injection (outside the cone of extraocular muscles) or sometimes retrobulbar injection (within the muscle cone) of Lignocaine. For a longer effect this is sometimes combined with Marcaine (bupivacaine).

Drugs and Contact Lenses

As a rule, contact lenses should not be worn when the eye is being treated with drops. The exception is when the contact lenses themselves are being used for some therapeutic purpose. Soft hydrophilic contact lenses may take up and store the preservative from some kinds of drop. The preservative benzalkonium chloride is especially liable to be absorbed onto a contact lens. When it is essential that drops are administered to a patient wearing contact lenses, it is often possible to prescribe in the form of single dose containers which do not contain a preservative.

Artificial Tears

Artificial tears provide one of a number of measures that are used to treat tear deficiency. Other measures include occlusion of the lacrimal puncta or the use of mucolytic agents such as acetylcysteine (5%) eye drops which are very effective as a mucolytic agent.

The first step is to make the diagnosis. Once a deficiency of tears has been confirmed then the mainstay of treatment is hypromellose or dextran eye drops, which are cheap and effective in most mild cases. Adsorptive polymers of acrylic acid can also give symptomatic relief. Polyvinyl alcohol is another compound present in a number of tear substitutes. It is useful in mucus deficiency

states Carbomers are high molecular weight synthetic polymers, and carmellose are also used as tear substitutes. Recently, a new agent, sodium hyaluronate (0.1%) has been shown to improve symptom relief and improve the ocular surface abnormalities in cases of severe dry eye. By their nature tear substitutes tend to adhere to the surface of the eye and in the conjunctival sac. For this reason their prolonged use is liable to give rise to preservative reactions. Preservative free preparations are often preferable. Some patients with a severe dry eye problem may need to instil the drops every hour or even more frequently.

Anti-Inflammatory Drugs and the Eye

Local steroids are widely used in the treatment of eye disease; systemic steroids are not used unless the sight of the eye is threatened. It must be remembered that systemic steroids give the patient a sense of well being which may give a false impression of the real benefit obtained. Furthermore systemic steroids can have serious and life threatening side effects such as vertebral collapse through osteoporosis, and perforated gastric ulcer. (Fig. 24.1) Systemic steroids are also diabetogenic, lead to weight gain, cataract and elevated intraocular pressure after prolonged use. More recently, the adverse event of central serous chorioretinopathy has also been described as an adverse event of systemic steroids.

Systemic steroids should only be prescribed by or on the recommendation of a specialist for inflammatory conditions of deeper ocular structures e.g. ciliary body, choroid, retina, optic nerve, orbital inflammation (specific or nonspecific), acute congestion or orbit in dysthyroid disease, sympathetic ophthalmia, giant cell arteritis (GCA).

Several non-steroidal immunosuppressants (also referred to as 'steroid sparing agents') are now available to the experienced specialist. The different categories include:

Steroids give a patient a feeling of well-being. . . .

Fig. 24.1 There might be a false impression of the real benefit obtained

- Calcineurin inhibitors e.g. ciclosporin (as above), tacrolimus (FK509)
- Antimetabolites e.g. azathioprine, methotrexate
- Purine synthesis inhibitors e.g. mycophenolate mofetil
- Monoclonal antibodies e.g. canakimub, basiliximab
- Alkylating agents e.g. cyclophosphamide
- Biologics including anti-TNF drugs e.g. adalimumab, etanercept
- IL-6 inhibitors, including tocilizumab
- Non-steroidal anti-inflammatory agents e.g. flurbuprofen (Froben) preferred as treatment for scleritis.

Local steroids should also be applied with caution, and it is a good rule always to have a specific reason for giving them. That is to say, they should not be prescribed just to make red eyes turn white without a clear diagnosis. The reasons for this are twofold: first, local steroids enhance the multiplication of viruses, especially herpes simplex; secondly, they can cause glaucoma in certain predisposed individuals. In such individuals, the instillation of one drop of steroid may cause a temporary rise of intraocular pressure. The most potent steroid in this respect is dexamethasone followed by betamethasone, prednisolone and hydrocortisone. It has been claimed that rimexolone, clobetasone and fluometholone are relatively safe in this respect. Topical steroids may cause posterior subcapsular cataracts, in a time and dose related manner. Delays in corneal epithelial healing, and in the extreme, corneal melt due to inhibition of collagen synthesis may complicate topical steroid use.

Intravitreal injections of high concentrations of steroids (fluocinolone, dexamethasone or triamcinolone) are now available for the treatment of macular oedema due to diabetes (diabetic macular oedema), and retinal vein occlusions, as well as in the treatment of uveitis. Their use in uveitis is obvious. In macular oedema, these steroids aim at antagonizing non-VEGF inflammatory pathways in the pathogenesis of the oedema, as well as some of the VEGF pathway. Each drug has its specific duration of activity, and therefore frequency of administration. Dexamethasone has a very short duration (approximately 2–3 h) in the eye normally. The impregnation of dexamethasone into polyglycolic acid vehicle (as in Ozurdex implant) significantly lengthens the duration of action to 3–6 months. Similarly fluocinolone implant has a 2–3 year duration of action in the eye. These pharmacologic treatments are particularly useful in eyes where the oedema has affected the fovea and immediate surrounding area, so that laser photocoagulation is not recommended or will be damaging to the vision.

Recently, a number of non-steroidal anti-inflammatory drugs (NSAIDs) have been made available in topical form (diclofenac [Voltarol], Ketorolac [Acular], flurbiprofen [Ocufen], bromfenac [Yellox], and nepafenac [Nevanac] to reduce our dependence on topical steroids. They have been shown to be of use in the treatment of post-cataract surgery inflammation and in reducing the pain after excimer laser surgery and corneal abrasions. They are also useful in severe keratitis in dry eye disease, where they suppress cell mediated immune reaction by blocking inflammatory molecule release.

Diagnostic Agents Used the Eye

Fluorescein drops or paper strips are used to stain areas of epithelial defect on the ocular surface: cornea or conjunctiva. Single use preparations are preferable as multi use preparations serve as a good culture medium for bacteria, especially Pseudomonas aeruginosa.

Local anaesthetic agents are used to assist ocular examination including checking of intraocular pressures, other examination as necessary, or for surgical anaesthesia e.g. for intravitreal injections or pre-cataract surgery. These include:

1. Cocaine 2% or 4%—powerful anaesthetic drop by takes 5 mins to work. May induce temporary clouding of corneal epithelium, pupil dilation, and delirium.
2. Tetracaine (Amethocaine) 0.5% or 1%—rapid effect, anaesthesia in 1 min. No pupil dilation but stings on administration and produces vasodilation. May cause dermatitis, and more disruption of corneal epithelium. It may be used as combination with fluorescein for tonometry.
3. Oxybuprocaine (Benoxinate) 0.4%—slower acting but no irritation or corneal damage. May be used as combination with fluorescein for tonometry.
4. Proxymethocaine (Ophthaine) 0.5%—provides rapid anaesthesia in 20 s. It does not sting, and has a weak to medium effect and short term action. It may be used as combination with fluorescein for tonometry. It has significant allergy rate.
5. Lignocaine 2%. It may be used as combination with fluorescein for tonometry.

6. Fundus angiography with fluorescein and indocyanine green have been previously described.

Corneal Protection in Unconscious Patients or Patients with Exposed Eyes

Protecting the eyes in unconscious patients is important because absent blink reflex and constant exposure of eye leads to dryness of cornea and conjunctiva. The natural blink reflex which moves lubricating tears over the surface of the eye normally is absent in the unconscious patient, or persons who have exposed eyes as in Bell's palsy. Such exposure and inadequate lubrication increases the risk of ocular infection and corneal ulcerations.

Eye protection could be achieved with adequate lubrication with (a) Lacrilube, a bland ophthalmic ointment, and (b) Chloramphenicol ointment especially if infection is suspected, (c) Gel tears or other viscous eye gel (e.g. Carbomer Gel).

Retinal Pharmacotherapy: Anti-Angiogenic Drugs and the Eye, and Intraocular Steroids

Uncontrolled angiogenesis (growth of new blood vessels) is a common finding in many potentially blinding conditions such as proliferative diabetic retinopathy, central or branch retinal vein occlusion, neovascular age-related macular degeneration (nAMD) and retinopathy of prematurity. Inhibiting their growth offers us the hope of dramatically reducing the number of patients going blind each year. It is now accepted that the angiogenic response is caused by elevated levels of a cytokine called Vascular Endothelial Growth Factor (VEGF) produced by abnormal or ischaemic cells within the eye. Attempts to reduce the levels of VEGF and hence turn off the angiogenic drive have involved intravitreal injections of anti-

VEGF antibodies or oligonucleotide aptamers which bind VEGF. This has been particularly useful in nAMD where the treatment of choice is intravitreal injections of anti-VEGF therapies. Blocking all isoforms of VEGF-A (as with aflibercept, bevacizumab, or ranibizumab, brolucizumab), have been shown to have better efficacy than blocking selected isoforms like VEG-165 (as with pegaptanib). Other new therapies block 2 pathways (VEGF and Angiopoietin 2), and may provide better outcomes than just VEGF blockage in retinal vascular diseases. More details of these therapies are provided in Chap. 19.

An alternative mechanism of treatment is the physical destruction of preformed new vessels. A type of treatment (called Photodynamic Therapy) for nAMD has seen the use of a light activated dye, injected intravenously, which preferentially localises in the choroidal neovascular membrane (CNV). Activation of the dye by light of a specific wavelength causes thrombosis and destruction of blood vessels harbouring the dye. Treatment of patients with one particular subtype of nAMD (classic with no occult blood vessels) has shown stabilization of vision in 60-70% of cases. This treatment is used less often since the advent of intravitreal anti-VEGF therapies, which have much better outcomes. However, it is still recommended in eyes with a particular type of nAMD called idiopathic polypoidal choroidopathy (IPCV), where combination of PDT with intravitreal anti-VEGF drugs seem to provide better outcomes.

In other intraretinal neovascular disease such as proliferative diabetic retinopathy (PDR), pan-retinal laser photocoagulation is still preferred as it more permanently switches off the VEGF drive compared to multiple injections of anti-VEGF agents. However, in rubeosis iridis/noevascular glaucoma, and ROP, anti-VEGF therapies have significant therapeutic roles.

Macular oedema due to different diseases, including diabetic retinopathy (diabetic macular oedema [DMO]), and retinal vein occlusions, have significant increase in VEGF as well as non-VEGF inflammatory cytokines released into the eye. As such blocking these VEGF and non-VEGF pathways help reduce the macular oedema. Pharmacological treatments for DMO target reducing vascular leak in the macula once it has occurred, they do not attempt to treat the underlying pathology. These pharmacological treatments are aimed at antagonizing VEGF (pegaptanib, ranibizumab, aflibercept and bevacizumab) or non-VEGF inflammatory pathways with steroids (fluocinolone, Ozurdex, triamcinolone).

Vitreomacular Traction

Ocriplasmin is a recombinant protease enzyme that breaks laminin and fibronectin bonds at the vitreoretinal interface. It therefore serves as a pharmacological therapy for traction at the vitreoretinal interface resulting in visual distortion and macular hole formation. Ocriplasmin is now licensed in the treatment of vitreomacular traction (VMT), including when there is macular hole of <400u in size. It is, however, not effective if there is significant epiretinal membrane associated with the VMT or the macular hole is large. The treatment requires intravitreal injection. As the drug is an enzyme, it has to be stored at a particular temperature and used within a short time of thawing and re-formulation.

Damage to the Eyes by Drugs Administered Systemically

There are a number of drugs, which if given in excessive doses, can lead to severe visual handicap and blindness. Some of these are still available on prescription.

Chloroquine and hydroxychloroquine in excessive doses can lead to pigmentary degeneration of the retina and blindness. These were commonly used anti-malarial treatments. However the emergence of resistance by the malaria parasite has resulted in much reduced use for that indication. Chloroquine sulphate which is more toxic than hydoxychloroquine is now less commonly used. Hydroxychloroquine is currently used by rheumatologists because of its significant anti-inflammatory effect. Certain antipsychotic drugs may also cause fundus pigmentation in excessive doses; melleril and chlorpromazine have been incriminated in this respect in the past. Recently, a number of cases of uveitis have been reported in patients using bisphosphonates for the treatment and prevention of osteoporosis. Interestingly, sudden visual loss has been reported in a number of patients taking the oral anti-inflammatory COX 2 inhibitors (Celecoxib and Rofecoxib). The vision has returned to normal upon cessation of treatment.

Steven-Johnson's syndrome (S-JS) is a rare but severe adverse event affecting the eyes, skin and mucous membranes. Drugs associated with S-JS are sulphonamides and derivatives (including acetazolamide), azithromycin, lamotrigine, carbamazepine, allopurinol, diclofenac and nevirapine. It should be remembered that different infections can also trigger S-JS, particularly viral and bacterial infections (see Chap. 21).

Apart from causing glaucoma in some patients, systemic steroids are thought to increase the rate of formation of cataracts. Ethambutol and isoniazid may cause optic atrophy. Sometimes excessive doses of quinine are taken as an abortifacient and as the patients regain consciousness they are found to be blind from quinine toxicity. Methyl alcohol is toxic to the ganglion cells of the retina and blindness is a hazard of meths drinkers. It sometimes contaminates crudely prepared alcoholic beverages leading to unexpected loss of vision. Other drugs with potential ophthalmic symptoms and signs include tamoxifen and digoxin. The list of drugs with ocular side effects is large and the reader should consult a specialised textbook for more information. Nowadays disasters and indeed lawsuits should be avoidable if the drug literature is checked before prescribing an unfamiliar drug.

Summary

- This chapter summarises the different drugs used by the ophthalmologist, and their effects locally and systemically. As well it describes how systemically administered drugs can affect the eyes of the user.
- Several different drugs are used for diagnosis and treatment of eye diseases.
- Some of these are administered locally (topically) whilst others may be administered intravitreally, by other local routes (sub-Tenon's, subconjunctival) or systemically.
- Some of these locally administered drugs may have systemic side effects, e.g. 10% phenylephrine.
- Other drugs administered systemically may have undesired ocular effects, e.g. Steven-Johnson Syndrome with sulphonamide derivatives.
- Typically, antibiotics may be delivered locally as treatment for superficial ocular infections. However, other routes are required for intraocular infections because of the poor bioavailability of topically applied medications.
- Parasympathetic and sympathetic agonists dilate the pupil, whilst parasympathetic agonists constrict the pupil.
- Drugs may reduce intraocular pressure by reducing the production of aqueous humour (e.g. beta blockers, alpha$_2$ adrenergic agonists or carbonic anhydrase inhibitors), by increasing the drainage of aqueous humour at the anterior chamber angle (e.g. pilocarpine), or increase uveoscleral outflow (prostaglandins or prostanoids).
- Several drugs are now available as topical medications for the treatment of allergic eye disease.
- Tear replacement drops are important in improving ocular lubrication.
- Intravitreal injections of anti-VEGF drugs and steroids are recent welcome additions to ophthalmic drug therapies.

Part V

Visual Impairment

Blindness

25

Abstract

This chapter considers the incidence and causes of blindness and the various artificial aids available for the visually impaired.

Blindness marks the failure or inefficacy of ophthalmological treatment. Once a patient becomes permanently blind, he or she may be lost from the care of the ophthalmologist. This means that the ophthalmologist may not have personal experience of the size of the problem and may not be in a position to experience the relative incidences of different causes of blindness. The keeping of accurate statistics is of great importance, and in order to keep statistical records it is necessary to have a clear definition of blindness. Many people who dread blindness imagine having no perception of light in each eye. Fortunately this situation is uncommon, but many people are severely debilitated by visual loss.

In this country the major problem is amongst the elderly where visual loss is often combined with defective hearing. Sensory deprivation is thus a major scourge at the present time, the problem is undoubtedly going to be much worse as the proportion of elderly people increases.

Definition

In Britain the statutory definition of blindness refers to persons who 'are so blind as to be unable to perform any work for which eyesight is essential'. When a patient's vision falls below this level then registration as a visually impaired person can be considered. This is a voluntary process, which allows the patient access to the social services for the visually impaired as well as certain tax concessions. Registration is usually initiated in the hospital clinic. Some patients are referred by their general practitioners or social workers for registration by the ophthalmic specialist. A special form is completed and copies go to the patient, the general practitioner and the social services department.

The ophthalmologist can certify a patient with poor eyesight as either severely sight impaired(blind) or sight impaired(partially sighted) by completing the Certificate of Visual Impairment(CVI) in England and Wales.(BPI in Scotland and A655 in Northern Ireland).

Certain guidelines are laid down when considering blind registration; the visual acuity should be less than 3/60, but if the field of vision is very constricted then the visual acuity may be better than this. Patients whose vision is not bad enough for blind registration but nonetheless have significant visual impairment can have their name placed on the partially sighted register. In these patients the binocular vision should normally be worse than 6/18. Patients sometimes erroneously claim the benefits of the partially sighted because they have only one eye, even though the good eye is normal. When the vision with one or both eyes is 6/18 or better, the patient is not usually considered to be partially sighted. When one eye is completely lost through injury or disease, then the amount of incapacity is set for medico-legal purposes at about 10%. In actual fact the amount of incapacity depends a great deal on the age of the patient. A child may adapt to a remarkable degree to being one eyed, even to the extent of being able to perform with skill at ball games. Adults who become one eyed find difficulty in judging distances or performing fine manual tasks. More importantly, a number of occupations are specifically barred to those whose vision is poor in one eye.

Benefits for the Visually Handicapped

There is no blind pension in the United Kingdom but those registered blind have a special income tax allowance and some exemptions from deductions from income support. Those patients with more severe visual impairment can have parking concessions and a free NHS sight test as well as rail cards and bus passes. Disability living allowance may be available for blind people under the age of 65 years but for the over 65 s only those both blind and deaf can qualify. Those seeking these concessions should consult an expert in the field. There are a number of voluntary organisations that run clubs, social centres and supply various other aids and benefits. For example, the Royal National Institute for the Blind (RNIB) provides a comprehensive range of services including the popular talking book service. They also supply regular funds for research into the causes of blindness.

The system of registration applies equally to children. In this instance, registration calls attention to the need for special educational requirements. These can include a specialist resource teacher, low visual aids, and other special sup-

plies and equipment. If necessary, special schooling may need to be considered.

Standards of Vision for Various Occupations

The standards for various occupations can vary from year to year and are more or less exacting, depending on the occupation. In Britain, in order to drive a private motor vehicle, one must be able, in good daylight, to read a number plate with glasses or contact lenses at 20 m. A full field of vision is also required, and this must extend at least 120° horizontally and 20° above and below. The field is measured by perimetry using a standard target. It is assumed that any healthy person applying to drive has a normal field of vision but if the driver has any eye condition that might lead to visual handicap then he or she must declare it. The driver and vehicle licensing centre may then ask for a report from an ophthalmologist or an optometrist. Double vision is a bar to driving, if it cannot be corrected by prisms in the glasses or the wearing of an eye patch.

Colour Blindness

This is not blindness in any sense of the word and indeed some colour blind individuals are unaware of any problem until their colour vision is tested. Eight percentage of the male population suffers from some form of congenital colour blindness. This is usually in the form of 'red-green blindness'. Inheritance of this type of defect is sex-linked so that unaffected female carriers pass the gene to 50% of their sons. The screening of school children for colour blindness is now widely practiced because of the occupational implications. The Ishihara test is the simplest and the best test for congenital colour blindness. Occupations which entail the reading of coloured warning lights or the matching of colours usually demand some form of colour vision test on entry. It is an advantage to the child to be aware of any defect during the early years of schooling.

Incidence and Cause of Blindness

About two million people in the United Kingdom are living with significant sight loss and the number is predicted to double by 2050. About 360,000 people in the UK are registered blind or partially sighted.

In the Western World blindness in children is largely due to hereditary retinal dystrophies, disorders of the central nervous system and congenital anomalies. In adults aged 20–60 years the major causes are diseases of the retina including diabetic retinopathy and optic atrophy. Over the age of 60 years macular degeneration, glaucoma and cataract are the important problems.

In Africa and Asia, the causes of blindness are rather different; many children become blind from corneal scarring associated with vitamin A deficiency and measles. Cataract is the most important cause in adults but in certain areas, for example southern Sudan, onchocerciasis and trachoma are still a serious problem.

It is apparent that the problems of blindness in Europe and North America are very different from those in poorer parts of the world where much could still be done by improving standards of nutrition and living conditions.

Aids for the Visually Impaired

The most widely recognised aid and symbol of blindness is the white stick. It is also one of the most useful aids because it identifies the patient as blind and encourages others to give assistance. Many blind people are concerned that they appear ill mannered when failing to recognise someone and are grateful for some indication of their handicap. Many different electronic devices have been tried but by and large these are only useful to younger patients who can make full use of them. Scanning systems are now available which when moved across the page can read out the page. Most blind patients are unable to afford this type of aid. Many of these devices rely on the patients hearing to identify an audible warning signal, but most blind people prefer to use their undistracted sense of hearing as an important clue to their whereabouts. Guide dogs are specially trained by the Guide Dogs for the Blind Association and the patient must also take part in the training. Some young people find that a guide dog can expand their mobility to a great degree. Certain tactile aids are also useful, the best known of which is Braille. This system of reading for the blind was introduced from France more than 100 years ago. The letters of the alphabet are represented by numbers of raised dots on stiff paper. See Fig. 25.1 Blind children can learn Braille very rapidly and develop a high reading speed. Some adults find that their fingers are not sufficiently sensitive and this applies especially to diabetics. Books in Braille are now available in many different languages. Tape recordings of books and newspapers are now very popular amongst blind and partially sighted of all ages. The Talking Book Service provides a comprehensive library for the use of the visually disabled.

There are numerous other gadgets, which can be helpful to the blind and partially sighted; a popular one is the device that can indicate whether a teacup is full or not. For those with some residual vision, a special telephone pad with large numbers on it can be very helpful. Other ingenious devices range from relief maps which can be felt by the blind person to a telephone which speaks back through the earpiece the digit that has just been pressed. Research has also been carried out on aids that signal the position of objects by means of electrical stimuli to the skin and even by means of implanted electrodes in the visual cortex.

One important advance has been voice synthesis by computers. Many current models have this facility, so that the user can hear emails and programs are available to allow printing in Braille. Just as important is the fact that the patient can now speak to the computer and give commands to control equipment or appliances.

In spite of these advances, the elderly visually handicapped patient may benefit most from someone who is prepared to give the time to read out letters or books. Some voluntary local societies can provide this service.

When the patient has a visual acuity of better than 6/60, then much can be achieved by the use

To make numbers in braille we put this special numeral symbol ⠼ before the letters **A** to **I** for numbers **1** to **9** so A = 1, B = 2 and so on. **J** is used for **zero**.

So **6** is the numeral symbol followed by the braille letter 'F' like this:

And the number **160** is like this:

Fig. 25.1 Embossed dot system of the Braille Alphabet

of optical magnification. An ordinary hand magnifying glass is the simplest and may often be the most effective form of assistance. If this is not adequate and the patient has been a keen reader, then a telescopic lens may be fitted to a spectacle frame with advantage. These multi-lens systems are known as low visual aids and hence the popular 'LVA' clinics in Eye departments for the testing and provision of these items. Apart from special telescopic lenses, closed circuit television aids are now available: a small television camera is held over the page and a magnified view of the written material is presented on a television screen.

The well being of a blind or partially sighted person may be greatly enhanced by relatively simple social measures. Advice in the home about the use of gas or electricity may be important and the patient can be made aware of the availability of local social clubs for the blind or keep fit classes and bus outings. An elderly patient who plays the piano may be helped by the provision of an enlarged photocopy of a favourite piece of music. In spite of all these various possibilities, one must not forget that the simplest

and most useful reading aid for a partially sighted person is a good light directed onto the page. The distance of the bulb from the page is as important as the wattage of the bulb.

Artificial Eyes

These may be made of glass or plastic moulded to the shape of the eye socket and painted to match the other eye. Usually they are removed and washed at night by the patient and replaced the following morning. A slight degree of discharge from the socket is the rule but excessive discharge may indicate that the socket is becoming infected. This in turn may be due to roughening of the artificial eye with wear. Under these circumstances arrangements should be made for the prosthesis to be replaced or polished. It should always be born in mind that a patient with an artificial eye may have had the eye removed because it contained a malignant tumour, in which case one must consider the possibility of local or systemic spread of the tumour. A well made artificial eye is almost undetectable to the untrained eye but normal movements of the eye may be restricted. Nowadays the use of orbital prostheses deep to the conjunctiva and attached to the eye muscles gives greatly increased movement. After many years and after renewing the artificial eye on several occasions the eye may appear to sink downwards and this problem can be repaired surgically.

Surgical removal of an eye (enucleation) is considered in the following circumstances:

- When the eye is blind and painful
- When the eye contains a malignant tumour
- When the eye is nearly blind and sympathetic ophthalmitis is a risk following a perforating injury

Before having an eye removed, the patient must be made fully aware of all the advantages and disadvantages. A general anaesthetic is needed and the patient remains in hospital for one or two nights after the operation. It is common practice to fit the socket with a transparent plastic 'shell' for a few weeks until the artificial eye is fitted.

Having read this chapter you should be able to answer the following questions:

1. What is the incidence of blindness in the United Kingdom?
2. Name some the aids that can be provided for the visually impaired.
3. How is blindness recorded in this country?
4. Why is it important to test children for colour blindness?

Further Reading

Ophthalmology: An Illustrated Text 4th Edition 2018
- M. Batterbury

The Oxford Handbook of Ophthalmology 2018
- Denniston and Murray

Atlas of Clinical Ophthalmology E- book, 3rd Edition 2005
- David J. Spalton, Consultant Ophthalmologist, St Thomas' Hospital, London, UK.
- Roger A Hitchings, Consultant Ophthalmologist, Moorfields Eye Hospital, London, UK.
- Paul Hunter, Consultant Ophthalmologist, Kings College Hospital, London, UK.
- Mosby Ltd. 2005.

Kanski's Clinical Ophthalmology: A Systematic Approach, by John Salmon MD FRCS FRCOphth 2019
- Elsevier 2019.

The Eye 5th Edition 2020
- John Forrester, Professor of Ophthalmology, University of Aberdeen, UK
- Andrew Dick Professor of Ophthalmology, University of Bristol, UK
- Paul McMenamin Director of the Centre for Human Anatomy Education, Monash University, Melbourne, Victoria, Australia.
- Fiona Roberts, Consultant Ophthalmic Pathologist, Southern General Hospital, Glasgow, UK.
- Eric Pearlman, Director, Institute of Immunology, Departments of Ophthalmology and Physiology, University of California, Irvine California, USA.
- Elsevier Health Sciences

Parsons' Diseases of the Eye 23rd Edition
- Elsevier

N. R. Galloway et al., *Common Eye Diseases and their Management*,
https://doi.org/10.1007/978-3-031-08450-8

Index

A

Abnormalities of refraction, 201
Abnormally constricted pupil, 248
Abnormally dilated pupil, 247
Acetylcholine, 264
Acne rosacea, 235
Acquired immune deficiency syndrome (AIDS),
    230, 231
Actinomycosis, 37
Acute angle closure glaucoma
    pathogenesis and natural history, 111
    signs, 112, 113
    symptoms, 111
    treatment, 113, 114
Acute dacryocystitis, 37, 38
Acute glaucoma, 70
Acute haemorrhagic conjunctivitis, 53
Acute iritis, 70, 71, 82
Acute keratitis, 71
Adenoviral conjunctivitis, 52, 53
Age-related macular degeneration (AMD), 74, 179,
    182–185, 189, 192
Aids for the visually impaired, 275, 276
Alkylating agents, 267
Allergic eye disease, 265
Amblyopia of disuse, 76, 127, 202
Anaemia, 81, 224
Anatomy of the eye
    blood supply, 11, 12
    compartments, 8
    extraocular muscles, 14
    eyelids, 13, 14
    inner layer, 8, 10, 11
    intraocular fluids, 8
    lacrimal apparatus, 14
    middle layer, 7, 9
    optic nerve, 12, 13
    outer layers, 7–9
    segments, 8
    visual pathways, 13

Aniridia, 200
Anterior uveitis
    causes, 166, 167
    complications, 166
    heterochromic iridocyclitis, 168
    management, 167, 168
    signs, 165, 166
    symptoms, 164
Anti-inflammatory drugs, 266, 267
Antimetabolites, 267
Arcuate scotoma, 106
Arcus senilis, 180
Argyll Robertson pupils, 248
Artificial eyes, 276, 277
Artificial tears, 266
Atopic conjunctivitis, 53, 54
Automated refraction, 160, 161
Autosomal dominant, 256
Autosomal recessive, 255

B

Background retinopathy (BGDR), 208
Bacterial conjunctivitis, 51, 52
Basal cell carcinoma, 46
Basic genetic mechanisms, 254, 255
Behcet's disease, 172
Benefits for the visually handicapped, 274
Bioinformatics, 254
Birdshot chorioretinopathy, 174
Blepharitis, 43, 44
Blindness, 3, 5, 273, 274
Bowman's membrane, 56

C

Calcineurin inhibitors, 267
Capillary haemangioma, 45
Carbachol (carbamylcholine), 264
Cardiff Acuity Chart, 156

Cataract, 5, 74–77, 193
  ageing process, 92, 93
  diabetes, 93
  lens, 91, 92
  management
    cataract operation, 98, 99
    convalescence, 100, 101
    fluctuation, 97
    focus/multifocal implants, 97, 98
    patient age, 98
    plastic intraocular implant, 97
    time spent in hospital, 100
    traumatic cataract, 99
  secondary to disease, 93
  signs
    ophthalmoscopy findings, 95, 96
    reduced visual acuity, 95
    retinal function, 96
    routine eye examination, 97
    slit lamp microscopy, 96
  symptoms, 94, 95
  trauma
    congenital factors, 94
    contusion, 93
    perforation, 93, 94
    radiation, 94
    toxicity, 94
Cavernous haemangioma, 138, 141
Central retinal vein occlusion, 114
Central serous retinopathy, 75
Certificate of completion of training (CCT), 6
Chemical injuries, 151
Chemosis, 216
Child's eye, 198
Chlamydia conjunctivitis, 52
Chloramphenicol, 262
Choroidal melanoma, 135, 136
Choroidal metastases, 136
Choroidal neovascularisation, 184
Choroidal neovascular membrane (CNV), 269
Chromosomal abnormalities, 259
Chromosome mapping, 254
Ciliary injection, 68
Cluster headache, 81
Colour blindness, 274
Colour vision, 21, 22
Congenital cataract, 201
Congenital disc anomalies, 239
Congenital nystagmus, 199, 200
Conjunctiva, 9, 14
  benign lesions, 140
  malignant lesions, 141
Conjunctival congestion, 216
Conjunctivitis
  acute, 68
  acute haemorrhagic conjunctivitis, 53
  adenovirus, 52, 53
  aetiological factors, 50
  allergic reaction, 53, 54
  bacterial conjunctivitis, 51, 52
  causes, 51, 68, 69

  chlamydia, 52
  chronic, 68
  corneal/intraocular inflammation, 68
  cultures, 50
  Herpes simplex, 53
  inflammation, 49
  microscopy, 50
  molluscum contagiosum, 53
  Phthirus pubis, 53
  secondary, 54–56
  signs, 50
  symptoms, 50
  trachoma, 52
Connective tissue diseases, 234
Contact lens
  cosmetic lens, 86, 87
  side-effects, 86
  therapeutic lens, 87
  types, 85
Contusion, 93, 145–147
  choroid, 147
  cornea, 146
  lens, 147
  optic nerve, 148
  retina, 147
  vitreous, 147
Convergence insufficiency, 83
Cornea, 8, 9, 13, 15
Corneal degeneration, 62, 63
Corneal disease, 63
Corneal dystrophies, 62
Corneal foreign body
  incidence, 56
  signs and symptoms, 56
  treatment, 57
Corneal oedema, 63
Corneal sensation, 63, 64
Corneal ulceration, 216
  acanthamoeba, 59
  causes, 58
  corneal nerve supply, 61
  due to bacteria, 59
  due to direct trauma, 58, 59
  due to exposure, 61
  virus infection, 59–61
Cosmetic lens, 86, 87
Craniopharyngioma, 203
C-reactive protein (CRP), 195
Crystallins, 92

D
Dacryocystitis, 37, 38
Deformities of the eyelids, 194
Demyelination, 132
Dermoid cyst, 45, 141
Diabetes mellitus, 114, 206
  anterior chamber, 207
  background retinopathy, 208
  cornea and conjunctiva, 207
  eyelids, 206

iris, 207
lens, 207, 208
ocular movements, 206
prognosis, 215
proliferative diabetic retinopathy, 210
retina and vitreous, 208
treatment, 210
Diabetic macular oedema (DMO), 210, 213, 214
Diabetic maculopathy, 210
Dialysis, 120
Digenic (polygenic) inheritance, 258
Double vision, 248–250
Down's syndrome, 93
Drug toxicity, 203
Drusen, 183

E
Ebola virus disease (EVD), 234
Ehlers-Danlos syndrome, 235
Endophthalmitis, 175
Epicanthus, 199
Episcleritis, 69, 176
Erythrocyte sedimentation rate (ESR), 195
Eserine, 5
Exophthalmos, 142
Exposure keratitis, 216
Extraocular muscles, 14
Eye clinic liaison Officer (ECLO), 4
Eye disease, elderly, 181, 182
Eye examination
    colour vision, 22
    external eye and lids, 23
    globe, 23–25
    ophthalmoscope, 25–28
    pupil examination, 22, 23
    spectacles, 22
    visual acuity, 20, 21
    visual filed, 21
Eyelids, 9, 13, 14
    allergic disease, 44
    benign tumours, 44, 45
    blepharitis, 43, 44
    blepharospasm, 41
    dry eye
        causes, 38
        diagnosis, 38
        management, 39
        Schirmer's test, 39
        slit lamp examination, 39
        tear film break-up time, 39
    ectropion, 40
    entropion, 40
    epicanthus, 40
    excessive secretion of tears, 38
    impaired drainage of tears
        acute dacryocystitis, 37, 38
        lacrimal passageway, 35–37
    ingrowing eyelashes, 42
    injuries, 46, 47
    lagophthalmos, 41

    malignant tumours, 46
    meibomian gland infection, 42, 43
    molluscum contagiosum, 44
    normal eyelids, 39, 40
    orbital cellulitis, 44
    ptosis, 41, 42
    redundant lid skin, 41
    styes, 43
Eye screening, 254

F
Failing vision
    abnormal fundus, 74
    in one eye, sudden visual loss, 75
    normal fundus, 73, 74
    systemic disease, 74, 75
    treatable causes, 75, 76
    untreatable causes, 76, 77
Fortifications, 80
Foundation years, 6
Fundus fluorescein angiography
        (FFA), 184

G
Gasserian ganglion, 81
Gene therapy, 259, 260
Geographic atrophy, 183
Giant cell arteritis, 80, 81, 132
Glass contact lens, 85
Glasses, 130
Glaucoma, 74, 76, 193, 194, 264, 265
    acute angle closure glaucoma
        pathogenesis and natural history, 111
        signs, 112, 113
        symptoms, 111
        treatment, 113, 114
    congenital/developmental glaucoma,
        115, 116
    intraocular pressure
        maintenance, 103, 104
        measurement, 104
        normal elevation, 103
    NPG, 110
    POAG
        cardinal signs, 105, 106
        incidence, 105
        pathogenesis and natural history, 105
        symptoms, 105
        treatment, 106–110
    primary glaucoma, 114
    secondary glaucoma
        abnormalities in lens, 115
        drug-induced glaucoma, 115
        to trauma, 115
        to tumours, 114
        to uveitis, 114
        to vascular disease, 114
    surgery, 214
Goldmann tonometry, 104

H
Haemangioma, 143
Haemorrhages, 238
Hay fever conjunctivitis, 53
Headache
    blood vessels, 80, 81
    bones, 82
    cerebrospinal fluid pressure, 80
    changes in blood, 81
    drugs, 83
    eyes, 82, 83
    history, 79
    meninges, 82
    nerves, 81, 82
    post-traumatic headache, 83
    sinusitis, 83
Hemianopia, 75
Hereditary optic atrophy, 203
Herpes simplex conjunctivitis, 53
Herpes zoster ophthalmicus, 64, 65
Hess screen, 132
Histoplasmosis, 171
Horner syndrome, 248
Human leucocyte antigens (HLA), 164
Hydrocephalus, 203
Hydroxmethylmethacrylate (HEMA), 85
Hypermetropia, 31–33
Hypertension, 80, 218
Hypoxic brain injury, 203

I
Incidence and causes of blindness, 273, 275
Intermediate uveitis, 168
Intracranial angioma, 81
Intracranial tumours, 74
Intraocular foreign body, 148, 149
Intraocular pressure
    maintenance, 103, 104
    measurement, 104
    normal elevation, 103
Intraretinal microvascular abnormalities (IRMA), 209
Ischaemic optic neuropathy, 223

K
Kaposi sarcoma, 138
Keratoacanthoma, 138
Keratoconus, 62

L
Lacrimal apparatus, 14
Lacrimal obstruction, 54, 199
Lacrimal passageway, 35–37
Lacrimal puncta, 36, 39
Lagophthalmos, 41
Leber's hereditary optic neuropathy (LOHN), 240, 258
Leucocoria, 202
Leukaemias, 225

Lid deformities, 54
Lid swelling, 216
LogMAR, 157, 158, 161
Long sight, 31–33
Lymphoproliferative disease, 143

M
Macula, 11
Macular degenerations, 203
Magnetic resonance imaging (MRI), 27
Malignant hypertension, 218
Malignant melanoma, 46
Malignant tumours, eyelids
    basal cell carcinoma, 139
    squamous cell carcinoma, 139
Marfan syndrome, 234
Marginal ulcer, 59
Median longitudinal fasciculus (MLF), 244
Meibomian cysts, 137
Melanoma of iris, 137
Migraine, 80, 81
Mitochondrial inheritance, 258
Molluscum contagiosum, 44, 137
Monoclonal antibodies, 267
Moulded scleral lens, 85
Multifactorial diseases, 259
Multiple sclerosis, 243, 244
Myasthenia gravis, 132, 250
Myokymia, 41
Myopia, 31–33
Myopic chorioretinal degeneration, 77

N
Narrow angle glaucoma, 82
Nasolacrimal duct, 36, 37
Neovascular glaucoma, 71
Non-steroidal anti-inflammatory agents, 267
Normal disc, 237, 238
Normal pressure glaucoma (NPG), 110
Nystagmus, 244

O
Objective refraction, 160
Ocriplasmin, 269
Ocular coherence tomography (OCT), 28
Ocular muscle imbalance, 133
Oculotoxic drugs, 75
Onchocerciasis, 229
Ophthalmia neonatorum, 202–203
Ophthalmology
    career in, 5, 6
    clinical specialisation, 3
    degenerative changes, 3
    history, 4, 5
    patient communication, 4
Ophthalmoscope, 4, 5, 23, 25–28
Optical coherence tomography (OCT), 180

Optic atrophy, 200, 203, 239, 241, 251
Optic disc, 105
    congenital disc anomalies, 239
    normal disc, 237, 238
    pale disc, 239–241
    swelling, 241, 242
Optic nerve, 9, 11–14, 17
Optic neuritis, 242
Optic radiation, 245
Optic tract, 245
Optokinetic drum, 159
Orbit, 141, 142
Orbital fracture, 132
Orbit injuries, 150

P
Paget's disease of bone, 82
Pale disc, 239–241
Papilloedema, 242, 251
Papilloma, 44, 137
Paralytic ectropion, 40
Parasympathetic antagonists, 263
Perforation, 93, 94, 148
Phakomatoses, 203
Photodynamic therapy (PDT), 189
Physiology of eye
    accommodation, 16
    aqueous humour, 15
    ciliary body, 16
    cornea, 15
    eyelids, 14
    lens, 16
    retina, 16, 17
    tear film, 14, 15
    vitreous, 15
Pilocarpine, 264
Pingueculum, 140
Platelet derived growth factor (PDGF), 192
Port delivery system (PDS), 191
Post herpetic neuralgia, 81
Posterior uveitis
    causes, 170
    management, 170
    signs, 169
    symptoms, 169
Posterior vitreous detachment (PVD), 120
Post-meningitis, 203
Preferential looking, 156
Presbyopia, 31, 32, 180
Presbyopic headaches, 83
Primary open angle glaucoma (POAG), 179
    cardinal signs, 105, 106
    incidence, 105
    pathogenesis and natural history, 105
    symptoms, 105
    treatment, 106–110
Proliferative diabetic retinopathy (PDR), 209
Proliferative vitreoretinopathy (PVR), 124
Proptosis

    haemangioma, 143
    infection, 143
    pseudoproptosis, 142
    thyrotoxicosis, 142
    trauma, 143
Pseudoxanthoma eleasticum, 235
Pterygium, 55, 140
Ptosis, 41, 42, 199
Pupil, 263
Purine synthesis inhibitors, 267

R
Radiational injuries, 150
Radiation cataract, 94
Raeder's paratrigeminal neuralgia, 81
Red eye
    acute glaucoma, 70
    acute iritis, 70, 71
    acute keratitis, 71
    conjunctivitis
        acute, 68
        causes, 68, 69
        chronic, 68
        corneal/intraocular inflammation, 68
    episcleritis, 69
    neovascular glaucoma, 71
    scleritis, 70
    subconjunctival haemorrhage, 68
    virtual consultations, 67
Refraction, 160
Refractive headache, 82
Registration, 273
Retina, 9–12, 16, 17
Retinal artery occlusions, 221, 222
Retinal breaks, 118, 119
Retinal detachment, 74, 76
    classification, 118, 119
    exudativeretinal detachment, 122
    incidence, 117, 118
    pathogenesis, 118
    rhegmatogenous
        breaks in, 119
        mechanism of, 120
        prognosis, 124
        prophylaxis, 122
        PVD, 120
        retinal breaks formation, 120
        retinal degeneration, 119
        retinal surgery, 122–124
        vitreous, 119
        with trauma, 120
    signs and symptoms, 120, 121
    subretinal fluid, 117
    tractional retinal detachment, 121, 122
Retinal pigment epithelium (RPE), 183
Retinal vein occlusions (RVO), 220, 221
Retinoblastoma, 136
Retinopathy of prematurity, 202
Retrobulbar neuritis, 74, 77

Reverse-transcriptase polymerase chain reaction
       (RT-PCR), 233
Rhabdomyosarcoma, 141
Royal College of Ophthalmologists, 6

S
Sarcoidosis, 172
Sclera, 8, 9
Scleritis, 70, 176
Screening, 199, 202
Seborrhoeic keratosis, 138
Severe acute respiratory syndrome coronavirus 2
       (SARS-CoV-2), 232
Sex-linked recessive, 256, 257
Sheridan Gardiner test, 157
Shingles of eye, 64, 65
Short sight, 31–33
Sickle cell disease, 227, 229
Silico-analysis, 254
Simultaneous macular perception, 126
Slit lamp microscope, 3
Snellen chart, 157
Soft contact lens, 85–87
Spectacles, 22, 160
       automated refraction, 160, 161
       objective refraction, 160
       subjective refraction, 160
Spring catarrh, 54
Squamous cell carcinoma, 46
Squint, 125, 126, 201
       adults, 131, 133
       childhood, 127, 128, 130, 131
       ocular muscle imbalance, 133
Stargardt disease, 256
Stereopsis, 126
Steven-Johnson's syndrome (S-JS), 235, 236, 270
Stickler syndrome, 235
Striate cortex, 245
Stroke, 195
Stycar test, 157, 159
Styes, 43
Subarachnoid/subdural haemorrhage, 81

Subconjunctival haemorrhage, 49, 68
Subjective refraction, 160
Subretinal fluid, 117
Sympathetic agonist, 263
Sympathetic ophthalmia, 149, 174
Syphilis, 172
Systemic diseases, 205

T
Telangiectatic haemangioma, 138
Temporal arteritis, 75, 194, 195
Therapeutic lens, 87
Thyroid eye disease, 132, 215–217
Thyrotoxicosis, 250
Toxocariasis, 171
Toxoplasma gondii, 170, 171
Trachoma, 52
Trichiasis, 42
Trigeminal neuralgia, 81
Tuberculosis, 171

U
Uvea, 9, 11, 15
Uveitis, 163, 164, 203

V
Vascular endothelial growth factor (VEGF), 184, 268
Vernal conjunctivitis, 54
Visual acuity, 20, 21, 50, 155, 156, 158, 198, 199, 202
       children, 156–157
       testing, 156
Visual field, 21, 105, 106
Visually evoked potential (VEP), 28
Vitreomacular traction (VMT), 180, 269
Vitreo-retinal surgery, 214
Vitreous detachment, 180

X
Xanthelasma, 45, 138

Printed in the United States
by Baker & Taylor Publisher Services